Comprehensive Aquatic Therapy

Second Edition

Andrew J. Cole, M.D.
Northwest Spine & Sports Physicians, PC
Bellevue, WA
Clinical Associate Professor
Department of Rehabilitation Medicine
University of Washington School of Medicine
Seattle, WA

Bruce E. Becker, M.D.
Medical Director
St. Luke's Rehabilitation Institute
Spokane, WA
Clinical Professor
Department of Rehabilitation Medicine
University of Washington School of Medicine
Seattle, WA

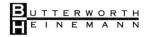

An Imprint of Elsevier

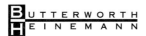

An Imprint of Elsevier

The Curtis Center
Independence Square West
Philadelphia, Pennsylvania 19106

Comprehensive Aquatic Therapy   0-7506-7386-9
Copyright © 2004, Elsevier Inc. (USA). All rights reserved.

No part of this publication may be reproduced or transmitted
in any form or by any means, electronic or mechanical,
including photocopying, recording, or any information storage and
retrieval system, without permission in writing from the publisher.
Permissions may be sought directly from Elsevier's Health Sciences
Rights Department in Philadelphia, PA, USA: phone: (+1) 215 238 7869,
fax: (+1) 215 238 2239, e-mail: healthpermissions@elsevier.com.
You may also complete your request on-line via the Elsevier Science
homepage (http://www.elsevier.com), by selecting 'Customer Support' and
then 'Obtaining Permissions'.

NOTICE

Medicine is an ever-changing field. Standard safety precautions must be followed, but as new research and clinical experience broaden our knowledge, changes in treatment and drug therapy may become necessary or appropriate. Readers are advised to check the most current product information provided by the manufacturer of each drug to be administered to verify the recommended dose, the method and duration of administration, and contraindications. It is the responsibility of the treating physician, relying on experience and knowledge of the patient, to determine dosages and the best treatment for each individual patient. Neither the Publisher nor the editor assumes any liability for any injury and/or damage to persons or property arising from this publication.

The Publisher

Previous editions copyrighted 1997

Library of Congress Cataloging-in-Publication Data

Comprehensive aquatic therapy/edited by Andrew J. Cole, Bruce E. Becker; with 23
  contributing authors.— 2nd ed.
    p.; cm.
  ISBN 0-7506-7386-9
    1. Hydrotherapy. I. Cole, Andrew J., 1958-II. Becker, Bruce E.
    [DNLM: 1. Hydrotherapy. 2. Rehabilitation—methods. WB 520 C737 2003]
  RM811.C675 2003
  615.8'53—dc21   2003048177

Acquisitions Editor: Rolla Couchman
Publishing Services Manager: Joan Sinclair
Project Manager: Mary Stermel

Printed in the United States of America

Last digit is the print number: 9 8 7 6 5 4 3 2

To Carl Samuelson who leads with grace, dignity, and humor. A coach who teaches lessons for life.

A.J.C

I express profound gratitude to my friend and wife Carol, who has provided unstinting support, proofreading, and physical and emotional sustenance throughout our 35 years of marriage, and to our children Adrianne and Derek with heartfelt apologies for the time stolen from them to pursue my own projects. To my father, Erhart Becker, I give thanks for providing me with a true role model for optimism, enthusiasm, and integrity. I know that my mother's spirit has aided my career from above in a great many ways. To the energies and dedication of the many mermadams and mermen who have supported both the creation and the sales of this text, I am forever indebted.

B.E.B

Contents

Contributing Authors		vii
Preface		xiii
Acknowledgments		xv

1. **Aquatic Rehabilitation: A Historical Perspective**   1
   Jonathan Paul De Vierville

2. **Biophysiologic Aspects of Hydrotherapy**   19
   Bruce E. Becker

3. **Facility Design and Water Management**   57
   Alison Osinski

4. **The Halliwick Concept**   73
   Johan F. Lambeck, Fran Coffey Stanat, and Douglas W. Kinnaird

5. **Watsu**   99
   Harold Dull and Peggy Schoedinger

6. **Equipment Options and Uses for the Aquatic Therapy Pool**   115
   Marilou Moschetti

7. **Aqua Running**   137
   Robert P. Wilder and David K. Brennan

8. **Aquatic Rehabilitation for the Treatment of Neurologic Disorders**   151
   David M. Morris

9. **Spine Pain: Aquatic Rehabilitation Strategies**   177
   Andrew J. Cole, Michael Fredericson, Jim Johnson, Marilou Moschetti, Richard A. Eagleston, and Steven A. Stratton

10. **Hydrotherapeutic Applications in Arthritis Rehabilitation**   207
    Bruce E. Becker and Gwendolyn Garrett

11.	**Aquatic Strategies in Musculoskeletal Pain** *Joseph T. Alleva, Thomas H. Hudgins, and Marti Biondi*	227
12.	**Pediatric Aquatic Therapy** *Teresa M. Petersen*	239
13.	**Aquatic Therapy: From Acute Care to Lifestyle** *Bruce E. Becker and Juliana Larson*	289
14.	**Hydrotherapy and Pressure Ulcers** *Chester H. Ho and David T. Burke*	307
15.	**Staff Training and Development in Aquatic Therapy** *Ruth I. Meyer*	325
16.	**The Lyton Model: An Interdisciplinary Model of Care** *Lynette Jamison and Charlotte Norton*	341
17.	**Legal Aspect of Aquatic Therapy** *Annie Clement*	351

Contributing Authors

Joseph T. Alleva, M.D.
Senior Attending
Department of Physical Medicine
Evanston Northwestern Healthcare
Assistant Professor
Northwestern University
Evanston, IL
Aquatic Strategies in Musculoskeletal Pain

Bruce E. Becker, M.D.
Medical Director
St. Luke's Rehabilitation Institute
Spokane, WA
Clinical Professor
Department of Rehabilitation Medicine
University of Washington School of Medicine
Seattle, WA
Biophysiologic Aspects of Hydrotherapy, Hydrotherapeutic Applications in Arthritis Rehabilitation, Aquatic Therapy: From Acute Care to Lifestyle

Marti Biondi, P.T.
Physical Therapist
Evanston Northwestern Healthcare Rehabilitation
Evanston, IL
Aquatic Strategies in Musculoskeletal Pain

David K. Brennan, M.Ed.
President
Houston International Running Center
Clinical Assistant Professor
Department of PM&R
Baylor College of Medicine
Houston, TX
Director of Education and Training
SwimEx, LLC
Warren, RI
Aqua Running

David T. Burke, M.D., M.A.
Assistant Professor
Harvard Medical
Director, Inpatient Traumatic Brain Injury Rehabilitation Program
Spaulding Rehabilitation Hospital
Boston, MA
Hydrotherapy and Pressure Ulcers

Annie Clement, Ph.D, J.D., B.S., M.A.
Professor
Barry University
Miami Shores, FL
Legal Aspects of Aquatic Therapy

Andrew J. Cole, M.D.
Northwest Spine & Sports Physicians, PC
Bellevue, WA
Clinical Associate Professor
Department of Rehabilitation Medicine
University of Washington School of Medicine
Seattle, WA
Spine Pain: Aquatic Rehabilitation Strategies

Jonathan Paul De Vierville, Ph.D., M.S.S.W.
Professor of History, The Humanities and Interdisciplinary Studies
Department of Social and Behavioral Sciences
St. Philip's College
Director, Alamo Plaza Spa at the Menger Hotel
San Antonio, TX
President, The Hot Wells Institute
Aquatic Rehabilitation: A Historical Perspective

Harold Dull, M.A.
Founding Director
Worldwide Aquatic Bodywork Association
Middletown, CA
Watsu

Richard A. Eagleston, M.A., P.T., A.T.C.
Consultant
Stanford University Men's Swimming
Owner/Chief Physical Therapist
S.T.A.R. Physical Therapy
Redwood City, CA
Spine Pain: Aquatic Rehabilitation Strategies

Michael Fredericson, M.D.
Associate Professor
Division of Physical Medicine and Rehabilitation
Department of Orthopedic Surgery
Stanford University Medical Center
Stanford, CA
Spine Pain: Aquatic Rehabilitation Strategies

Gwendolyn Garrett, M.S., O.T.R.
Aquatic Therapy of Virginia
Newport News, VA
Hydrotherapeutic Applications in Arthritis Rehabilitation

Chester H. Ho, M.D.
Staff Physician
Spinal Cord Injury/Disorders Unit
Louis Stokes Cleveland Department of Veterans Affairs Medical Center
Department of Physical Medicine and Rehabilitation
Case Western Reserve University
Cleveland, OH
Hydrotherapy and Pressure Ulcers

Thomas H. Hudgins, M.D.
Affiliate Staff
Evanston Hospital
Evanston, IL
Lake Forest Hospital
Lake Forest, IL
Aquatic Strategies in Musculoskeletal Pain

Lynette Jamison, M.O.T., OTR/L, C.P.O.
Director
Aquatics and Rehabilitation
Desert Pain Institute
Owner/Consultant
Future Waves Aquatics Consulting
Phoenix, AZ
The Lyton Model: An Interdisciplinary Model of Care

Jim Johnson, M.D.
Sports Medicine Physician
Southern Sports Medicine
USA Swimming National Team Physician
Nashville, TN
Spine Pain: Aquatic Rehabilitation Strategies

Douglas W. Kinnaird, B.A., N.C.T.M.B., A.T.R.I.C.
Massage Therapist, Specialist in Aquatic Therapy and Rehabilitation
Therapy Pool Program
Mittleman Jewish Community Center
Founder/Instructor
Kinnaird Seminars
Presenter
Aquatic Therapy and Rehab Institute
Portland, OR
The Halliwick Concept

Johan F. Lambeck, B.P.T.
Physiotherapist
Aquatic Rehabilitation Consultant
Malden, Netherlands
The Halliwick Concept

Juliana Larson, B.S., L.M.T.
Owner
Aquatic Solutions
Cedar Key, FL
Aquatic Therapy: From Acute Care to Lifestyle

Ruth I. Meyer, M.Ed., R.K.T.
Therapist
Spectrum Physical Therapy Health and Wellness
Charlottesville, VA
Staff Training and Development in Aquatic Therapy

David M. Morris, M.S., P.T.
Associate Professor
Department of Physical Therapy
University of Alabama at Birmingham
Birmingham, AL
Aquatic Rehabilitation for the Treatment of Neurologic Disorders

Marilou Moschetti, B.Sc., P.T.A.
AquaTechnics Consulting Group
Aptos, CA
Equipment Options and Uses for the Aquatic Therapy Pool, Spine Pain: Aquatic Rehabilitation Strategies

Charlotte Norton, D.P.T., M.S., A.T.C., C.S.C.S.
Consultant
Building Bridges
Sacramento, CA
The Lyton Model: An Interdisciplinary Model of Care

Alison Osinski, Ph.D.
Owner
Aquatic Consulting Services
San Diego, CA
Facility Design and Water Management

Teresa M. Peterson, P.T., M.S., P.C.S.
Owner
Aquatic Physical Therapy, L.L.C.
Overland Park, KS
Instructor, Pediatric Physical Therapy
University of Kansas Medical Center
Kansas City, KS
Pediatric Aquatic Therapy

Peggy Schoedinger, P.T.
Consultant and Lecturer/Owner
International Aquatic Therapy Seminars
Aquatic Therapy Innovations, Inc.
Boulder, CO
Watsu

Fran Coffey Stanat, Ph.D.
Director
Therapeutic Recreation Program
School of Allied Health Professions
University of Wisconsin-Milwaukee
Milwaukee, WI
The Halliwick Concept

Steven A. Stratton, Ph.D., P.T., A.T.C.
Stratton Rehab
San Antonio, TX
Spine Pain: Aquatic Rehabilitation Strategies

Robert P. Wilder, M.D., F.A.C.S.M.
Associate Professor
Department of Physical Medicine and Rehabilitation
The University of Virginia
Charlottesville, VA
Aqua Running

Preface

The aquatic environment has provided therapeutic benefit throughout the millennia. Most early aquatic venues were derivatives of natural locations: mineral pools, ocean waters, streams, and springs. The development of specific aquatic rehabilitation techniques arose largely from the evolution of earlier techniques translated into new aquatic venues. Techniques had to be modified to suit mineral spring temperatures, variations in saline or mineral content which altered buoyancy and required modifications in treatment methods, and advances in science and materials which allowed and suggested a broader range of treatment options. This evolutionary trend has continued to the present.

Health care became more formally centered within the hospital environment during the twentieth century, especially in North America; a decreasing reliance was placed upon the spa as a health care option. While many hospitals had therapeutic pools, and most had hydrotherapy departments with Hubbard tanks and whirlpool baths, treatment in the aquatic environment was a peripheral part of health care. The use of aquatic rehabilitation techniques did not grow, and often, the advantages of water as a treatment medium were forgotten or ignored in the press of time and energy within the health care system.

As health care reimbursement became more and more controlled by the third party payment system, treatment methods such as aquatic rehabilitation tended to be neglected because other techniques could be used which were economically more efficient, even while less effective. Aquatic therapy was placed at a disadvantage because during a treatment session, many clinical effects are achieved, but the billing systems forced the practitioner to pick only one effect per session, or to bundle the charge. For example, during a typical aquatic session of a hip fracture patient, the patient will be exposed to hydrostatic pressure, which drives out edema around the fracture site and in the distal limb while increasing circulation to the fracture site. At the same time, the patient will be moving the limb through an increasing range of motion, while exerting muscle force to strengthen the muscles across the hip joint and protect the strength elsewhere. The same patient will be initiating walking with the forces of gravity reduced by water buoyancy while working on gait training and balance activities. But the therapist cannot bill for each beneficial effect, instead having to choose an arbitrary most important choice, or to bundle the treatment charge under "pool therapy." A single session in the pool might achieve many treatment benefits, all in a shorter time and at lower cost than the alternative of choosing many treatments that can each be billed individually. Typically, it has been much more profitable to pick the latter course. Thus, there has been an economic force behind the decline in aquatic therapeutics. This decline has been aggravated by the decrease in curriculum time in medical education and physical therapy in aquatic therapeutic rationale and technique.

During the second half of this century, fewer hospitals included pools as a part of their construction because of expense and maintenance. Physical therapy departments devoted less space to hydrotherapy departments, because of the diminishing role hydrotherapy has had in contemporary health care. Rehabilitation hospitals usually included pools, and often used these pools for group activities and sometimes for recreational purposes for rehabilitation patients, but there was little crossover between the community pool and the therapeutic pool, and virtually no crossover between the other aquatic rehabilitation venues in use in hospitals and the community.

As a consequence, a communication gap has developed between these various facilities, and between the personnel responsible for the care of the public in each. Physical therapists have tended to practice in isolation, therapeutic recreation personnel have developed their own programs, organizations such as the Red Cross have created programs on their own, and overall there has been minimal interaction with the health care system. A Babel of systems, techniques, and turf barriers has evolved as a result. Where intellectual cross-fertilization should exist to the general betterment of society, this has been too infrequently the case.

The society as a whole has not been well served by this fragmentation. Because the aquatic environment has such a broad margin of therapeutic safety, and because it can be used in the management of a wide range of issues, from the formal medical management of specific diseases to the recreational use by multigenerational populations, better coordination is in order. The continuum of care from acute disease management to general health and well-being can be aided by the aquatic environment. The current gaps in understanding of the physiologic benefits of water, treatment techniques, and methods to mesh the health care system with the community do not serve the public well.

Aquatic facilities are expensive to build and maintain. At the same time, health care is widely viewed as too expensive. Scarcely an issue of the evening paper is published without a reference to changes in the health care system to decrease costs. Thus, it is perhaps reasonable that the logical direction of aquatic therapy should be to narrow the physical and communication gaps between the health care system and the community pool, to extend the hospital into the community, and vice versa.

There is another important element at play here. Even the most casual visitor to the aquatic therapy environment will notice an important difference from almost any other treatment venue: the sound of laughter. There is something within the human soul that is liberated upon immersion. Patients with acute illnesses, those with severely disabling conditions, and children in pain can all be seen smiling and relaxed in the pool. Those familiar with Ron Howard's movie "Cocoon," will remember the seniors at play in the pool, suddenly lifted from their geriatric status into the mental frame of rowdy children. There is no official medical term for this phenomenon, but only the most callous health care provider would deny its value in the therapeutic process, and as reflected in some of the contents of this edition, the important mind-body connection provided by aquatic therapy is becoming understood.

During the years since the first edition of this book was written, there have been many signs of movement in the growing understanding of the importance and broad applicability of aquatic therapy. In developing the second edition of this book, the authors have responded to the requests of a broad range of aquatic professionals who felt that there was a need to summarize and update the effects of the aquatic environment on human physiology, to bring forward new advances in treatment methodologies, and describe the current state of the aquatic rehabilitation art. In so doing, we have attempted to relate the scientific underpinnings which are the foundation of all aquatic therapies and at the same time build these foundations into the treatment rationales which are in current use. We hope that we have succeeded in creating a reference that will facilitate the transfer of knowledge of the great number of biologic processes that are affected by the aquatic environment. At the same time, we hope to enable aquatic practitioners to develop their own methods and techniques built upon this scientific understanding, and built upon the heads and shoulders of the careful and visionary treatment innovators who went before them.

The aquatic environment has tremendous utility in these times of health care containment: to transfer medical treatment efficiently into the community setting, to build fitness and conditioning as a lifestyle, to rebuild the community pool into a health and wellness center integrated with the health care system would be a great service to the population. But this is not truly a revolutionary idea: one only has to examine the design of the most advanced ancient Roman baths to realize that society has come this way before. Thus, we have begun to close the circle historically, adding a great deal of science and technology along the way to better understand the processes and reasons for aquatic therapy. Let us all work together toward this closure.

Andrew J. Cole, M.D.
Bruce E. Becker, M.D.

Acknowledgments

There are a great number of individuals who have facilitated the creation of the second edition of this book. Our parents perhaps were the central people in the development of our interest in aquatic therapeutics. For Bruce, it was because they followed the aquatic and physical therapy recommendations of the Sister Kenny Hospital staff during his recovery from poliomyelitis as a child in Minneapolis. He will remain grateful for life. For Andy, it was because of his parents commitment to exercise and aquatic sports that created so many meaningful childhood memories. Our adult learning about aquatic rehabilitation has been fostered by many individuals. Drs. Luis deLerma, Herman Flax, Jens Henrickson, Chester Wong and Robert Christopher were all instrumental in the early days of the American Society of Medical Hydrology, supporting Dr. Sidney Licht in keeping the organizational flames alive through the years of bridging the gap between the therapy world and formal medicine, while linking to the established strong traditions of the International Society of Medical Hydrology. Their support of the organization, and assistance during our years as presidents of the organization have been tremendously helpful. The Aquatic Therapy and Rehabilitation Institute Aquatechnics Consulting organizers and instructors have been a tremendous inspiration throughout many years, and we cherish their friendship and help. Many are represented herein.

Prior to publication of the first edition, and certainly since, there have been many individuals both inside the USA and out, who have been of tremendous value both academically and spiritually. Dr. Helmut Pratzel has provided a wealth of understanding of the properties of water, and Dr. Yuko Agishi and his many Japanese colleagues have created an entire scientific body of aquatic physiology research that would have been very difficult to create within the financially challenged medical research system of the USA. The efforts of our colleagues and friends who are contributors to this second edition are stellar, and we have gained greatly through their professional efforts. We hope after the editorial prodding that goes into a text such as this that they will remain our friends!

Our wives Carolyn and Carol, have been tremendously supportive and helpful during the many nighttime hours spent in this second edition's creation and tremendously useful in proofing and guiding our efforts. Their love and forgiveness have been critical. We would also like to thank Joseph M. Ihm, M.D., and Robert L. Cooper, M.D. for their many hours spent proofreading the final copy.

Chapter 1
Aquatic Rehabilitation: A Historical Perspective

Jonathan Paul De Vierville, PhD, MSSW

A NEW BRANCH ON AN OLD TREE

Aquatic rehabilitation is a new name for a treatment method with ancient roots. Over the centuries, health care practitioners have used various terms for the therapeutic and rehabilitative benefits conferred by water. Aquatic rehabilitation is a late-20th century term that describes a scientific theory, a medical rationale, and a set of clinical procedures using water immersion for the restoration of physical mobility and physiologic activity, and, at times, for effecting psychological transformation.

As a recently developed medical treatment modality, aquatic rehabilitation has a relatively brief history. When linked with the lengthy history of healing waters, thermal baths, health resort medicine, and spa therapies, however, aquatic rehabilitation serves as a contemporary affirmation of the classic medical traditions that used healing water pools. In this sense, contemporary aquatic rehabilitation can trace its origins from the first civilizations.

ORIGINS OF AQUATIC THERAPY

Humans, especially the sick and suffering, have long resorted to springs, baths, and pools for their soothing and healing properties. Taking the waters, soaking in baths and pools, and resting at places called spas played an important social and spiritual role in the river valley civilizations of Mesopotamia, Egypt, India, and China. Bathing pools were widely used for individual, religious, social renewal, and healing rituals. Healing water rituals also appeared in ancient Greek, Hebrew, Roman, Christian, and Islamic cultures. Ancient civilizations used the waters for cleaning the earthly body of disease and cleansing the spiritual body of sin. These cultures taught that clean bodies and pure souls facilitated seasonal as well as eternal renewal, which in turn ensured cultural regeneration.

Swiss cultural historian Sigfried Giedion made the following observation:

> The bath and its purposes have held different meanings for different ages. The manner in which a civilization integrates bathing within its life, as well as the type of bathing it prefers, yields searching insight into the inner nature of the period.... The role that bathing plays within a

culture reveals the culture's attitude toward human relaxation. It is a measure of how far individual well-being is regarded as an indispensable part of community life.[1]

Giedion explains the bath and its role in two types of regenerative processes: individual and social. Individual bathing is a private hygienic act of body care known as an *ablution*. The other type of regenerative process is social bathing, a receptive, relaxed, and restorative activity that enhances wellness for the whole being and embodies the "broad ideal [of] total regeneration."[1]

THE SPA CONCEPT

Much of the current field of aquatic rehabilitation has its roots in the European and early American spa world. Etymologically, *spa* is traced from the Latin verb *spargere*, to pour forth. Roman legions built their camps at hot springs, where healing waters "poured forth." The modern word *spa* found its way into the English language through the old Walloon word *espa*, which referred to a fountain. From *espa* the English derived *spaw*. In 1326, at a little village located in the Ardennes range, the name *Spa* was used to identify some hot mineral springs discovered to possess therapeutic and medicinal values. Shortly thereafter, pools were built at Spa, Belgium. Two hundred and twenty-five years later, William Slingsby discovered the sulfur springs of Tewhit near Harrogate, England, and compared these natural sulfur mineral fountains to those at Spa, Belgium.

In the 1950s, Dr. Sidney Licht, a founding member of the American Society of Medical Hydrology and Climatology, defined a spa as a "place where mineral containing waters flow from the ground naturally, or to which [they are] pumped or conducted, and [are] there used for therapeutic purposes."[2] Similarly, Dr. Walter S. McClellan, the first medical director of the Saratoga Spa in Saratoga Springs, NY, considered a spa "a place or location where nature has provided natural healing agents such as mineral waters or peloids, at which provisions have been made in physical plant and equipment for the administration of treatments which utilize[s] these agents, and where the program is carried out under medical control."[3] Thus, the historical definition of the spa recognizes an important social institution that provides a time and place for activities, leisure, relaxation, healing, and renewal. The spa parks like those at Saratoga and other spa towns with springs spawned development of the foundations of contemporary aquatic rehabilitation.

GREEK, ROMAN, AND MEDIEVAL SPA CULTURES

Social bathing as a component of individual and cultural recreation was an important part of the cultures of the ancient Greeks and Romans. The Greeks believed in the relationship between the gymnastic invigoration of the body and the academic stimulation of the mind (Figs. 1-1 and 1-2). The buildings at Delphi (334 BC) included the gymnasium, *xystos* (track), and *palaestra* with its *loutron* (cold water washroom), and *ephebeum*. The *ephebeum*, the large main room, was used for educational and social functions. Similar to Delphi, the Sanctuary of Zeus at Olympia shows the large gymnasium in close proximity to the *palaestra*, with its *loutron*. Other bathing arrangements of the era resembled those at the Greek colony (310-280 BC) of Gela (Sicily), where individual tubs are set in a line and in a circle.[4]

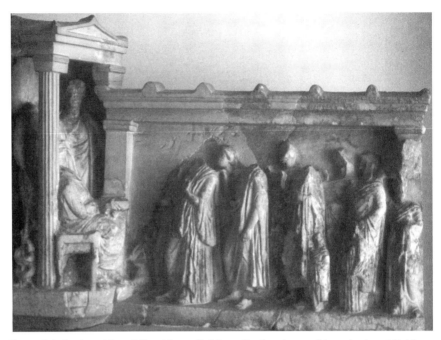

Figure 1-1. Ancient (circa 340 BC) bas relief from the Sanctuary of Aesculapius at Epidarus, Greece.

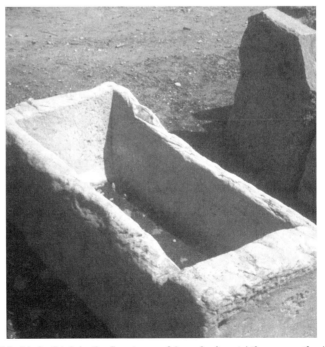

Figure 1-2. Marble bathtub in the Sanctuary of Aesculapius at Athens near the Acropolis.

4 COMPREHENSIVE AQUATIC THERAPY

Parallel to current practice, bathing followed exercise and was believed to have therapeutic value.

Whereas the Greeks considered bathing an added function to the gymnasium, the Romans considered bathing a central social function to accompany activities that might include exercise in a gymnasium. Roman culture elevated bathing practices to a more practical, formal, educational, social, and technically refined level (Fig. 1-3). Roman *thermae*, including hot-air baths, frigid pools, and relaxation areas, functioned as important social and civil institutions and enabled usage that was believed to be medically beneficial. The physician Galen had his office in the baths of Hadrian.

The Roman *thermae* contained multiple rooms and pools with varied temperatures and an *ambulacrum* with space for libraries, lecture rooms, art and sculpture galleries, multipurpose meeting and ceremonial halls, shaded parks and promenades, small theaters, indoor athletic halls, and, occasionally, sports stadiums. Behind the scenes were the furnaces and service areas for wood, food, and laundry. The first public baths in Rome and possibly the first in the series of imperial *thermae* are believed to be the Baths of Agrippa, built in 25 BC.[4]

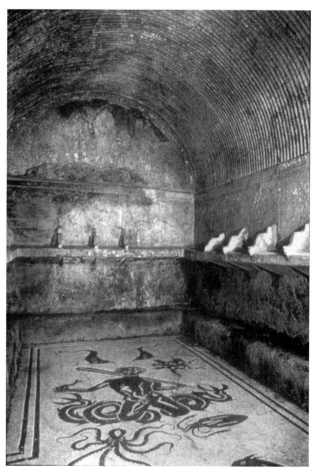

Figure 1-3. Roman bath and mosaic at Pompeii.

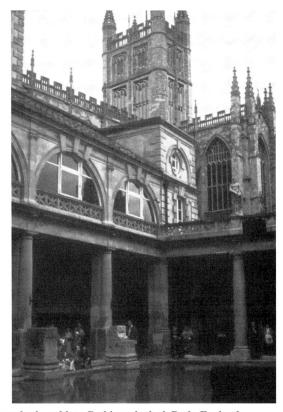

Figure 1-4. Roman bath and late Gothic cathedral, Bath, England.

Following the decline of the Western Roman Empire, Byzantium carried on the *thermae* traditions in the East. Islamic culture later replaced the active games and athletics with scrubs and massages, which became a central part of the traditional Turkish bath. Russian culture combined hot vapor baths with cold plunges. The Russian steam bath may be one of the oldest forms of social bathing for physical, spiritual, and cultural regeneration.

In Europe during the Middle Ages, grand healing pools were built around thermal springs in Poretta, Italy; Bath, England; and Spa, Belgium, as well as Baden-Baden and Aachen in Germany (Fig. 1-4). As early as 740 AD in Switzerland, the Benedictine Abbey of Pfäfers served as the spiritual and cultural center of Switzerland. Here the mountain monks operated the baths of Pfäfers, where during the Renaissance the new humanists came to meet and talk. In 1535, Theophrastus of Hohenheim, better known as Paracelsus, practiced his healing arts at Bad Pfäfers. By the 19th century, Bad Ragaz in Switzerland had developed into a major health resort spa, where today the aquatic rehabilitation procedure known as the Bad Ragaz ring method is taught and practiced. Similar aquatic histories and traditions are found at other European spas, including Aix-les-Bains, Evian-les-Bains, Vichy, Baden-Baden, Motecatini Terme, Albano, San Pellegrino, Karlsbad, Marienbad, and Franzbad (Fig. 1-5). These sites have served European medicine for centuries, and even today many are part of standard traditional health care practice.

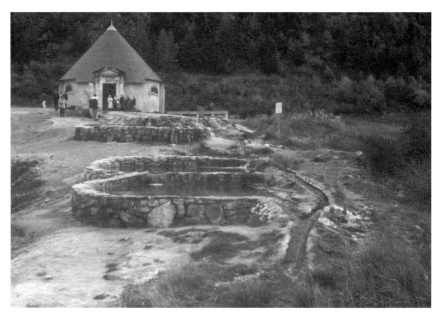

Figure 1-5. Mountain baths from the Middle Ages, France.

GROWTH OF AQUATIC THERAPY IN AMERICA

The European history of aquatic traditions is lengthy, as is America's. New World natives practiced similar hot air and cold plunge baths in the sweat lodge, which served both medical and religious purposes. Since Ponce De Leon's search and De Soto's trek through the New World forests, America's healing waters have been discovered, lost, and rediscovered with each generation. In the 1600s, the English, Dutch, and French colonists built their stone huts and wooden tubs near wilderness healing springs frequented by Indians. During the 1700s, natural philosophers such as Drs. John De Normandie and Benjamin Rush traveled to the colonial mineral springs and thermal pools to analyze the waters for their chemical and medicinal virtues. In Virginia, Thomas Jefferson rode his horse to the distant Warm Springs Valley and made notes on the healing mineral springs and pools (Fig. 1-6). Jefferson used Palladio's ancient Roman drawings to design the Sweet Springs spa in West Virginia.

In the decades before the Civil War, major health reforms swept the nation, and numerous hydropathic establishments, institutes, and medical colleges were built for the practice of the *water cure* (cold water bathing). Health reformers, including Dr. and Mrs. Shew, Dr. Russell Trall, Dr. Nichols, and Mary Gove-Nichols wrote lengthy books on bathing practices, and spa doctors traveled to distant frontier springs. Others, such as Dr. Thomas Goode of the Homestead in Virginia and Dr. John Jennings Moorman of the Greenbrier in West Virginia, developed notable medical reputations for their aquatic treatments (Fig. 1-7). Western pioneers, such as Hiram Abiff Whittington at Hot Springs, Ark, constructed large thermal pools for traveling invalids.

During the era of Reconstruction, Dr. George G. Walton analyzed many newly discovered frontier springs and constructed an elaborate scientific classification system of the springs based on geography, climatology, mineralogy, chemistry, and

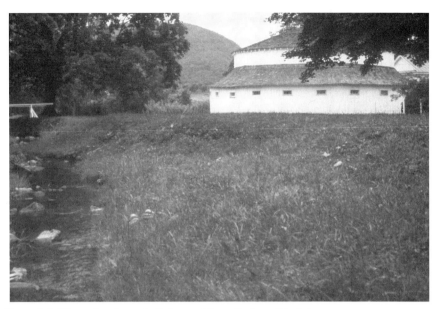

Figure 1-6. Women's octagon bath house, Warm Springs, Virginia.

geology. In 1880, the American Medical Association (AMA) Committee on Sanitaria and Springs published its first national report on sanitaria. The AMA committee classified the nation's 646 known springs and mineral water pools. Several years later, Dr. Albert Charles Peale classified 2822 active therapeutic springs. By 1896, 19 spa doctors using the healing waters and thermal pools at Hot Springs had published their medical theories and cases in the *Hot Springs Medical Journal*.

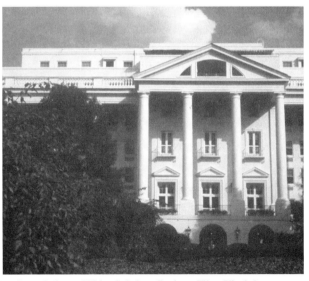

Figure 1-7. The Greenbrier at White Sulphur Springs, West Virginia.

AMERICAN SPAS IN THE TWENTIETH CENTURY

At the turn of the century, medical men such as Simon Baruch, John Harvey Kellogg, and Guy Hinsdale regularly conducted clinical hydrotherapeutic experiments and prescribed what were termed *balneotherapeutics*. They also recommended climatotherapeutics and sent their patients to mountain springs where clean air and sunshine provided healthy environments. Baruch established the American medical standards for hydrotherapy in his *Principles and Practice of Hydrotherapy* (Fig. 1-8). Kellogg, who directed the Battle Creek Sanitarium in Michigan, published an enormous volume on hydrotherapy, which included his scientific theories and practices of hydrotherapy based on a systematic but iconoclastic and controversial physiologic system for internal and external aquatic treatments. After World War I, Dr. H. H. Roberts published an examination of the therapeutic value of America's health resorts and spas for rehabilitation.[5] In 1920, Simon Baruch published his last book, *An Epitome of Hydrotherapy*.

Although most spa doctors wrote about and prescribed the internal and external curative benefits of water, baths, and pools, they usually placed limited emphasis on water exercise. Most bathing activities in America were passive. As early as 1911, however, Dr. Charles LeRoy Lowman was using therapeutic tubs to treat patients with cerebral palsy and spastic conditions. Lowman, who founded the Orthopaedic

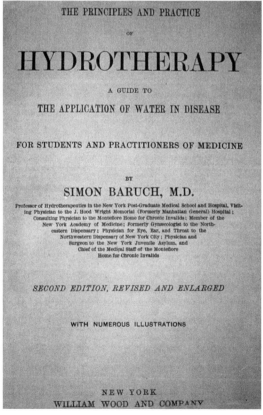

Figure 1-8. Title page for Dr. Simon Baruch's book *The Principles and Practice of Hydrotherapy*.

Hospital in Los Angeles, Calif, in 1913 (now Rancho Los Amigos), visited the Spaulding School for Crippled Children in Chicago, where he observed paralyzed patients exercising in a wooden tank. On his return to California, he transformed the hospital's lily pond into two therapeutic pools. One fresh-water pool was used for therapy with paralyzed patients and patients with poliomyelitis; the other pool was filled with salt water and was used to treat patients with infectious diseases. He also made a motion picture showing the various conditions treated with pool therapy.[6] At Warm Springs, Ga, LeRoy Hubbard developed his famous tank, and, in 1924, Warm Springs received its most famous patient for aquatic therapy, Franklin D. Roosevelt. Still a private citizen, Roosevelt traveled to Georgia, where he exercised his withered legs. A decade later, newsreels showed the crippled President Roosevelt performing therapeutic water exercises, which encouraged the medical acceptance of aquatic rehabilitation.

SPA DESIGN, RESEARCH, AND THE DEPRESSION YEARS

Before the Great Depression, America's spas experienced rapid expansion. When the stock market crashed, spas did not immediately feel the impact. In fact, the publicly owned spas, such as Saratoga Spa at Saratoga Springs and Hot Springs, benefited from the Depression: More people visited spas for therapeutic reasons, and the wealthy, who could no longer afford travel to Europe, chose American pools.[7] At the Homestead, Drs. Frank Hopkins and Melitus Jarman described the expanded Hot Springs Spa as a place in America where a professional medical staff administered the ancient "Aesculapian art."[8]

At Saratoga, financier Bernard M. Baruch, Roosevelt's friend and the son of Simon Baruch, headed a special commission. The Baruch Commission was formed with the assistance of the New York Academy of Medicine and comprised a geologist from Columbia University, a committee of five physicians, and Dr. Franz Groedel, a notable European balneologist. Groedel, later a founder and president of the American College of Cardiology,[9] was then a professor at the State University, Frankfurt-am-Main, Germany, and director of the Kerckhoff Institute at Bad Nauheim. The Commission planned a scientific American spa[10] and studied spa design, natural treatments, and efficient operations based on sound medical and scientific care for chronically ill patients, especially those with cardiac, vascular, and circulatory ailments.[11] Groedel's work at Saratoga and subsequent scientific lectures provided a major medical contribution to American health resort medicine, spa therapy, and aquatic rehabilitation.[12] The Commission selected McClellan as medical spa director.[10] His first task at Saratoga Spa was to design a new spa research laboratory, and he recruited help from Dr. W. E. Fitch, author of the 1927 comprehensive volume, *Mineral Waters of the United States and American Spas*. Fitch was the medical director at French Lick Springs Hotel and Spa in Indiana, which was staffed and equipped with the best available hydrotherapeutic department. (It was at French Lick Spa during the 1931 summer National Governors Convention that Governor Franklin Roosevelt initially gathered support for his presidential bid.)

Also in 1931, Fitch, McClellan, and several scientific directors, general managers, and others met at French Lick Spa with the purpose of organizing "an association which would be of mutual benefit to everyone interested in the advancement of Medical Hydrology in this country."[13] Participants reviewed a half-century of

American spa programs. Their discussion anticipated spa therapy and aquatic rehabilitation for the following 50 years.[13] Shortly thereafter, Groedel came to New York to help design the Saratoga Spa.

During the Depression years, investigators researched the physical, psychiatric, thermal, mechanical, chemical, mineral, electrical, and radioactive qualities of the American spa waters, and medical organizations held special meetings and conducted spa tours. A wealth of information, research, and articles on health resort medicine, spa therapy, and pool treatments appeared in the professional journals of that time. At Northwestern University Medical School in Chicago, Dr. John S. Coulter, the first full-time academic physician in physical medicine, presented lectures on physical therapy, which he placed within the history of spa medicine.[14] In Boston, Dr. Rebekah Wright, a psychiatrist employed by the Massachusetts Department of Mental Diseases, researched the use of water for its psychotherapeutic effects. In her book, *Hydrotherapy in Hospitals for Mental Diseases*, Wright described 32 aquatically based procedures used to achieve sedative, stimulating, anodyne, hypnotic, eliminative, and antipyretic effects on the body.[15] In 1933, America's healing waters were officially recognized with the establishment of the Simon Baruch Research Institute of Balneology at Saratoga Spa and the printing of a series of scientific bulletins. At Hot Springs National Park in Arkansas, another group of spa doctors, including Louis G. Martin,[16] Euclid Smith,[17] George B. Fletcher,[18] and Nelda King,[19] physical therapist at the Maurice Baths, researched and practiced pool therapy and underwater physiotherapy. In 1936, Roosevelt traveled by special presidential train to Hot Springs, where he visited the Army and Navy Hospital and Bath House Row. The same year, Dr. Albert W. Wallace described America's health resort spas and their full medical potential in the *Journal of the American Medical Association (JAMA)*.[20] He listed the following 10 universal spa features:

1. Proper use of mineral springs and climates
2. Competent medical supervision
3. Proper dietary regimen
4. Systematic rest
5. Regulated exercise
6. Proper knowledge of the patient's reserve and limits
7. Spa therapies, including physical, electric, heliotherapeutic, and hydrotherapeutic procedures administered by competent attendants
8. Planning and regulation of the patient's day
9. Elevation of the morale
10. Development of a proper perspective (patient's and doctor's) toward the patient's disease

Spa medicine at that time used large pools and tanks. In the basement pool of the Maurice Bath House in Hot Springs, a warm swimming pool was installed in the 1930s for underwater physical therapy exercises and pool therapy treatments for patients with chronic arthritis.[17] By 1937, Lowman had published *Technique of Underwater Gymnastics: A Study in Practical Application*, in which he detailed pool therapy methods of specific underwater exercises that "carefully regulated dosage, character, frequency, and duration for remedying bodily deformities and restoring muscle function."[6] This was one of the earliest American publications on what has evolved into aquatic rehabilitation, and it was a landmark effort to quantify the aquatic regimen.

At the Fifteenth Congress of Physical Therapy in 1936, Groedel,[21] McClellan,[22] and Behrend[23] presented papers on spa medicine research. As a result of the Sixteenth Congress, a three-page editorial on American health resorts appeared in the *Archives of Physical Therapy, X-Ray and Radium*, and a Committee on Spas and Health Resorts in the United States was formed.[24] The committee's first action was to establish a formal outline for a national survey.[24a] Physicians subsequently toured spas at French Lick, Battle Creek, and Mount Clemens in Michigan, and Glens Springs, Richfield Springs, Sharon Springs, and Saratoga Springs in New York. In 1937, a resolution was drafted calling for the AMA to establish a council on spas and health resorts.[24] Dr. Bernard Fantus convinced Morris Fishbein, editor of *JAMA*, to publish a special article requesting that the AMA "study the vital importance of active medical programs for spas and health resorts."[26] The following year, a second spa tour group visited Bedford Springs, Penn, the Homestead, the Greenbrier, and French Lick, ending its tour at the Seventeenth Congress in Chicago, where the Committee on Spas and Health Resorts presented a full report.[27,28] The AMA understood the therapeutic significance and growing interest in spas and appointed its own committee, but the trustees did not like the historical reputation of America's spas and insisted that the only suitable term was *health resort*, not *spa*. *JAMA* published numerous articles affirming the value of "health resort" therapy for "chronic disabling conditions, including those affecting the heart and circulation, rheumatic disorders, ailments of the stomach, intestinal tract, gallbladder and liver, nervous conditions, certain disorders of the skin and some metabolic diseases."[28] Even *Medical Economics* published an article on the medical and economic implications of spa medicine.[29]

WAR, PHYSICAL MEDICINE, AND SPA REHABILITATION CENTERS

The Depression and later the medical consequences of World War II benefited American spas. In 1941, there were a total of 8826 mineral springs at 2717 different locations with 321 spas and health resort facilities,[30] but there were no major national organizations or certification or accrediting bodies. Medicine was changing with increased specialization and was generally organized along organ systems. Although Drs. Coulter and Frank H. Krusen led the organization of the American Academy of Physical Medicine in 1938, no specialty included the multidisciplinary practice of health resort medicine, spa therapy, and aquatic rehabilitation as a central theme. Even though the AMA did define certain minimum health resort standards based on established scientific procedure, references in the medical literature, especially to spa therapy and natural therapeutic agents and resources, were generally ignored.

Dr. Henry Sigerist, a leading medical historian of that time and founder of the *Bulletin of the History of Medicine*, tried to keep the waters flowing by writing about the history of American spas.[31] But 1941 was a time for war, not for spa organizing or teaching. The war forced major changes on America's spas and their treatment methods. The Army, the Navy, and the Veterans Administration commandeered some of the best spas and turned them into military hospitals for physical therapy and rehabilitation programs.[32] Despite the war, *JAMA* published a special series of 18 articles on health resort therapy between October 1943 and May 1947.

After the war, a new Commission on Physical Medicine was established and was chaired by Krusen. A member of the AMA Health Resort Committee and a rigorous scientist, Krusen was skeptical about health resort medicine and spa therapy, although he was a firm believer in the therapeutic value of medical hydrology as a part of a grander concept. He promoted physical medicine and rehabilitation, a subject he taught at the Mayo Clinic. Krusen, the first to use the term *physiatrist*, played a key role in the development of postwar physical medicine and rehabilitation, especially as a newly developed medical specialty.

The Commission on Physical Medicine Subcommittee for Medical Hydrology and Health Resorts reported on the future of spa health resorts as rehabilitation centers.[33] The report assessed the needs for basic research, teaching, clinical practice, and rehabilitation in the field of hydrotherapy as related to physiologic changes that occurred in the circulation, respiration, metabolism, and body chemistry during water treatments. Several American spas offered medically supervised regimens, and a few orthopedic and mental hospitals practiced hydrotherapy, but scientific research was sparse. The military hospitals at Hot Springs, Ark; Glenwood Springs, Colo; and Saratoga Springs, NY, operated institutional spa rehabilitation centers. The report recommended the establishment of spa rehabilitation centers throughout the country at health resorts. Besides treating war veterans, spa rehabilitation centers also treated patients injured in industrial jobs, patients having chronic degenerative diseases, and patients in posthospital convalescence. Unfortunately, the Committee on Physical Medicine did not include these recommendations in its final report. The interest and organizational support for health resort medicine, spa therapy, and aquatic rehabilitation had diminished significantly by the war's end.

POSTWAR POOLS AND MEDICAL HYDROLOGY

Postwar American culture focused on the powers of science and technology, and relatively few physicians remembered how earlier civilized cultures used and revered the regenerative powers of healing waters. During the early 1950s, as poliomyelitis affected nearly 58,000 Americans annually, the National Foundation for Infantile Paralysis supported the corrective swimming pools and hydrogymnastics of Lowman and the therapeutic use of pools and tanks for the treatment of poliomyelitis. But with the development of the Salk vaccine and the subsequent reduced incidence of poliomyelitis in the later 1950s, the medical perception of need for complex aquatic therapy regimens waned, and pools became far less important to hospital practice. Pools went into disrepair, and therapists began to lose interest in, and understanding of, the old techniques. The advances made immediately before and during the war years, followed by the increased technical sophistication gained during the polio era, began to fade.

By 1962, however, Drs. Licht, Herman Flax, Sigmund Foster, William Erdman, Lucille Eising, J. Wayne McFarland, Jens Henriksen, and Richard Gubner recognized the need for torchbearers to keep medical hydrology knowledge alive. They organized the American Society of Medical Hydrology and Climatology (ASMH) as the North American affiliate for the International Society of Medical Hydrology and Climatology (ISMH). Since 1921, the ISMH, as the World Congress for Health Resort Medicine and Spa Therapy, has been meeting every 4 years around the world. ISMH has a long-established international history and publishes statutes and standards for health resort medicine and spa therapy. The Thirty-Second World

Congress of ISMH in 1994 was held in Bad Wörishofen, Germany, the historical spa town of Father Sebastian Kneipp, one of the legendary figures in modern medical hydrology (Fig. 1-9). The Thirty-Third World Congress of ISMH in 1998 was held in Karlovy Vary, Czech Republic, and the Thirty-Fourth World Congress of ISMH in 2002 was held in Budapest, Hungary.

The late 1960s and early 1970s were a golden time in American basic science research. Research funds were plentiful as the country attempted to move into space. During this period of Space Age research, as Dr. Bruce Becker points out, scientists "began to study the effects of weightlessness through research in water, the only environment that could approximate the effects of space flight."[34]

In 1969, Neil Armstrong first walked in the lunar environment. In the same year, several other historic events occurred relating to aquatic environments, therapies, and rehabilitation. In January, the first issue of the *Medical Hydrology Quarterly* appeared under the editorship of Henriksen. This issue contained a report on Dr. V. R. Ott's lecture on spa cardiac rehabilitation to the 1968 ASMH annual meeting, in which he made the following observation:

> The need for spa courses today seems as vital as in those olden times when spa vacations were stipulated in marriage contracts of wealthy citizens and when people believed that bathing in mineral wells was diving into a miracle fountain and becoming rejuvenated by decades. Present medicine should not neglect the possibilities of adapting an age-old principle to modern science and to the philosophy of rehabilitation.[35]

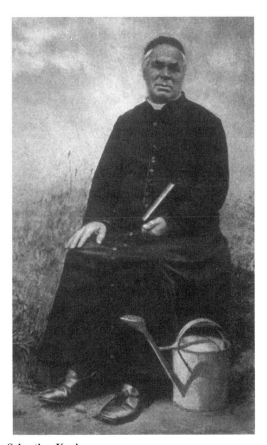

Figure 1-9. Father Sebastian Kneipp.

AQUATICS, FITNESS AND HEALTH SPAS ORGANIZE

What was written in the 20th century still holds true today in the 21st century and for future research, development, education, and practice of comprehensive aquatic therapies and rehabilitation. In recent years the increasing public interest combined with the long neglect of formal training in the principles of aquatic rehabilitation began to create a hunger in professionals working in the area, especially among professionals interested in alternative, complementary, and spa medicine. Interest grew within the American Physical Therapy Association (APTA). The Aquatic Exercise Association (AEA) was established in the mid-1980s to provide professional development, services, and products related to aquatic fitness and aquatic therapy industries for allied health care professionals, including physical and occupational therapists, kinesiotherapists, recreational and aquatic therapists, and aerobics instructors. AEA publishes *The AKWA Letter* and offers workshops and certification programs for aquatic instructors and pool specialists. A related organization, the Aquatic Therapy and Rehabilitation Institute (ATRI), has labored to develop multidisciplinary standards for aquatic therapy. It is important to note the differentiation between AEA's focus on aquatic *exercise* and ATRI's focus on aquatic *therapy*. Together, the AEA and ATRI host an Annual Aquatic Symposium with many workshops conducted in aquatic environments as well as formal classroom instruction. Organizations such as these play important roles in further development and expansion of American comprehensive aquatic rehabilitation. Paralleling the growth of these organizations has been the development of a large special interest section within the APTA, led by several of the contributors to this book.

During the later decades of the 20th century an increased sense of speed and stress spread through society, and the public began to seek healthful spaces of sanctuary and solace. Planning a vacation for one's health became more important, especially among the high-strung but aging Baby Boomer population. To meet this new health need, in 1989 Bernard Burt assembled a list of health resorts in the first edition of *Fodor's Health and Fitness Vacations*.[36] Taking a vacation for health reasons was not a new concept nor was a list of resorts and spas, telling travelers where they could find the needed health resources. What was new and important about Burt's guide was its listing of health resort and spa resources, not only by region but also by the types of fitness programs and health spa treatments. The book lists 12 categories of programs, including luxury pampering, life enhancement, weight management, nutrition and diet, stress control, holistic health, spiritual awareness, preventive medicine, "taking the waters," sports conditioning, youth camps for weight loss, and nonprogram resort facilities. Although it is useful for health seekers looking for wellness and fitness, the book contained little information on the affiliation of programs with formal medicine and therapy. The public had responded to medicine's disregard for spa medicine by viewing established medicine as irrelevant to the New Age concept of wellness.

In 1991, the International Spa and Fitness Association organized its first international conference and trade exposition, dubbed "The Ultimate Workout." In attendance were 150 delegates from 20 states and 10 countries, including spa owners, managers, marketing and public relations directors, nutritionists, chefs, massage therapists, estheticians, trainers, consultants, travel agents, government officials, airlines, and equipment and supply vendors. But conspicuously absent from this group was any significant representation from the medical establishment. The scientific rationalization and specialization since the 1950s had engineered a divorce between the mind and the body, with medicine assuming responsibility for and focusing on the physical body.

At the end of the century, however, a general shift began to appear with informal personal values of health care, wellness, and prevention along with the formal medical attitudes toward health, disease, and healing systems. This change came first in the form of widespread health consumer interest in alternative, complementary, and integrative medicines. In the 1990s a newly formed Office of Complementary and Alternative Medicine at the National Institutes of Health began funding cooperative efforts with state university medical schools and other public health care organizations. These new holistic medical and integrative health programs addressed various public concerns focused around innovative medical attitudes and values. One of the seminal works to appear in the mid-1990s was Andrew Weil's *Spontaneous Healing*.[37] Aquatics is not mentioned specifically in Weil's work, but what is important for the history of comprehensive aquatics is his prescription for the reform of medical education, especially in the rehabilitative context and in terms of lifestyle management, healthy living, sustainability, and longevity.

Seen from our larger historical context, however, the radical medical reform Weil proposes is not all that new or revolutionary. If we look back at the origins and reflect on the history of comprehensive aquatics, we can see what Weil was really endorsing—a rediscovery, recovery, and renaissance of the ancient Asklepian medicine and Hygeian lifestyle. Weil provides contemporary faces for an ancient tradition. Also, we can see similarities and comparisons between the 19th century Kur system and principles of Father Kneipp and the 21st century prescriptions of Dr. Weil.

What is radical and really revolutionary for the future of comprehensive aquatics is "The Longevity Revolution" as announced in 1998 by Theodore Roszak in *America the Wise*.[38] A major and fundamental shift in modern demographic patterns is providing numerous seeds for basic cultural change. Roszak sensed a majority of a "New People" in middle and senior age (ages 50 to 100 years) who place less emphasis on survival of the youthful fittest and more value on wisdom, compassion, and longevity. Here emerges a "deep ecology of wisdom," in which the increased number of elders with their informed search for natural and well-balanced lifestyles shift the general public's perception and understanding of health care, illness, and rehabilitation. In other words, as the 80 million plus Baby Boomers get older, their health consumer and patient demands are transforming the medical market needs and services. Evidence of this perceptual change already was observed and documented in the surveys and studies conducted in the 1990s by Eisenberg of Harvard Medical School.[39]

Naturally accompanying this population shift of perception is a deeper attention, sensitivity, and awareness for the place, process, and functional use of water and aquatics in both health and disease. These public health concerns are evidenced in the widening use of bottled drinking waters along with extensive new designs and construction for home relaxation showers, whirlpool baths, herbal hot tubs, floating pools, and water parks. Comprehensive aquatics is reemerging as a new form of spa culture that reaches across the full range of health care and medicine.

Further evidence of this spreading interest in aquatics is witnessed by the numerous health and lifestyle, wellness, and spa conferences for both professionals and consumers. For example, The International Spa Association Education Foundation now suggests the use of Ten Domains by which contemporary spa culture can be evaluated and better understood, comprehensively. The Ten Domains include the following:

1. The Waters: Baths, Hydrotherapies and Aquatics
2. Foods: Nutrition and Diets
3. Movement: Exercise and Fitness
4. Body Work: Massage and Touch
5. MindBody: Spa Psychology's and Meditation
6. Natural Therapeutic Agents: Aesthetics and Skin
7. Environments: Local, Regional and Global Climates, Seasons and Ecology
8. Cultural and Social: Leisure, Recreation, Tourism and the Arts
9. Management: Operations, Marketing and Communications
10. Space-Time/Energy: Chronobiology, Life Style Patterns and Kurs

The Ten Domains are designed to assist professional practitioners at all levels of study, experience, and practice to see the full range, scale, and scope of historically well-established spa and aquatic philosophies, principles, and procedures.[40]

AN AQUATIC RENAISSANCE

Aquatics as applied to health and rehabilitation is experiencing a renaissance. Many professional groups and organizations are interested in America's healing waters. Besides those already mentioned, this list includes the American Academy of Physical Medicine and Rehabilitation, with its own special-interest aquatic rehabilitation group, the American Congress of Physical Medicine and Rehabilitation, the Council for National Cooperation in Aquatics, the National Museum and Educational Center for Allied Healthcare Professionals, the American Kinesiotherapy Association, the National Spa and Pool Institute, and the American Red Cross with its Water Safety Instructor Certification.

This renaissance has parallels in most areas of scientific interest. A waxing of enthusiasm is followed by development of a field, which is, in turn, followed by waning interest and consolidation of some of the gains achieved, with loss of some others. The current rebirth of aquatic therapy signals a new milestone along a road that began in ancient times with Aesculapius and the *thermae* of Rome and continued through Byzantium, Russia, and Europe, leading to modern corporate American medicine. The belief in the therapeutic effects of water continues today. The cultural perceptions, ideas, and theories are reflected in the value placed on the aquatic environment. Contemporary aquatic rehabilitation is rediscovering and redefining the aquatic traditions established earlier in this century by medical hydrology, health resort medicine, and spa therapy.

American health care practitioners are looking again at the aquatic environment as a safe, effective, and inexpensive way of using water to preserve health and treat disease. In this way our civilization will reconnect to the ancient aquatic traditions of healing, rejuvenation, and repair.

REFERENCES

1. Giedion S: Part VII: The mechanization of the bath. In Giedion D (ed): Mechanization Takes Command, A Contribution to Anonymous History. Oxford: Oxford University Press, 1948, p 628.

2. Licht S (ed): Medical Hydrology. The Physical Medicine Library, vol 7. Baltimore: Waverly, 1963, p 437.
3. McClellan WS: Spa therapy. Interne Oct:674, 1946.
4. Yegül F: Baths and Bathing in Classical Antiquity. Cambridge, Mass: MIT Press, 1992, pp 9, 49, 490.
5. Roberts HH: The therapeutic value of the spas and health resorts of America. Med Rec 95:321, 1919.
6. Lowman CL: Technique of Underwater Gymnastics: A Study in Practical Application. Los Angeles: American Publications, 1937, p 4.
7. Conte RS: The History of the Greenbrier, America's Resort. Charleston, WVa: Pictorial Histories, 1989, p 121.
8. Cohen S: The Homestead and Warm Springs Valley, Virginia: A Pictorial Heritage. Charleston, WVa: Pictorial Histories, 1984, p 17.
9. Franz M: Groedel Memorial Meeting Bulletin. American College of Cardiology, October–November 1951.
10. Groedel FM: The Mineral Springs and Baths at Saratoga Springs. Saratoga, NY: Saratoga Springs Commission, 1932, pp 2, 5.
11. McClellan WS: What is being done at New York State's great enterprise: Saratoga Springs. J Am Med Hydrol 1:27, 1932.
12. Publications of Saratoga Spa, no. 1. Saratoga, NY: Saratoga Springs Authority, 1935.
13. The American Society of Medical Hydrology: Working Committee Minutes of Meeting Held at French Lick Springs Hotel, December 4, 1931. Available in the archives of The American Society of Medical Hydrology.
14. Coulter JS: Physical Therapy, vol 7. The CLIO Medica Series of Primers on the History of Medicine. Chicago, Ill, 1932.
15. Wright, R: Hydrotherapy in Hospitals for Mental Diseases. Boston: The Tudor Press Inc., 1932.
16. Martin LG: Under Water Physiotherapy and Pool Therapy. Presented with motion pictures before the 58th Annual Session of the Arkansas Medical Society at Hot Springs National Park, Ark, May 2–4, 1933.
17. Smith EM: Hydrotherapy in arthritis, underwater therapy applied to chronic atrophic arthritis. Paper presented before the 14th Annual Session of the American Congress of Physical Therapy, Kansas City, Mo, September 11, 1935. Also presented at the Annual Meeting of the American Therapeutic Society, Atlantic City, NJ, June 4–5, 1937.
18. Fletcher GB: Underwater or pool treatment of certain conditions of muscles, nerves and joints. Read before the Tri-State Medical Society, Marshall, TX, November 9, 1939.
19. King N: Pool therapy. Paper presented at the Garland County-Hot Springs Medical Society, Hot Springs, Ark, January 12, 1932.
20. Wallace AW: The modern health resort, an appraisal of its possibilities. JAMA 107:419, 1936.
21. Groedel FM: Physiologic effect of carbon-dioxide baths on the circulatory system. Arch Phys Ther X-ray Radium 18:457, 1937.
22. McClellan WS: The Saratoga Spa, its place in the treatment of rheumatic disorders. Arch Phys Ther X-ray Radium 18:468, 1937.
23. Behrend HJ: Modern hydrotherapy. Arch Phys Ther X-ray Radium 18:146, 1937.
24. American health resorts [editorial]. Arch Phys Ther X-ray Radium 18:509, 1937.
24a. McClellan, WS: Personal communication, 1936.
25. McClellan WS: A history of the American spa. Mimeographed unpublished manuscript, p 11, 1959. Found at Hot Springs Library, Hot Springs, Ark.
26. Fantus B: Our insufficiently appreciated American spas and health resorts. JAMA 110:40, 1938.
27. McClellan WS: Unpublished program notes from 1938 Spa Inspection Tour of American Spas Committee.
28. McClellan WS: Report on spas and health resorts. Arch Phys Ther X-ray Radium 20:42, 52, 1937.
29. McClellan WS: Spas, American style. Med Econ Oct:37, 1939.
30. Kovacs R: American spas. Med Rec 153:254, 1941.

31. Sigerist HE: American spas in historical perspective. Bull Hist Med 11:133, 1942.
32. McClellan WS: The utilization of health resorts for military reconstruction. JAMA 123:564, 1943.
33. Sigerist HE: Towards a renaissance of the American spa. Ciba Found Symp 8:333, 1946.
34. Becker B, Cole AJ: The Biological Aspects of Hydrotherapy. J Back Musculoskeletal Rehabil 4:255, 1994.
35. Henriksen JD: Spa cardiac rehabilitation. Med Hydrol Q 1:1, 1969.
36. Burt B: Fodor's Health and Fitness Vacations. New York: Fodor's Travel Publications, 1989.
37. Weil A: Spontaneous Healing. New York: Random House, 1995.
38. Roszak T: America the Wise, the Longevity Revolution and the True Wealth of Nation. New York: Houghton Mifflin, 1998.
39. Eisenberg DM, et al: Trends in Alternative Medicine Use in the United States, 1990–1997: Results of a Follow-up National Survey. JAMA 280:1569–1575, 1998.
40. International Spa Association Education Committee Report 2001.

Chapter 2
Biophysiologic Aspects of Hydrotherapy

Bruce E. Becker, MD

Since the earliest recorded history, water has always been believed to promote healing and to be useful in a broad range of medical ailments. As noted in Chapter 1, natural springs and water therapies became a central focus of many health-promoting establishments. Healers from all backgrounds have noted the effects of water on various medical problems. Through observation, centuries of trial and error, and scientific methodology, traditions of healing through aquatic treatments have evolved. Water has been found to exert a great many biologic effects. Over recent decades, the therapeutic external application of water, usually through immersion of part or all of the body for the purpose of obtaining these biologic effects came to be called *medical hydrology*.

Recent research into the rehabilitative aspects of aquatic therapies has been sparse. Were it not for two fortuitous aspects of aquatic immersion, very little current research would be available and the hapless practitioner would have to rely on the centuries of oral and written traditions for guidance, at the risk of being labeled an unscientific practitioner. The first fortunate stimulus for recent research was the recognition that aquatic immersion is an ideal method of studying cardiac, pulmonary, and renal responses to sudden changes in blood volume, an essential part of understanding how humans maintain normal function during physiologic change. The second circumstance was the recognition that aquatic immersion is an ideal environment to mimic weightlessness. As man prepared to enter the space environment, scientists needed to better understand the effects that space might have on the human organism. Critical basic science research was performed on essentially all biologic systems during aquatic immersion, so that the necessary understanding of physiology could be gained in preparation for man's first true total escape from gravity. Thus, as we prepared to send man into space, the ultimate technologic environment, we found answers in what was our first environment: thermoneutral total body immersion. As a consequence of these two driving forces to understand human physiology, aquatic rehabilitation has a wealth of basic science research as a foundation, indeed a better and broader foundation than that available for many other rehabilitative techniques.

Aquatic immersion has profound biologic effects, extending across essentially all homeostatic systems. These effects are both immediate and delayed, and they allow water to be used with therapeutic efficacy for a great variety of rehabilitative problems. Aquatic therapies are beneficial in the management of patients with musculoskeletal problems, neurologic problems, cardiopulmonary diseases, and many other conditions. In addition, the margin of therapeutic safety is wider than that of almost any other treatment milieu. Knowledge of these biologic effects can aid the skilled rehabilitative clinician.

AQUATIC PHYSICS

Water is composed of oxygen and hydrogen. One atom of oxygen bonds with two atoms of hydrogen to form a molecule of water (H_2O) with a molecular weight of 18. The nearest approach of water molecules occurs in ice, in which state they are separated by 0.276 nm. The radius of the molecule is 0.138 nm. The molecules are bonded triangularly, with the hydrogen atoms separated by an arc of 104 degrees, 31 seconds, and separated from the oxygen atom by 0.0958 nm. This angle is greater than the expected 90 degrees because of the incomplete sharing of electrons between the oxygen and hydrogen atoms, creating a partially ionized state. The physical configuration of these bonded molecules creates an open electrical field, which creates affinity for many other chemical substances, hence water's tremendous solubility.[1]

Matter commonly exists at normal Earth temperatures in three states: solid, liquid, and gas. A solid maintains a consistent shape and size, which typically does not change without significant force. In contrast, liquids readily alter shape but typically retain volume despite force. Gases are the least fixed, lacking a fixed shape and size. Both liquids and gases have the ability to flow, and because flow properties depend more on density than on any other factor, both are referred to as fluids. Although water is used therapeutically in all its forms, this chapter deals only with water in its liquid form.

Nearly all of the biologic effects of immersion are related to the fundamental principles of hydrodynamics. An understanding of these principles makes the medical application process more rational.

STATIC PROPERTIES OF WATER

Density and Specific Gravity

Density is defined as mass per unit volume, and is given the Greek letter ρ (rho).[2] The relationship of ρ to mass and volume is characterized by the formula:

$$\rho = \frac{m}{V}$$

where m is the mass of a substance whose volume is V. Density is measured in the international system by kilograms per cubic meter and occasionally as grams per cubic centimeter. A density given in the latter format must be multiplied by 1000 to equal the former. Density is a temperature-dependent variable, although this is much less so for solids and liquids than for gases. Water reaches its maximum density at 4°C. Water has the unusual property of becoming more dense above the freezing point; typically, as liquids freeze they become more dense. This property of water is important, because if water were typical, as it froze into ice, it would sink into the mass of still-liquid water, thus allowing lakes to freeze from the bottom, killing off most of the biomass within. The density of salt water varies considerably, from ocean to ocean, up to the Dead Sea, which has a density greater than 1.16.[3]

In addition to density, substances are defined by their specific gravity, the ratio of the density of that substance to the density of water. Water has a specific gravity equal to 1 at 4°C (because this number is a ratio, it has no units). Although the human body is mostly water, the body's density is slightly less than that of water and averages a specific gravity of 0.974, with males averaging higher density than females. Lean body mass, which includes bone, muscle, connective tissue, and organs, has a typical density near 1.1, whereas fat mass, which includes both essential body fat plus fat in excess of essential needs, has a density of about 0.9.[4] Highly fit and muscular males' specific gravities tend to be greater than 1, whereas the specific gravity for an unfit or obese male might be considerably less. Consequently, the typical human body displaces a volume of water weighing slightly more than the body, forcing the body upward by a force equal to the volume of the water displaced.

Hydrostatic Pressure

Pressure is defined as force per unit area, where the force, F, by convention is understood to act perpendicularly to the surface area, A.[2] This relationship is expressed as

$$P = \frac{F}{A}$$

The standard international unit of pressure is called a pascal, abbreviated Pa, after the French scientist Blaise Pascal, and is measured in newtons per square meter. Other common measurement units are dynes per square centimeter, kilograms per square meter, millimeters of mercury (mm Hg) per foot, and pounds per square inch (psi).

Fluids have been found experimentally to exert pressure in all directions, as swimmers and divers know. If a theoretic point is immersed in a vessel of water, the pressure exerted on that point is equal from all directions. If unequal pressure were being exerted, the point would move until the pressures on it were equalized.

Pressure in a liquid increases with depth and is directly related to the density of the fluid. If a theoretic point is immersed to a distance, h, below the surface, the force exerted on the point is due to the weight of the column of fluid above it. The formula F (force) = m (mass) × g (the acceleration of gravity) defines the force and is equal to ρ (density) × A (area) × h (the height of the column of fluid). Thus, pressure is expressed as

$$P = \frac{F}{A} = \rho \frac{Ahg}{A}$$

By canceling out A, we find that

$$P = \rho g h$$

Therefore, pressure is directly proportional to both the liquid density and to the immersion depth when the fluid is incompressible, as water is at the depths used in therapeutic environments. Sometimes it is useful to know the pressure differential between two immersed points separated by a vertical distance, h. This pressure differential may be calculated by the adapted formula:

$$\Delta P = \rho g \Delta h$$

where Δ is the change in pressure and depth. Because *P* responds not only to the fluid depth but also to any force exerted on its surface, the pressure of the earth's atmosphere is an important contributor to the total force from immersion. Water exerts a pressure of 22.4 mm Hg/foot of water depth, which translates to 1 mm Hg/1.36 cm (0.54 inch) of water depth. Thus, a body immersed to a depth of 48 inches is subjected to a force equal to 88.9 mm Hg, which is slightly greater than diastolic blood pressure. This is the force that aids the resolution of edema in an injured body part.

Buoyancy

Immersed objects have less apparent weight than the same object on land because a force opposite to gravity is acting on the object. This force is called *buoyancy*, the upward force generated by the volume of water displaced. Buoyancy arises from the fact that pressure in a fluid increases with depth. A cylinder immersed vertically in water (Fig. 2-1) has more force exerted on its bottom surface than on its top surface. A cylinder with height h has top and bottom surfaces with area A and is immersed in a liquid with density ρ_f. Because the pressure on the top of the cylinder is equal to $\rho_f g h_1$, where g is the force of gravity and h_1 is the top surface depth, the force developed is $F_1 = P_1 A$, which is equal to $\rho_f g h_1 A$ and is a downward force. A force pushing up on the bottom surface of the cylinder is calculated by similar means.

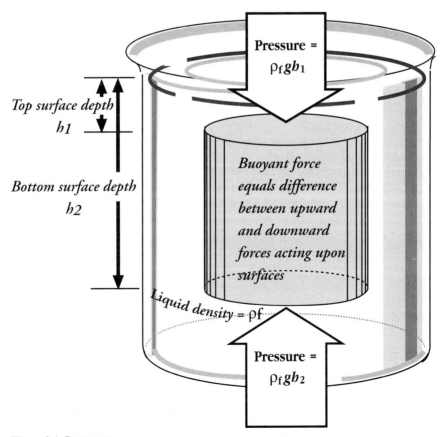

Figure 2-1. Buoyancy.

This force equates to $F_2 = P_2 A = \rho_f g h_2 A$. The net force is called the *buoyant force* F_B, and it pushes up with the magnitude:

$$\begin{aligned} F_B &= F_2 - F_1 \\ &= \rho_f g A (h_2 - h_1) \\ &= \rho_f g A h \\ &= \rho_f g V \end{aligned}$$

where $V = Ah$ is the volume of the cylinder. Because ρ_f is the density of the liquid,

$$\rho_f g V = m_f g$$

defines the weight of fluid of comparable volume to the cylinder volume. Thus, the buoyant force F_B is equal to the weight of the fluid displaced. This principle, discovered by Archimedes, explains why we float, why water can be used as a laboratory for weightlessness, and why water can be used to advantage in the management of medical problems requiring weight off-loading. The principle applies equally to floating objects. A human with specific gravity of 0.97 reaches floating equilibrium when 97% of his or her volume is submerged.

CENTER OF BUOYANCY VERSUS CENTER OF BALANCE

The product of a force and a distance over which the force acts is called a *moment*, and it may also be called *torque*. Although the terms are technically equivalent, *torque* is often used with reference to rotational motion. The fact that the force of buoyancy is an upward force leads to important consequences in the therapeutic aquatic environment. Center of gravity is a point at which all force moments (the magnitude of forces with their respective directions of action) are in equilibrium. For a human being standing in the anatomic position, the center of gravity is located slightly posterior to the midsagittal plane and at the level of the second sacral vertebra because the human body is not uniform with respect to density (e.g., the lungs are less dense than the lower limbs). The center of gravity is really the physical aggregate of the centers of gravity of all the body parts.

The center of buoyancy is defined as the center of all buoyancy force moments. Consequently, the human center of buoyancy is in the midchest (Fig. 2-2). When both centers are aligned in a vertical plane, only vertical vector forces are apparent, which may produce a compressive or distractive force on the body. When these points are not aligned vertically, a rotational force results. This force is defined by the horizontal displacement of centers and the vector magnitude difference between the upward force on the center of buoyancy and the downward force on the center of gravity. This torque force may assist a floating human in maintaining an upright head-out posture, or, when buoyancy devices are used, may tend to float a person face down (supine). These same forces affect a limb and become a vector continuum as the limb moves through water.

BUOYANCY AND JOINT LOADING

As the body is gradually immersed, water is displaced, creating the force of buoyancy. This takes the weight off the immersed joints progressively, and with neck

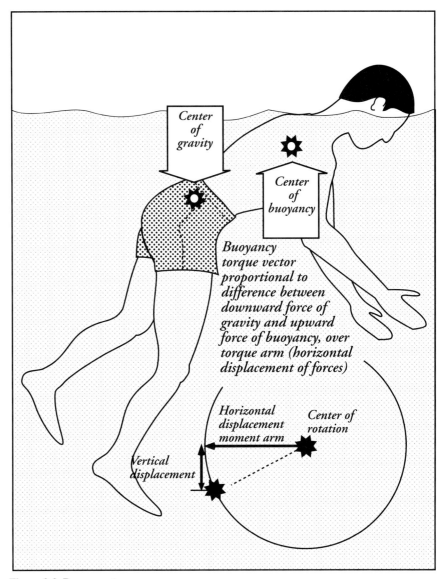

Figure 2-2. Buoyancy torque.

immersion, only about 15 pounds of compressive force (the approximate weight of the head) is exerted on the spine, hips, and knees. A person immersed to the symphysis pubis has effectively off-loaded 40% of his or her body weight, and when further immersed to the umbilicus, approximately 50%. Xiphoid immersion off-loads body weight by 60% or more, depending on whether the arms are overhead or beside the trunk (Fig. 2-3).[54] A body suspended or floating in water essentially counterbalances the downward effects of gravity with the upward force of buoyancy. This effect may be of great therapeutic utility. For example, a fractured pelvis may not become mechanically stable under full-body loading for a period of many weeks, but with water immersion, gravitational forces may be partially or completely offset so that only muscle torque forces act on the fracture site, allowing

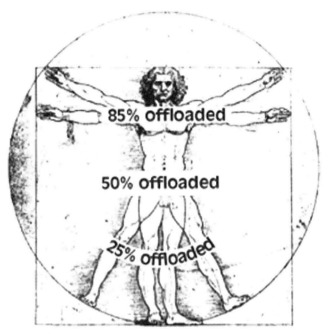

Figure 2-3. Buoyancy off-loading by immersion depth.

active assisted range-of-motion activities, gentle strength building, and even gait training.

Refraction

When light passes from one medium to another, it encounters a boundary layer and generally undergoes a change at this interface. Part of the incident light is reflected at the boundary, and the portion passing into the new medium may change direction. This bending is referred to as *refraction* and is governed by specific properties of the material, particularly the speed of light in the material, and the angle of incidence of the light beam. This phenomenon was studied in the early 1600s by Willebrord Snell, who discovered a consistent relationship between θ (theta), the angle of incidence, and n, the index of refraction. This relationship, called *Snell's law*, is expressed as follows:

$$n_1 \sin \theta_1 = n_2 \sin \theta_2$$

where θ_1 is the angle of incidence, θ_2 is the angle of refraction, and n_1 and n_2 are the respective indices of refraction in air and water, respectively.[2] Thus, if light enters a medium where n is greater (and speed is less), the beam of light is bent toward the normal (perpendicular to the interface). Conversely, when light exiting a medium of high n enters a medium of low n, such as air, it deviates from the normal.

Consequently, from the pool edge, a person standing in waist-deep water appears to have foreshortened trunk and legs, and this foreshortening increases with the distance from the observer to the immersed person, given that both are on the same plane, as the angle of the incident light θ increases. In a therapeutic environment, it requires experience and careful attention to recognize the difference between the appearance of a body part location and its true position.

Surface Tension

The surface of a liquid acts like a membrane under tension. Thus, a drop of water may hang on the end of a straw, and a needle heavier than water may float on the surface of a glass of water, suspended from this membrane-like barrier. This is because the attraction between adjacent molecules of water is circumferential everywhere except at the surface, where the attraction bonding is parallel to the surface. Surface tension is defined as the force F per unit length L that acts across any line in a surface and tends to pull the surface open.[2] Surface tension is denoted by the Greek letter γ (gamma), and the force equation is

$$\gamma = \frac{F}{L}$$

Work must be done to increase the surface area of the fluid. Consequently, in the absence of a force input, fluids tend to be shaped in ways that minimize the surface area. A raindrop assumes a shape that offers the minimum surface area consistent with the drop's volume, speed, and temperature.

TIME-DEPENDENT PROPERTIES

Water in Motion

Water in motion is a complex physical substance. In fact, despite centuries of study, many aspects of fluid motion are still incompletely understood. The major principles of flow are known and can be applied to general activities.

Flow Motion

Water in motion has several characteristics. When water moves smoothly, with all layers moving at the same speed, the water is said to be in *laminar* or *streamline flow*. In this type of movement, all molecules are moving parallel to each other and their paths do not cross. Typically, laminar flow rates are slow because when water moves rapidly even minor oscillations create uneven flow and parallel paths are knocked out of alignment. When this latter condition occurs another type of pattern develops, called *turbulent flow*. In turbulent flow, flow patterns arise that run dramatically out of parallel and may even set up paths running in opposite directions. These paths, called *eddy currents*, look like whirlpools in response to obstacles in the flow path or to irregularities in the surface of flow-directing vessels. Examples of irregularities are the eddy holes that appear behind boulders in fast-moving streams and eddy currents that form in the bloodstream inside arteries encrusted with cholesterol plaque. Turbulent flow absorbs energy at a much greater rate than streamline flow, and the rate of energy absorption is determined by the internal friction in the fluid. This internal friction is called viscosity. The major determinants of water motion are viscosity, turbulence, and speed.

Viscosity

Water at room temperature and through most of the range of its most common therapeutic uses is a liquid. Liquids share a property called *viscosity*, which refers to the magnitude of internal friction specific to the fluid. Different fluids possess varying amounts of molecular attraction within the fluid, and as layers of fluid are set into motion, this attraction creates resistance to movement and is detected as friction. Energy must be exerted to create movement, and, as in the first law of thermodynamics, energy is never lost but rather transformed and stored as potential or kinetic energy. Some energy is transformed into heat, some is transformed into kinetic energy, and some may be stored as energy by increasing surface tension. Fluids are in part defined by individual viscosity, expressed quantitatively as the coefficient of viscosity, which is designated by the Greek letter η (eta). With a greater coefficient, the fluid is more viscous, and more force is required to create movement within the fluid. This force is proportionate to the number of molecules of fluid set in motion and the velocity of their movement. Because velocity is described as distance over time, viscosity is the first time-dependent property of water. Thus, the equation that expresses this relationship must define the volume of the fluid in motion (F), where A is the area, l is depth, and v is the velocity of the motion:[2]

$$F = \eta A \frac{v}{l}$$

Solving this equation for η, we find that $\eta = Fl/vA$. The standard international unit of measurement of viscosity is newton seconds/m^2 (this is equivalent to a pascal-second [Pa•s]). In the centimeters/gram/second (cgs) system, the measurement is dyne-seconds per square centimeter. One unit is called a *poise,* after the French scientist J. L. Poiselle (1799–1869), who studied the physics of blood circulation. Often, coefficients are stated in centipoise (one-hundredth of a poise) (Table 2-1).

Laminar Flow

As water moves smoothly within a vessel, the speed of movement changes with the size of the vessel. The flow rate is defined as the mass of water (m) moving past an imaginary point per a unit of time t: m/t.[2]

$$\frac{\Delta m}{\Delta t} = \rho_1 \frac{\Delta V_1}{\Delta t} = \rho_1 A_1 \frac{l_1}{\Delta t} = \rho_1 A_1 v_1$$

Table 2-1. Coefficients of Viscosities for a Variety of Fluids

Fluid	Temperature (°C)	Coefficient of Viscosity η (Pa·s)
Water	0	1.8×10^{-3}
Whole blood	37	4×10^{-3}
Blood plasma	37	1.5×10^{-3}
Engine oil (SAE 10)	30	200×10^{-3}
Glycerin	20	1500×10^{-3}
Water vapor	100	0.013×10^{-3}

Pa·s: Pascal-seconds.

where ρ_1 represents fluid density at a point in space 1, V_1 represents the volume of water, v_1 represents the velocity of flow, and l_1 represents the length of water column of area A_1. As water moves past a subsequent point 2, the same volume of water with area A_2 and length l_2 may need to increase or decrease velocity to adapt to vessel area changes because water is essentially incompressible.

Poiselle developed an equation that describes the laminar flow of an incompressible fluid through a tube of fixed internal radius and length:[2]

$$Q = \frac{\pi R^4 (P_1 - P_2)}{8 \pi L}$$

Q (the volume rate of flow) is directly proportional to the pressure gradient and inversely proportional to the viscosity and is also proportional to the fourth power of the tube radius. Therefore, if the tube doubles in radius, flow volume increases by a factor of 16. This equation only holds true for laminar flow, however, and only provides an approximation of turbulent flow volumes.

Turbulent Flow

Flow volumes lessen when turbulence occurs, largely due to the significant rise in internal friction in the fluid. The onset of turbulent flow is a function of fluid velocity, but it is also related to fluid density, viscosity, and enclosure radius. Laminar flow is compared with turbulent flow in Figure 2-4. The transition from laminar to turbulent flow often occurs abruptly. This transition point is characterized by a formula incorporating these factors and is called the *Reynolds number (Re)*, after the English physicist Sir Joshua Reynolds. This number is calculated by the formula:

$$Re = \frac{2 \tilde{v} r \rho}{\eta}$$

where $\tilde{v}$ is the average fluid velocity, ρ is fluid density, and r is the radius of the tube in which the fluid is flowing.[2] Typically, Reynolds numbers greater than 2000 produce turbulent flow.

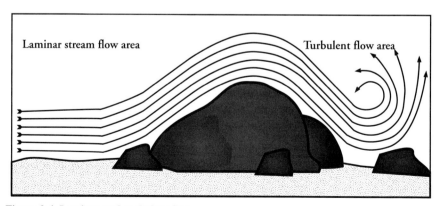

Figure 2-4. Laminar and turbulent flow.

Drag Contribution

When an object moves relative to a fluid, it is subjected to the resistive effects of the fluid. This force is called drag force and is due to fluid viscosity and turbulence when present. It is defined by a second Reynolds number:[2]

$$Re' = \frac{vL\rho}{\eta}$$

where v equals the velocity of the object relative to the fluid. Although the Reynolds formulas are similar, the results are different. A 1-mm object moving through water at 1 mm/sec has a Reynolds number of 1. When this formula produces a Reynolds number equal to or less than 1, the flow is usually laminar, and the force needed to move through the fluid is directly proportional to the speed of the object. The viscous force F_v is directly proportional to the object speed:

$$F_v = kv$$

where k is the second Reynolds number. The magnitude of k depends on the size and shape of the object and on the fluid viscosity. If the object is a sphere, this k is equal to

$$k = 6\pi r\eta$$

With faster movement, higher Reynolds numbers are produced, and the drag force begins to increase as the square of the velocity. The force required to move through water thus becomes

$$F_d = kv^2$$

where F_d is drag force and k is the Reynolds number. Streamlining reduces the resultant Reynolds number. The speed needed to produce Reynolds numbers between 1 and 10 produces turbulence behind the object, known as a *wake*. At these speeds, the force increases with the square of the velocity, $F_v \propto v^2$. As the speed increases yet further, with Reynolds numbers around 106, there is an abrupt increase in drag force. This force is due to turbulence produced not only behind the moving object but also in the layer of fluid passing over the object, known as the *boundary layer*.

Resistance Effects

Water is intermediate in viscosity as liquids go, but it still presents much resistance to movement. Under turbulent flow conditions, this resistance increases as a log function of velocity and depends on the shape and size of the object. The greatest surface area drag in a swimming person is the head, although the negative pressure following the swimmer causes the greatest force resisting forward movement. There is turbulence produced by the moving body surface areas, and a drag force produced by the turbulence behind. Viscosity, with all its attendant physical properties, is a quality that makes water a useful strengthening medium. Viscous resistance increases as more force is exerted against it, but that resistance drops to zero almost immediately on cessation of force because there is only a small amount of inertial moment. (Viscosity effectively counteracts inertial momentum.) Thus, when a rehabilitating person feels pain and stops movement, the force drops precipitously and water viscosity damps movement almost instantaneously. This allows great control of strengthening activities within the envelope of patient comfort. Calculation of these forces has been done and a mathematical model has been developed using a prosthetic leg model.[5]

Because much aquatic rehabilitation usefulness comes from the movement of a person through water, it is worth understanding the variables involved in propulsion. The work involved in overcoming drag force equals the product of the magnitude of the drag force times the displacement. Because drag depends on the square of the velocity, w_d, the work done in joules equals

$$w_d = F_d d = kv^2$$

where d equals the displacement, k is the Reynolds number, and v is the velocity.[2] Power refers to work done per unit time. In this instance, the power to overcome drag, P_d, equals the drag force times the velocity, and thus,

$$P_d = F_d v = kv^3$$

so that the power to overcome drag at a given speed depends on the Reynolds factor and the cube of the velocity. In water walking, a person can use ground reaction forces to move forward, and thus inertia and viscous resistance are the essential factors. In swimming, propulsion depends on thrust, which is achieved through attempts to propel water backward, thus gaining forward movement according to Newton's third law of motion: To every action there is an equal and opposite reaction. The mass of water propelled backward (m_1) is given a velocity change (Δv_i) and thus an impulse equal to $m_1 \Delta v_i$. Because this happens in stroke-by-stroke and kick-by-kick increments, the mean propulsive force equals

$$F_p = \int_n^r F_p dt = \frac{1}{T} \sum m_i \cdot v_i$$

where F_p equals the force of propulsion, d equals displacement, and T equals time. The swimmer must not only transfer kinetic energy to the water through this change in velocity of the water but must also exert energy to overcome drag. Of course, the energy translated to the water being accelerated is lost to propulsion of the swimmer. Because water is viscous and resists with the log of velocity, with increasing swim effort, less energy may be wasted on water acceleration and more used on swimmer propulsion. Alas, with increasing swim speed, turbulent drag increases. The net effect is that stroke efficiency may increase at rapid speeds, but this efficiency is expended in overcoming drag.

THERMODYNAMICS

Specific Heat

Water is used therapeutically in all its thermal forms: solid, liquid, and gas. A major reason for its usefulness lies in the physics of aquatic thermodynamics. All substances on earth possess energy stored as heat. This energy is measured in a quantity called a *calorie*, abbreviated *cal*. A calorie is defined as the heat required to raise the temperature of 1 g of water by 1°C, for example, from 14.5°C to 15.5°C.

The energy required to raise the temperature of water varies slightly, even though this difference is less than 1% in the range of 0°C to 100°C. Sometimes the energy required to raise temperature is defined in kilocalories, the amount required to raise the temperature of 1 kg of water by 1°C. This unit by convention is termed a *Calorie* (with a capital C), abbreviated *Cal*. This is the unit in which food energy content is measured. The British system measures heat energy in British thermal units (BTU), the amount of energy required to raise 1 pound of water by 1°F. A mass of water possesses a definable, measurable amount of stored energy in the form of heat.

The amount of energy stored may be released in a change to a lower temperature, or additional energy may be required to raise temperature. The formula defining the quantity of energy required or released is

$$Q = mc\Delta T$$

where m equals the mass of water, c equals the specific heat capacity of the fluid, and ΔT equals the change in temperature.[2] The work required to produce this energy is called the *mechanical equivalent of heat* and is measured in joules (J). One calorie is equivalent to 4.18 J. A body immersed in a mass of water becomes a dynamic system. If the temperature of the water exceeds the temperature of the submerged body, the system equilibrates to a different level, with the submerged body warming through transference of heat energy from the water, and the water cooling through loss of heat energy to the body. By the first law of thermodynamics, the total heat (and thus energy) content of the system remains the same. Energy applied to this system raises the kinetic energy of some of the molecules, and when high-kinetic-energy molecules collide with lower-kinetic-energy molecules, they transfer some of their energy, raising and equilibrating the total energy of the system.

Again, by cgs system definition, water is defined as having a specific heat capacity equal to 1. In contrast, air has a significantly lower specific heat capacity (0.001). Thus, water retains heat 1000 times more than an equivalent volume of air does (Table 2-2).

Thermal Energy Transfer

The therapeutic utility of water depends greatly on both its ability to retain heat and its ability to transfer heat energy. Exchange of energy in the form of heat occurs in three ways: conduction, convection, and radiation. Conduction may be thought of as occurring through molecular collisions over a small distance. Convection

Table 2-2. Various Heat Capacities

Substance	Specific Heat c_p
Water (15°C)	1.00
Ice (−5°C)	0.50
Steam (110°C)	0.48
Ethyl alcohol	0.58
Protein	0.40
Human body (avg.)	0.83
Mercury	0.033
Air	0.001

requires the mass movement of large numbers of molecules over a large distance. Liquids and gases are generally poor conductors but good convectors. Radiation transfers heat through the transmission of electromagnetic waves. Conduction and convection require contact between the exchanging energy sources. Radiation does not. Conduction occurs in the absence of movement, but convection requires that energy transfer occurs through movement of one source across the other. The rate of radiant energy transfer from a body is proportional to the fourth power of its temperature in degrees Kelvin. It is also proportional to surface area, to the emissivity of the material, and to the distance between the energy-radiating and energy-absorbing bodies.

Heat transfer across a gradient is measured by the amount of heat in calories transferred per second across an imaginary membrane. The ability of substances to conduct heat varies widely. Water is an efficient conductor, transferring heat 25 times faster than air.

Metals and water tend to conduct heat well, and gas or gas-containing materials (e.g., cork, glass, wool, and down) conduct heat poorly (Table 2-3). The latter are thus good insulators, whereas the former are good conductors. Human tissue without blood is a rather good insulator.

The human body produces considerable heat through the conversion of food calories into other energy forms. Only about 20% of this converted energy is used to do work, and the rest is converted into thermal energy. Core temperature would rise about 3°C per hour during light activity if not for the body's ability to dissipate heat. This dissipation process occurs through all heat transfer mechanisms, but by far the most important is convection, occurring through the flow of warm blood from the core to the skin and lungs, where contact with the cooler air occurs. Blood becomes a convective fluid that transfers heat to the surface. Because energy must be further dissipated, the body uses another mechanism, which allows energy loss through the latent heat of evaporation of sweat and respiratory loss, further cooling the skin. This mechanism is remarkably efficient because the evaporative loss of 2.5 mL of water cools the body 0.94°C (2°F). This fact is of considerable importance in scuba diving, where the humidity of inspired air approaches 0% humidity, and the temperature of surrounding water is always lower than that of the diver's body.[6] Consequently, even in warm ocean waters, the diver sustains significant heat loss through respiratory evaporative water loss, dropping core temperature in a short period of time. Typically, the compensatory mechanism used is the wet suit to insulate against heat loss through the skin, even though the respiratory loss cannot be prevented.

Table 2-3. Thermal Conductivity

Substance	Thermal Conductivity (k) (kcal/sec/m/°C)
Water (15°C)	1.4×10^{-4}
Air	0.055×10^{-4}
Human tissue (bloodless)	0.5×10^{-4}
Glass	2.0×10^{-4}
Silver	10×10^{-4}
Copper	9.2×10^{-4}
Down	0.06×10^{-4}
Cork, glass, and wool	0.1×10^{-4}

Heat transfer increases as a function of velocity. Thus, a swimmer loses more heat when swimming rapidly through cold water than does a person standing still in the same water. Fortunately for the swimmer, heat is produced through exercise. Heat transfer is achieved through all three mechanisms—conduction, convection, and radiation—with transfer to an immersed human body, mostly occurring through conduction and convection, although heat loss from the body to the surrounding water occurs mostly through radiation and convection. This thermal conductive property, in combination with the high specific heat of water, makes the use of water in rehabilitation very versatile because water retains heat or cold while delivering it easily to the immersed body part.

These physiologic effects start immediately after immersion. Heat transfer begins, and as the specific heat of the human body is less than that of water, the body equilibrates faster than water does. Hydrostatic pressure effects begin immediately, although most of these effects are to cause plastic deformation of the body through time (e.g., blood displaces cephalad, right atrial pressure begins to rise, pleural surface pressure rises, the chest wall compresses, and the diaphragm is displaced cephalad).

FUNDAMENTAL BIOLOGIC ASPECTS OF AQUATIC THERAPY

Circulatory System

Water exerts pressure on the immersed body. The column of blood contained in the arterial system is under pressure generated by the left ventricle during systolic contraction, and normal blood pressure at rest is less than 130 mm Hg. Blood remains under pressure during diastole, the period of ventricular relaxation, because of the closure of the mitral valve, and the elastic properties of the arterial system sustain the pressure at 60 to 80 mm Hg on average in the normotensive adult. The diastolic pressure is largely determined by the autonomic nervous system—controlled peripheral vascular tree through smooth muscle within the vessel walls, creating peripheral resistance.

Pressure in the venous side of the circulation is much lower than pressure on the arterial side of the system. Venous pressures vary depending on the part of the body and its vertical relationship to the heart. Venous pressures are in part controlled by the system of valves, which prevent backflow. These one-way valves act to divide the large vertical column of venous blood into many short columns with little vertical height. These valves create much lower hydrostatic pressure gradients inside the vein and shorten the effective fluid column so that the maximum venous pressure is 30 mm Hg peripherally, decreasing steadily so that blood reaching the right atrium has a negative pressure (−2 to −4 mm Hg).[15] The role of these valves in maintaining a low-pressure system is critical, as can be observed when they fail, creating venous varicosities due to the lack of sufficient vessel wall strength to support the increased fluid column. This low-pressure gradient system that exists within the venous system is the driving force returning blood to the heart. Consequently, venous return is very sensitive to external pressure changes, including compression from surrounding muscles and certainly from external water pressure. Because an individual immersed in water is subjected to external water pressure in a gradient, which within a relatively small depth exceeds venous pressure, blood is displaced upward through this one-way system, first into the thighs, then into the abdominal cavity vessels, and finally into the great vessels of the chest cavity and into the heart. Venous return is enhanced by the shift of blood from the periphery to trunk vessels to thorax to heart. Central venous pressure begins to rise with immersion to the xiphoid and increases until the body is completely immersed. Right atrial pressure increases by 14 to 18 mm Hg with immersion to the neck, going from about −2 to −4 to 14 to 17 mm Hg.[7,8] When the whole body is immersed to the neck, the transmural pressure gradient of the right atrium increases significantly, measured by Arborelius and coworkers[7] at 13 mm Hg, going from 2 to 15 mm Hg. Extrasystoles may result, especially early in immersion.[7] There is an increase in pulse pressure as a result of the increased cardiac filling and decreased heart rate during thermoneutral immersion.[9,10]

Pulmonary blood flow increases with increased central blood volume and pressure. Mean pulmonary artery wedge pressure increases from 5 mm Hg on land to 22 mm Hg during immersion to the neck.[11] Most of the increased pulmonary blood volume is distributed in the larger vessels of the pulmonary vascular bed, and only a small percentage (≤5%) is at the capillary level. This is validated by the fact that the diffusion capacity of the lungs changes very little.

Central blood volume increased by 0.7 L during immersion to the neck when studied by the Arborelius group.[7] This represents a 60% increase in central volume, with one third of this volume taken up by the heart and the remainder by the great vessels of the lungs. Cardiac volume increases 27% to 30% with immersion to the neck.[12] But the heart is not a static receptacle. The healthy cardiac response to increased volume (stretch) is to increase force of contraction. As the myocardium stretches, an improved actin-myosin filament relationship is produced, enhancing the myocardial efficiency.[13] This increase in myocardial efficiency has been researched for nearly 70 years and is commonly referred to as *Starling's law*. Stroke volume increases as a result of this increased stretch. Although normal resting stroke volume is about 71 mL/beat, the additional 25 mL resulting from immersion equals about 100 mL, which is close to the exercise maximum for a sedentary deconditioned individual on land.[14] Mean stroke volume thus increases 35% on average with immersion to the neck.[11] There is both an increase and a decrease in end-systolic volume.[11] These changes are compared to preimmersion status in Figure 2-5.

Most of the changes are temperature dependent, with cardiac output rising progressively with increasing water temperatures. Weston and coworkers[13] found cardiac output to increase by 30% at 33°C and up to 121% at 39°C. There is considerable individual variance in the many studies assessing this phenomenon.

Stroke volume is one of the major determinants of the rise in cardiac output seen with training; heart rate response ranges remain relatively fixed.[14] In an untrained individual, maximum heart rate is commonly approximated by subtracting the individual's age from a pulse rate of 220 beats per minute (bpm). The upper limit in an untrained individual is only 10% to 15% less than that in a trained one. As heart rate increases beyond an optimal point, cardiac output begins to decrease due to shortening of the diastole, which reduces time for ventricular filling as well as reducing time for coronary blood flow in the left ventricle circulatory tree.[14] Maximum stroke volume is reached at 40% to 50% of maximum oxygen consumption, which equals a heart rate of 110 to 120 bpm on land. This is generally accepted as the rate at which aerobic training begins.[15]

As cardiac filling and stroke volume increase with progress in immersion depth from symphysis to xiphoid, the heart rate typically drops.[16] This drop is variable,

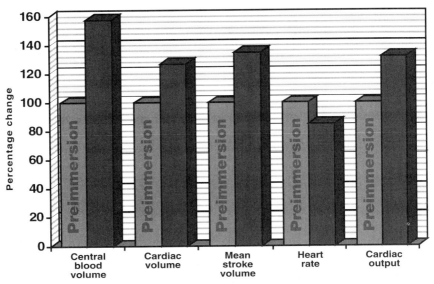

Figure 2-5. Cardiovascular changes after immersion.

with the amount of decrease dependent on water temperature. Typically, at average pool temperatures the rate lowers by 12% to 15%.[8] There is a significant relationship between water temperature and heart rate. At 25°C, heart rate drops approximately 12 to 15 bpm,[17] whereas at thermoneutral temperatures, the rate drop is less than 15%, and in warm water, the rate generally rises significantly, contributing to the major rise in cardiac output at high temperatures.[13] The reduction variability is related to decreased peripheral resistance at higher temperatures and increased vagal effects. A proposed diving response may be involved as well in colder temperatures.

Water-based exercise has often been said to be less effective than land-based exercise for improving cardiovascular fitness. Yet during exercise, maximal myocardial oxygen consumption efficiency (peak heart muscle efficiency) occurs with stroke volume increase because heart rate rise is a less efficient means of increasing output.[14] Stated another way, the most efficient way for the heart to deliver more blood is to increase stroke volume, because a heart rate increase places greater demands on myocardium. Energy is wasted at the onset of myocardial contraction, when the heart is contracting but moving no volume, and at the endpoint of contraction, when the heart is moving little volume and the myocardium is maximally contracted. The optimal length-tension relationship develops with increased stroke volume. Thus, as cardiovascular conditioning occurs, cardiac output increases are achieved with smaller increases in heart rate but greater stroke volumes. This is the reason that conditioned athletes are able to maintain lower resting pulses while maintaining similar cardiac outputs compared with matched deconditioned individuals.

In 1989, Gleim and Nicholas[19] found that oxygen consumption ($\dot{V}O_2$) was three times greater at a given speed of running (53 m/min) in water than on land. Thus, looking at the reverse effect, during water walking and running, only one half to one third the speed was required to achieve the same metabolic intensity as on land.[15] It is important to note that the relationship of heart rate to $\dot{V}O_2$ during water exercise parallels that of land-based exercise, although water heart rate averages 10 bpm less, for reasons discussed earlier.[19] Consequently, metabolic intensity in water, as on land, may be predicted from monitoring heart rate.

Cardiac output is the product of stroke volume times pulse rate per unit time. Because the ultimate purpose of the heart as an organ is to pump blood in response to physiologic demand, its best measure of performance is the amount of blood pumped per unit time. Submersion to the neck increases cardiac output by more than 30% in a sedentary individual.[7] Output increases by about 1500 mL/min, of which 50% is directed to increased muscle blood flow.[18] Normal cardiac output averages approximately 5 L/min in a resting individual. In a conditioned athlete, maximum output during very strenuous exercise is about 40 L/min, which is equivalent to 205 mL/beat times 195 bpm. Maximum output at exercise for a sedentary individual on land is approximately 20 L/min, which is equivalent to 105 mL/beat times 195 bpm.[14] Because immersion to the neck produces a cardiac stroke volume of about 100 mL/beat, a resting pulse of 86 bpm produces a cardiac output of 8.6 L/min and is already producing cardiac exercise. The increase in cardiac output appears to be somewhat age dependent, with younger subjects demonstrating greater increases (up 59%) than older subjects (up only 22%).[20] The increase is also highly temperature dependent, varying directly with temperature increase, from 30% at 33°C to 121% at 39°C.[13] Research has shown that conditioned athletes demonstrate an even greater increase in cardiac output than untrained control subjects during immersed exercise and that this increase is sustained for longer periods than in the untrained control group.[21] This fact may refute the myth that water exercise is not an aerobically efficient training method. In fact, these facts point to the possibility that it may be an ideal cardiovascular conditioning medium. However, although there is an emerging body of direct research data on water exercise–produced cardiac output, significant work needs to be done to delineate the effects of age, sex, temperature, and conditioning, to explain the significant individual response variations and to facilitate the most effective prescription of aquatic exercise dose and frequency. The total cascade of cardiovascular responses is summarized in Figure 2-6.

It is possible to measure the actual resistance seen by the left ventricle. This resistance derives from the formula $R = P_{sa} - P_{ra}/Q$, where P_{sa} is the mean arterial pressure, P_{ra} is the mean right atrial pressure, and Q is cardiac output. During immersion to the neck, systemic vascular resistance decreases by 30%.[7] Decreased sympathetic vasoconstriction produces this reduction, with peripheral venous tone diminishing by 30%, from 17 to 12 mm Hg at thermoneutral temperatures.[22] Total peripheral resistance lowers during the first hour of immersion and persists for a period of hours thereafter. This drop is related to temperature, with higher temperatures producing greater lowering, which consequently decreases end-diastolic pressures. Systolic pressures increase with increasing workload but appear to be approximately 20% less in water than on land.[13] Venous pressures also drop during immersion because less vascular tone is required to support the system. These vascular pressure responses to immersion are demonstrated in Figure 2-7. Much study has been done on the effect of immersion on blood pressure. Very short-term immersion (10 minutes) in thermoneutral temperatures has been found to very slightly increase both systolic and diastolic pressures, perhaps as part of the cool water accommodation process.[13] Other studies done in carefully controlled environments have found no effects or actual drops in pressures. In an important study for aquatic rehabilitation, Coruzzi and coworkers[23] found that longer immersion produced significant decreases in mean arterial pressure, with group I (sodium-sensitive) hypertensive patients showing even greater drops (−18 to −20 mm Hg) than normotensive patients and group II (sodium-insensitive) patients showing

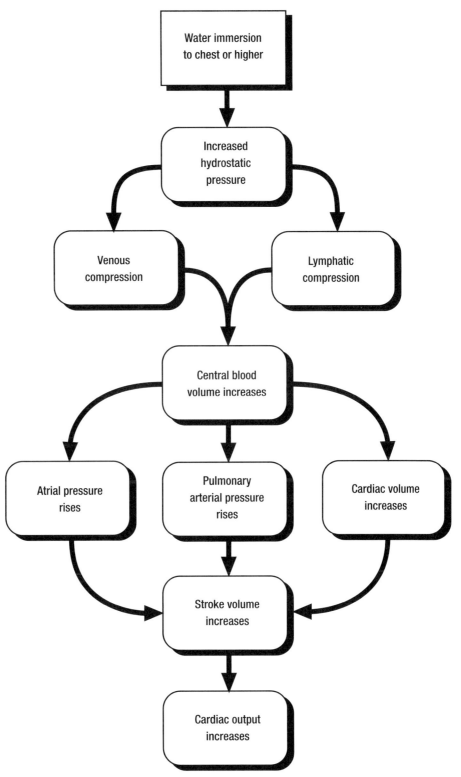

Figure 2-6. Schematic diagram of cardiovascular changes after immersion.

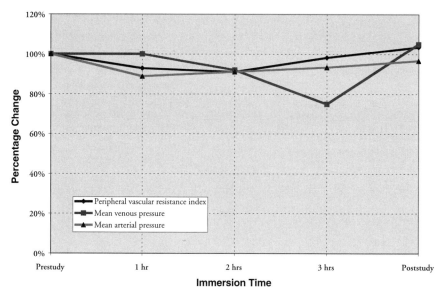

Figure 2-7. Vascular pressures during immersion.

smaller drops (−5 to −14 mm Hg). No studies have demonstrated consistent sustained increases in systolic pressure with prolonged immersion, although several have found no significant decreases. Based on a substantial body of research, the therapeutic pool appears to be a safe and potentially beneficial environment for both normotensive and hypertensive patients, in contrast to widespread belief.

Two recent studies have provided intriguing data to support the use of aquatic environments in cardiovascular rehabilitation after infarct and ischemic cardiomyopathy. Tei and coworkers[25] studied patients with severe congestive heart failure (ejection fraction means 25% ± 9%), under the hypothesis that in this clinical problem, the essential concern is the inability of the heart to overcome peripheral vascular resistance and that exposure to a warm environment causes peripheral vasodilatation, reducing vascular resistance and cardiac afterload. The researchers found that after a single immersion lasting 10 minutes in a hot water (41°C) bath, both pulmonary wedge pressure and right atrial pressure dropped by 25%, as did cardiac output and stroke volume. Both left ventricular and left atrial dimensions decreased significantly as well when measured echocardiographically 30 minutes after immersion.[24] The same investigators then initiated a month-long study of 56 patients with chronic heart failure (CHF) using warm water immersion or a sauna bath one to two times per day, 5 days a week, for 4 weeks and found improvement in ejection fractions of nearly 30% along with a reduction in left ventricular end-diastolic dimension, along with subjective improvement in quality of life, sleep quality, and general well-being.[25]

Relative Perceived Exertion Scales

For more than 30 years it has been recognized that the subjective experience of effort is closely related to measurable parameters of workload. Through these years, beginning in the early 1960s with the groundbreaking work of Borg[26–28] and later confirmed by many other researchers, this relationship has been carefully studied. It is now known that the inner perception of effort closely correlates with $\dot{V}O_2$, blood and muscle lactate, heart rate, and other objective measurements. Coefficients of correlation with heart rates have ranged from 0.8 to 0.9, and high levels have also been shown with all other measures of exertion. It is significant that relative perceived exertion (RPE) scores correlate closely with blood lactate.[28]

RPE scoring originated with Borg, who designed a rating scale to allow an individual to relate his or her effort level to a specific scale point, facilitating training consistency and measurement.[26] This scale used values ranging from 6 to 20 and was intended to represent pulse rate increase, with average resting pulse rate at 60 bpm, increasing to 200 bpm at maximum effort. Thus, a scale measurement was approximately equal to the heart rate divided by 10, although this numeric relationship should not be taken as sacred because many other variables affect heart rate on an individual basis. Borg cautioned against the use of RPE scales in cardiac rehabilitation settings because they had not been developed in the setting of known cardiac pathologic conditions. This scale has been modified in a number of ways by many, including Borg himself, who subsequently changed to a 10-point scale.[28] Many practitioners have successfully used this 10-point scale in the aquatic environment. It has been found that the metabolic costs of water-running are slightly less than treadmill running for equal RPE scores.[29] Wilder and Brennan[30] developed a variant of the Borg scale for water-running exercise programs: Their scale goes from 1 (light work) to 5 (extremely hard work).

Pulmonary System

The pulmonary system is profoundly affected by immersion of the body to the level of the thorax. Part of the effect is due to shifting of blood into the chest cavity, and part is due to compression of the chest wall itself by water. The combined effect is to alter pulmonary function, increase the work of breathing, and change respiratory dynamics.

A brief overview of pulmonary physiology aids understanding of the changes involved. When an individual is at rest, breathing comfortably, the normal excursion of air during inspiration and expiration is called *tidal volume*. At the endpoint of nonforced expiration, a volume of air remains in the lungs that can be expelled with increased effort. This volume is called *expiratory reserve volume* (ERV). ERV can be experienced by simply exhaling normally and then exhaling forcibly to the maximum amount. Even when this last volume has been expelled, air remains in the lungs that cannot be voluntarily expelled. This remainder is called *residual volume* (RV). The combination of ERV and RV is called *functional residual capacity* (FRC). This volume of residual air is believed to play a buffering role for blood oxygen and carbon dioxide saturation levels, preventing extreme fluctuation. At the end of comfortable inspiration, there is still room for more air to be inhaled; this is called *inspiratory reserve volume* (IRV). As one exercises and increases the need for oxygen, tidal volume increases, reducing both ERV and IRV. The combination of ERV and IRV plus tidal volume is called *vital capacity* (VC), which is a laboratory measurement of the maximum amount of air that can be inhaled and subsequently exhaled. These relationships are graphically demonstrated in Figure 2-8. VC varies widely according to stature, sex, and the individual. A low VC per body mass reduces the amount of oxygen potentially available for metabolism, whereas a large VC-to-body mass ratio increases aerobic potential.[4]

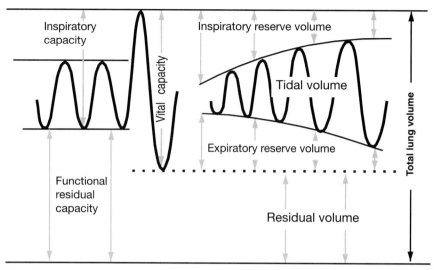

Figure 2-8. Pulmonary function divisions.

VC decreases about 6% to 9% for patients submerged to the neck compared with control subjects submerged to the xiphoid.[31,32] About 50% to 60% of this VC reduction is due to increased thoracic blood volume, and 40% to 50% is due to hydrostatic forces counteracting the inspiratory musculature.[31,32] Water temperature plays a large role in the amount of vital capacity reduction, with cold water producing a larger reduction than warm water, although whether this is due to increased peripheral vasoconstriction in cooler water temperatures with enhanced central blood volumes displacing air or to a peripheral effect upon the muscles of respiration is not known.[7,33,34] Certainly both may be involved. FRC reduces to about 54% of the normal value with immersion to the xiphoid.[32] Most of this loss is due to a reduction in ERV, which decreases by 75% at this level of immersion.[31] The change in this volume may be perceived readily at poolside: While sitting on the edge of the pool exhale normally, and then expel the rest of the reserve volume forcibly. Enter the water to neck level, and perform the same experiment; the difference is highly perceptible. Little air remains to exhale at the endpoint of relaxed exhalation. ERV is reduced to 11% of VC, equal to breathing at a negative pressure exceeding −20 cm of water.[32] There is scant loss of RV, which may remain the same or drop slightly.[7,33,35] Pressure on the rib cage shrinks the rib cage circumference by approximately 10% during submersion.[32] Figure 2-9 depicts the changes in pulmonary function during immersion.

The ability of the alveolar membrane to exchange gases is called diffusion capacity. Diffusion capacity of the lungs is reduced slightly during immersion to the neck, as is blood oxygen concentration as the lung beds become distended with blood shifted from the extremities and abdomen. Total intrapulmonary pressure shifts to the right by 16 cm of water, which causes airway resistance to the movement of air to increase by 58% or more because of reduced lung volume.[32] Expiratory flow rates are reduced, increasing the time needed to move air in and out of the lungs. Chest wall compliance is reduced due to the pressure of water on the chest wall, increasing pleural pressure to from −1 to +1 mm Hg,[11] and lung compliance itself is reduced by 45% during full-body immersion.[36–38]

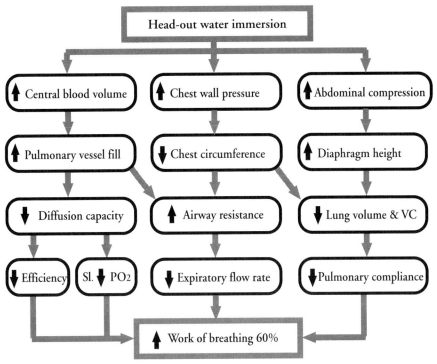

Figure 2-9. Schematic of immersion effects on respiration. (VC= vital capacity; PO$_2$ = partial pressure of oxygen.)

The combined effect of all these changes is to increase the total work of breathing when a person is submerged to the neck (Fig. 2-10). The total work of breathing for a tidal volume of 1 L increases by 60% during submersion to the neck. Of this increased effort, three fourths is attributable to an increase in elastic work (redistribution of blood from the thorax) and the rest to dynamic work (moving air against increased airway resistance and increased hydrostatic force on the thorax).[31,36–38] Most of the increased work occurs during inspiration and requires both primary and accessory muscles of respiration to come into play at higher workloads. Inspiratory muscle weakness is an important component of many chronic diseases, including congestive heart failure and chronic obstructive lung disease.[39] Because viscosity and flow rates under turbulent conditions enter into the elastic workload component of breathing as respiratory rate increases, there is an exponential workload increase with more rapid breathing, as during high-level exercise. Thus, for an athlete used to land-based conditioning exercises, a program of water-based exercise results in a significant workload challenge to the respiratory apparatus, primarily in the muscles of inspiration.[38] Inspiratory muscle fatigue seems to be a rate- and performance-limiting factor, even in highly trained athletes, and inspiratory muscle-strengthening exercises have proven to be effective in improving athletic performance in elite cyclists.[40,41] The challenge of inspiratory resistance posed during neck-depth immersion can raise the efficiency of the respiratory system if the time spent in water conditioning is sufficient to achieve respiratory apparatus strength gains. The author has had a number of elite athletes comment upon this phenomenon when they return to land-based competition after a period of intense water-based aquatic

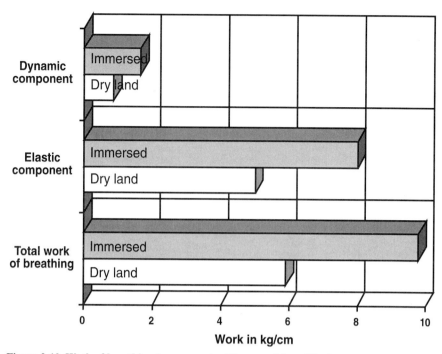

Figure 2-10. Work of breathing (energy costs of immersed breathing).

rehabilitation sufficient to strengthen the respiratory musculature. The common response is a perception of easier breathing at peak exercise levels, effects similar to the studies conducted with elite cyclists.

A 1994 study of individuals with CHF found an associated increase in respiratory muscle weakness, especially in the musculature of inspiration, and this weakness correlated closely with cardiac function.[42] It is postulated that this respiratory weakness may be a significant factor in the impaired exercise capacity seen in individuals with CHF. Because the added work of respiration during immersion occurs almost entirely during the inspiratory phase, it is intriguing to question whether a period of inspiratory muscle strengthening through immersed activity might improve exercise capacity in these individuals.

Aquatic therapy can be very useful in the management of patients with neuromuscular impairment of the respiratory system, such as that seen in spinal cord injury and muscular dystrophy. In a very small 1974 study done at the University of Washington on three patients with advanced muscular dystrophy, researchers found that the patients showed a steady increase in vital capacity during a 4-month period of twice-weekly therapy, but a significant decrease during a 3-week school break from therapy, which was reversed when therapy again was reinstituted, only to show a later decline during a spring break followed by recapture of the losses once therapy was reinitiated.[43] Although this was a small study, the observations noted are quite striking. A lengthy study of swimming training on cardiorespiratory fitness in spinal cord–injured individuals was done in the late 1970s in Poland. The authors found a more than 440% increase in fitness levels, compared with a 75% increase seen in spinal cord–injured patients in a standard land-based training program over the same period of time.[44]

Musculoskeletal System

Water immersion causes significant effects on the musculoskeletal system as well. The effects are caused by the compressive effects of immersion as well as reflex regulation of blood vessel tone. Conclusions in several of the studies previously quoted were that during immersion, it is likely that most of the increased cardiac output is redistributed to skin and muscle rather than to the splanchnic beds.[45] Resting muscle blood flow has been found to increase from a dry baseline of 1.8 to 4.1 mL/min/100 g of tissue with neck immersion.[46] In the same study, xenon clearance in the tibialis anterior, a measure of tissue perfusion, during immersion to the heart level was found to increase 130% above dry land clearance, essentially an increase identical to that in cardiac output during immersion. To this point, there have been no studies assessing the effect of immersion upon muscle blood flow during exercising conditions. Thus, we may only conclude that oxygen delivery is significantly increased during immersion at rest, as is the circulatory drive to remove muscle metabolic waste products, but it is reasonable to posit that blood flow during exercise is enhanced as well. To resist blood pooling in dry conditions, sympathetic vasoconstriction tightens the resistance vessels of skeletal muscle. Immersion pressure removes the biologic need for vasoconstriction, thus increasing muscle blood flow. Hydrostatic forces add an additional circulatory drive. Because water depth of 0.5 inch produces pressure of 1 mm Hg, immersion to only 36 inch of depth results in pressure that exceeds average diastolic pressure and acts to drive out edema and other metabolic end products. The hydrostatic effects of immersion, possibly combined with temperature effects, have been shown to significantly improve dependent edema and subjective pain symptoms in patients with venous varicosities.[47] Similarly, a rehabilitation program of hydrotherapy using contrasting temperatures produced both subjective improvement, systolic blood pressure increases in the extremities, and significant increases in ambulation in patients with intermittent claudication.[48]

Conditioning Effects

Controversy has existed regarding the utility of a program of water-based exercise in maintaining fitness in athletes who must be sheltered from the effects of gravity during recovery from an injury. For maintenance of cardiorespiratory conditioning in highly fit individuals, water running equals dry land running in its effect on maintenance of maximum $\dot{V}O_2$ when training intensities and frequencies are matched.[49] Similarly, when aquatic exercise is compared with land-based equivalent exercise in effect on maximum $\dot{V}O_2$ gains in unfit individuals, aquatic exercise is seen to achieve equivalent results, and when water temperature is low, the gains achieved are accompanied by a lower heart rate.[50] Lactate threshold more closely correlates to training performance than heart rate or $\dot{V}O_2$. Blood lactate has been found to shift to the left in relationship to oxygen uptake in both submaximal and maximal water running compared with dry land treadmill running.[51] Thus, water-based exercise programs may be used effectively to sustain or increase aerobic conditioning in athletes who need to keep weight off a joint, such as when they are recovering from an injury or when they are involved in an intensive training program in which joint or bone microtrauma might occur. A key question frequently raised is whether aquatic exercise programs have sufficient specificity to provide a reasonable training venue for athletes in this situation. Hamer and Morton[52] addressed this question and found that subjects in water-based running programs did have significant reductions in submaximal heart rates and improved performance on graded exercise tests compared with control subjects who did not exercise. It is probable that the musculoskeletal and neuromuscular challenges posed by the aquatic environment are sufficiently different than dry land challenges so that it is unlikely that aquatic training can substantially improve dry land performance in coordination skills, where reflex timing becomes a major part of the performance success.

Open Versus Closed Kinetic Chain Issues

An aquatic exercise program may be designed to vary the amount of gravity loading by using buoyancy as a counterforce. A joint that is moving against fixed resistance, such as the ground, forms a closed kinetic chain. Rehabilitative programs for specific joints may be more effective as either closed or open kinetic chain programs. Generally, if a joint with normal gravity loading has undergone extensive reconstruction, many rehabilitation specialists feel that closed chain exercises are preferable.

Shallow-water vertical exercises generally approximate closed chain exercise, albeit with reduced joint loading because of the counterforce produced by buoyancy. Deep-water exercises more generally approximate an open chain system, as do horizontal exercises, such as swimming. Paddles and other resistive equipment tend to close the kinetic chain. Aquatic programs, however, offer the ability to damp the force of movement instantaneously because of the viscous properties of water. Some differences are seen in biomechanical and neuromuscular interactions between agonist and antagonist muscles during immersed knee flexion/extension activities compared with similar land-based exercise movements, which are attributable to fluid viscosity.[53]

The effects of buoyancy and water resistance make possible high levels of energy expenditure with relatively little movement and strain on lower extremity joints.[54] Off-loading of body weight occurs as a function of immersion, but the water depth chosen may be adjusted for the amount of loading desired.[54] The amount of weight off-loading occurring through progressive immersion is shown in Figure 2-11. The spine is especially well protected during aquatic exercise programs, which facilitates early rehabilitation from back injuries.

The force exerted against the floor by the walking body is counteracted by the ground. This force is termed *ground reaction force* and may easily be measured through a force plate. It has been found to differ from walking on ground substantially during walking in chest-deep water.[55] Figure 2-12 shows the force plate tracing of the pressure during a gait cycle on dry land compared with chest-deep immersion. The forces generated are reduced in magnitude by more than 50%, are generated more slowly, and are transmitted over a longer time interval during water walking. Clinically, this means that less joint compression is produced and impact strain is diminished.

Renal and Endocrine Systems

Aquatic immersion has many effects on renal blood flow, on renal regulatory systems, and on endocrine systems (Fig. 2-13). These effects have been extensively

Biophysiologic Aspects of Hydrotherapy   45

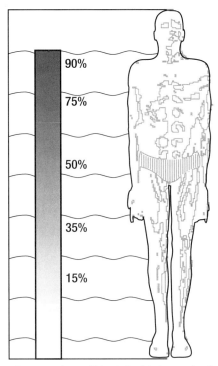

Figure 2-11. Percentage of body weight off-loaded with increasing immersion depth.

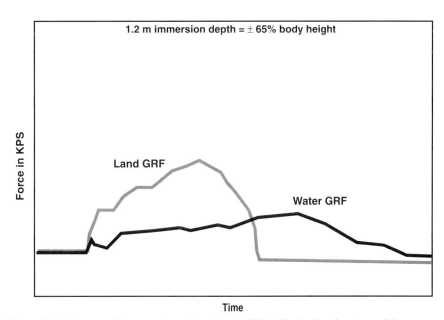

Figure 2-12. Comparative ground reaction forces (GRFs) for land and water walking. (KPS = kilopound-seconds.) (Adapted from Nakazawa K, Yano H, Miyashita M: Ground reaction forces during walking in water. In Miyashita M, Mutoh Y, Richardson AB, et al [eds]: Medicine and Science in Aquatic Sports/10th FINA World Sport Medicine Congress, Medicine and Sport Science, vol. 39. Basel: Karger, 1994, p 28.)

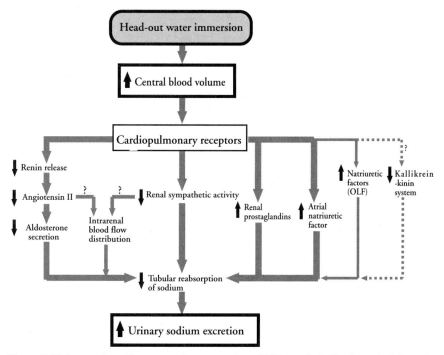

Figure 2-13. Immersion effects on sodium excretion. (OLF= ouabainlike factor.) (Adapted from Epstein M: Renal effects of head out immersion in humans: a 15-year update. Physiol Rev 72:577, 1992.)

studied. Epstein, one of the most skilled and prolific researchers of immersion effects on humans, published an exhaustive summary of these effects in 1992.[45] The flow of blood to the kidneys increases immediately on immersion. With neck-depth immersion, this volume expansion has been reported to equal a 10% increase in extracellular volume, an amount equal to 2 L of normal saline infusion.[56] This causes an increase in creatinine clearance (a measure of renal efficiency) initially on immersion.[57] Renal sympathetic nerve activity decreases due to the vagal response caused by left atrial distention, and this decrease in sympathetic nerve activity increases renal tubular sodium transport.[57] Calculated renal vascular resistance decreases by about one third.[13] Renal venous pressure increases almost 2-fold.[13] Sodium excretion increases 10-fold in individuals with normal total body sodium levels, and this sodium excretion is accompanied by free water, creating part of the diuretic effect of immersion. This increase in sodium excretion is a time-dependent phenomenon. Sodium excretion also increases as a function of depth up to chest-depth immersion and does not seem to increase further with neck-depth immersion.[58] Release of a humeral natriuretic factor occurs through distention of the atria, and the peptide produced, atrial natriuretic peptide (ANP), facilitates sodium excretion and diuresis. ANP relaxes vascular smooth muscle and inhibits production of aldosterone; it also appears to persist for a period of time after immersion. Potassium excretion also increases with immersion.[59]

Renal function is largely regulated by the hormones renin, aldosterone, and antidiuretic hormone (ADH). All of these hormones are greatly affected by immersion

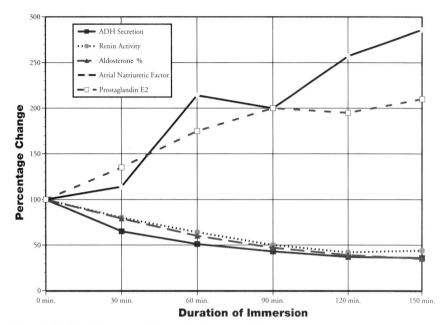

Figure 2-14. Renal hormone changes during immersion.

(Fig. 2-14). Aldosterone controls sodium reabsorption in the distal renal tubule and accounts for most of the sodium loss with immersion. Suppression begins on immersion, reaches maximum at 2 hours, but falls to 60% of maximum at 3 hours of immersion time. Aldosterone production is reduced to 80% of control at 30 minutes of immersion time, reaches 60% of control at 1 hour, and maximizes at 35% of control at 3 hours. ADH release is suppressed with immersion by 50% or more, which is the other major contributor to diuresis.[20,45] Another factor important in sodium regulation is ANP. ANP reduces the reabsorption of sodium in the distal renal tubular system, thus increasing urinary sodium content. Immersion produces a prompt and continuing increase in ANP.[58] Renal prostaglandin E secretion increases steadily through the first 2 hours of immersion and then drops gently over the next 3 hours.[45] Renin stimulates angiotensin, which in turn stimulates aldosterone release. Renin activity reduces by 20% of control at 30 minutes of immersion and 38% at 1 hour and maximizes at 62% of control at 3 hours of immersion. Plasma renin activity is reduced by 33% to 50% at 2 hours of immersion to the neck.[45]

Overall, immersion-induced central volume expansion causes increased urinary output accompanied by significant sodium and potassium excretion, beginning almost immediately on immersion, steadily increasing through several hours of immersion, and gently tapering off over subsequent hours. Figure 2-15 shows these time-dependent changes in urinary excretion. Of interest and practical significance is the fact that immersion seems to reduce normal thirst mechanisms in humans, so that even in volume-depleted individuals immersed in water to neck depth, normal

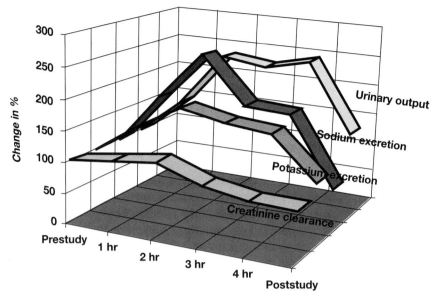

Figure 2-15. Renal function changes during immersion.

thirst mechanisms were masked.[60] Thus, it is essential for therapists immersed for lengthy periods each workday to exert effort to replenish fluid volumes, as the combination of increased diuresis and reduced thirst can create dehydration by the end of the workday.

The combined effect of the renal responses, the autonomic responses, and the cardiovascular responses on blood pressure has been studied intensively, with varying results. During sustained immersion in neutral-temperature water, blood pressure does not appear to change greatly. During neutral-temperature water immersion, patients with essential hypertension often show lowered blood pressure. Coruzzi and coworkers[23] found that more and than two thirds of their subjects with hypertension showed significant decreases in mean arterial pressure during an extended 2-hour immersion in thermoneutral temperature. These combined renal and sympathetic nervous system effects typically lower blood pressure in the immersed individual with hypertension during sustained immersion and create a period of lowered pressure for a period of hours thereafter.

Accompanying the renal hormone effects are changes in the autonomic nervous system neurotransmitters, called *catecholamines*, which act to regulate vascular resistance, cardiac rate, and cardiac force. The most important of these are epinephrine, norepinephrine, and dopamine. Catecholamine levels begin changing immediately upon immersion (Fig. 2-16).[61,62]

Thermoregulation

The ability of the body to adapt to a wide range of water immersion temperatures is quite striking, in view of the thermal properties of water as previously discussed. The maintenance of thermal homeostasis is primarily regulated by the preoptic area of the hypothalamus, but with inputs from skin temperature sensors as well as from

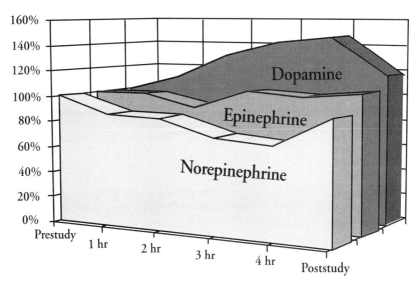

Figure 2-16. Catecholamine responses to immersion.

sensors that detect the rate of change in skin temperatures, allowing anticipatory control mechanisms to be activated.[63] The body has a large surface area to regulate heat loss or heat gain through the mechanisms of increasing or decreasing skin blood flow and through increased or decreased muscle activity such as shivering.[64] Blood pressure, both systolic and diastolic levels, does rise upon initial immersion in cooler water but in general does not change significantly over a quite wide range of temperatures once initial acclimatization occurs, although diastolic pressures seem to remain higher in cold water.[65–67] Typically, immersion in cold water (15°C) produces a period of slowed heart rate that begins to return toward baseline at around 10 minutes of immersion time and is followed by a period of slight heart rate increase that lasts for a brief period, falling again toward baseline.[68] In contrast, warm and hot water immersion (40°C and 41.5°C) produces a significant rise in heart rate, which parallels the rise in core temperature, whereas blood pressure tends to drop in warm water immersion versus changing little if at all in hot water immersion.[69] Cardiac output is increased during cool, neutral, and warm water immersion, although in cold water, it may rise less or remain the same during the initial equilibration phase.[68] Because heart rate is increased during warm water immersion whereas stroke volume is increased as in cool water, warm water immersion results in an increase in cardiac output compared with cool water immersion.[19,65,70] Total peripheral vascular resistance drops in thermoneutral temperatures and drops further yet in warmer temperatures but rises in cold water. Despite this, muscle blood flow is increased at all temperatures, although less so in cooler than in warm water.[65] Temperature does not seem to play a significant role in the perception of exertion, at least in young males exercising in cool and cold water, although competitive aquatic athletes consistently prefer cooler water temperatures for training and competition.[71,72]

In cooler and cold water, adaptive mechanisms rapidly come into play to preserve core temperature. These initially include vascular responses such as vasoconstriction and then move into heat production mechanisms such as shivering, which may become quite violent. With sufficient differential between core temperature and water temperature, these compensatory mechanisms cannot sustain core temperature.[66] In contrast, warm and hot water immersion allows fewer compensatory mechanisms to maintain core temperature. The major compensatory mechanisms, peripheral vasodilatation and increased cardiac output, that assist cooling in warm air temperatures work to counterpurposes in warm water, because they facilitate heat gain when the surrounding environment does not allow evaporative and radiant cooling. Immersion at 40°C (104°F), which is a common hot-tub temperature, produces a rectal (core) temperature rise, which equates to approximately 0.1°F/min of immersion.[69] This is not a problem in the neurologically intact human, because somatic awareness does not promote allowing a core temperature increase much beyond 1°C or even less. However, when alcohol or other drugs alter awareness, there is a serious risk of hyperthermia in a relatively brief period of time. There is also a risk when the metabolic ability of the tissues to respond is impaired, e.g., when vascular insufficiency is present. Pregnancy creates a special problem, because small increases in core temperature (1.5°C) have been noted to alter the growth of fetal neuronal tissue, although in the study quoted, the temperature increases were the result of the presence of infectious processes, which may not be entirely relevant to results of short-term warm water immersion.[73] There have been no reports of fetal abnormalities associated with short low-level increases in core temperature less than 38.9°C.[74] In general, pregnant women are quite sensitive to core temperature elevations and usually leave the hot tub well before core temperature increases are near teratogenic levels.[74] McMurray and coworkers[75–78] demonstrated the safe maintenance of core temperature during pregnancy when women performed aquatic exercises in 30°C water. A prudent guideline might be to limit hot-tub immersion in 40°C tubs to periods of less than 15 minutes for women in whom pregnancy is a consideration. Table 2-4 details physiologic responses to immersion temperatures.

Central and Peripheral Nervous Systems

Many effects have been observed anecdotally throughout centuries of aquatic environment use for health maintenance and restoration, but they are difficult to study. Predominant among these are the relaxation effect of water immersion and the

Table 2-4. Temperature Effects Upon Biologic Functions in Young Males

Fluid	Water Temperature		
	Cold (15°C)	Neutral (35°C)	Hot (44°C)
Heart rate	−15%	−15%	32%
Stroke volume	19%	39%	9%
Cardiac output	−1%	18%	44%
Systolic blood pressure*,†	19%	−8%	−17%
Diastolic blood pressure*,†	2%	−7%	−14%
Peripheral vascular resistance‡	−32%	−14%	−32%
Diuresis	365%	400%	225%
Muscle blood flow	80%	44%	4%

Data from Bonde-Petersen et al: Aviat Space Environ Med 63:346–350, 1992.
*Craig & Dvorak, J: Appl Physiol 21(5):1577–1585, 1966.
†Allison, et al: Mayo Clin Proc 68:19–25, 1993.
‡Nakamitsu, et al, J Appl Physiol 77(4):1919–1925, 1994.

effect that water immersion has on pain perception. Skin sensor nerve endings are affected, including temperature, touch, and pressure receptors. Sensory overflow has been suggested to be the mechanism by which pain is less well perceived when the affected body part is immersed in water. Pain modulation is consequently affected with a rise in pain threshold, which increases with temperature and water turbulence, producing the known therapeutic effect of agitated whirlpool immersion. In a 1994 study, researchers found a reduction in pain after bath therapy in patients with fibromyalgia undergoing 10 twice-weekly immersion sessions of 20 minutes' duration. Compared with a control group of patients receiving only Jacobson relaxation exercise, the bath patients noted less morning pain, and although the results were not statistically significant, they also noted a reduction in pain throughout the day, with improved sleep patterns.[79]

A relaxation effect is produced by a central process that is not understood, is probably multifactorial, and is produced within the reticular activating system deep within the brain. In research done to assess weightlessness and its effects upon humans in space, Mano and coworkers[80] found that sympathetic nervous system activity was suppressed during immersion. Sympathetic nervous system activity is associated with the alertness/arousal mechanism and the so-called "flight or fight" response. In an earlier quoted study, plasma dopamine has been noted to increase during immersion, and plasma dopamine levels correlate positively with mood state, although certainly there are many other factors at play in mood state maintenance.[62,81,82] Mood state has been found to improve after dry land exercise, but relatively little work has been done on this issue in an aquatic environment. Similarly, both anxiety and depression are reduced after dry land exercise and after aquatic exercise, but more research to test these effects needs to be done. Robiner,[83] in a warm water immersion study of 40 healthy volunteers of both sexes at the University of Minnesota, found a statistically significant reduction in anxiety, with DSM III anxiety symptoms falling by 40% from baseline measurements before immersion in a warm water whirlpool environment. Although lower in statistical significance, increases in well-being scores and lowered stress reaction scores were also noted. In contrast, Watanabe and coworkers[84] found that although a group of older persons exercising in an aquatic exercise program showed very significant decreases in anxiety scores, they did not score significantly lower than a group exercising on land who also showed significant decreases. Plasma catecholamine levels are known to increase during exercise and decrease after exercise; the amount of the increase decreases with the training effect, which may account for some of these psychological changes.[43] The normal heart rate has an inherent variability, which can be analyzed to assess the impact of respiration and autonomic nervous system activity. During relaxation states, this heart rate variability demonstrates an autonomic bias toward vagal or parasympathetic nervous system control, whereas during stressed states, sympathetic nervous system influence predominates. The heart rate variability pattern seen during immersion is that of vagal or parasympathetic control, indicating perhaps an inherent bias toward the relaxation state.[85]

Weight Control Issues

Aquatic exercise would seem to offer the safest and most protective environment for obese individuals due to the buoyancy effects of immersion, which minimize the risk of joint injury. With body weight reduced to essentially negligible levels, the immersed individual can exercise vigorously, and increases in $\dot{V}O_{2max}$ are seen in obese individuals over relatively short time periods.[86] The advantages of aquatic exercise include the heat-conductive effects of water, which greatly reduce the risk of heat stress when exercise is done in cooler pools. Individuals with significantly increased body fat percentages are also protected against core temperature loss in cooler pool temperatures.[86] Water exercise seems to have a fat-sparing quality because similar exercise intensities and durations do not produce similar body fat decreases.[87,88] It has been noted that elite aquatic distance athletes do not lower their body fat percentages to the same extent that elite track distance athletes do, corroborating this research. Nonetheless, aquatic exercise programs may be highly beneficial for the restoration of fitness in obese patients because of the protective effects against heavy joint loading found in the aquatic environment.[54] The ability to achieve an aerobic exercise level for sufficient time to produce a conditioning effect may be difficult in this population on dry land, and a program that begins in water and moves to land as strength, endurance, and tolerance builds may be the most effective method of achieving both conditioning and weight loss.

CONCLUSION

As the information in this chapter demonstrates, immersing the body in water produces many physiologic effects, which have been subjectively reported since nearly the beginning of recorded history, and the effects have been used therapeutically over centuries of medical history. Recent research has contributed to the understanding of the physiologic changes that create these therapeutic effects. There are, however, many areas that merit more study.

The cardiac effects produced by immersion are profound and salutary, both for the healthy heart and usually for rehabilitation of the heart. Through an understanding of the effects of the aquatic environment on cardiac workload, a program of progressive cardiac strengthening may be developed, so that function in even severely deconditioned or injured hearts may improve.

Equally important are the effects of immersion on the pulmonary system. Because the respiratory apparatus must work harder when immersed, respiratory muscle strengthening occurs, and the processes of respiration may be enhanced. A program of regular aquatic exercise should produce a significant training effect that is objectively and subjectively apparent. This effect has been studied in humans with spinal injuries and clearly does occur.[44,89]

The effects on the circulatory and autonomic nervous systems facilitate improvement in muscle blood flow, which results in enhanced oxygen delivery and blood glucose delivery to muscle tissue. Consequently, beneficial effects are produced both in normal muscle during exercising and in muscle and ligament structures during healing.

The effects of immersion on the renal system include promoting the excretion of metabolic waste products; assisting in the regulation of sodium, potassium, and water; and generally lowering blood pressure. The renal effects persist longer than the period of immersion, often lasting many hours or even days.

All of the above-mentioned effects are therapeutically useful. That these effects can occur in an environment that is clinically safe, promotes the reduction of pain, and is even pleasurable is unique. Aquatic rehabilitation is vastly underused. We have been lured by the appeal of high technology and advanced pharmacology, often at the cost of greater medical expense and more side-effect complications. A return to the roots of rehabilitation is appropriate.

These effects are also good reasons to use the aquatic environment in training and rehabilitation. However, much opportunity exists for further research to document the mechanisms producing the effects and study the most efficient means of achieving desired results in conditioning and therapy. In particular, research is needed on fat metabolism and water exercise, bone and calcium metabolism as a function of aquatic exercise, and management of hypertension through aquatic exercise.

Aquatic facilities are widely available, and public acceptance is already high, so there are tremendous potential public health benefits to be achieved through programs targeted at the most significant physiologic consequences of aging: hypertension, cardiovascular disease, arthritis and other joint pathologic conditions, and obesity and deconditioning. There are sound physiologic reasons for speculation that broader public participation in aquatic programs could lower the national health care budget while preserving improved function for the general population. Aquatic programs for achieving fitness and restoring function may be designed for a broad range of individuals through an understanding of the fundamental principles of aquatic physics and the application of those principles to human physiology.

REFERENCES

1. Kuroda PK: What Is Water?, In Licht S (ed): Medical Hydrology. Baltimore: Waverly, 1963, p 1.
2. Giancoli DC: Fluids in Physics. Principles with Applications, 2nd ed. Englewood Cliffs, NJ: Prentice-Hall, 1985, p 184.
3. Wardam B: Lowest point on earth is getting lower. In Jordan Times, Amman, Jordan, 2000.
4. Bloomfield J, Fricker P, Fitch K: Textbook of Science and Medicine in Sport, 5th ed. Champaign, Ill: Human Kinetics Books, 1992.
5. Poyhonen T, et al: Determination of hydrodynamic drag forces and drag coefficients on human leg/foot model during knee exercise. Clin Biomech (Bristol, Avon) 15:256–260, 2000.
6. Somers L, Diving Physics. In Bove AA, Davis JC (eds): Diving Medicine, 2nd ed. Philadelphia; Saunders 1990, p 9.
7. Arborelius M Jr, et al: Hemodynamic changes in man during immersion with the head above water. Aerosp Med 43:592–598, 1972.
8. Risch WD, et al: The effect of graded immersion on heart volume, central venous pressure, pulmonary blood distribution, and heart rate in man. Pflugers Arch 374:115–118, 1978.
9. Gabrielsen A, Johansen LB, Norsk P: Central cardiovascular pressures during graded water immersion in humans. J Appl Physiol 75:581–585, 1993.
10. Gabrielsen A, et al: Arterial pulse pressure and vasopressin release during graded water immersion in humans. Am J Physiol 278:R1583–R1588, 2000.
11. Arborelius M Jr, et al: Regional lung function in man during immersion with the head above water. Aerosp Med 43:701–707, 1972.
12. Risch WD, et al: Time course of cardiac distension with rapid immersion in a thermo-neutral bath. Pflugers Arch 374:119–120, 1978.
13. Weston CF, et al: Haemodynamic changes in man during immersion in water at different temperatures. Clin Sci 73:613–616, 1987.
14. Schlant RC, Sonnenblick EH: Normal physiology of the cardiovascular system. In Hurst J (ed): The Heart. New York: McGraw-Hill, 1986, p 51.
15. McArdle WD, Katch FI, Katch VL: Functional capacity of the cardiovascular system. In Exercise Physiology. Malvern, Penn, Lea & Febiger, 1991, pp 330–331.
16. Haffor AS, Mohler JG, Harrison AC: Effects of water immersion on cardiac output of lean and fat male subjects at rest and during exercise. Aviat Space Environ Med 62:123–127, 1991.

17. Evans BW, Cureton KJ, Purvis JW: Metabolic and circulatory responses to walking and jogging in water. Res Q 49:442–429, 1978.
18. Dressendorfer RH, et al: Effects of head-out water immersion on cardiorespiratory responses to maximal cycling exercise. Undersea Biomed Res 3:177–187, 1976.
19. Gleim GW, Nicholas JA: Metabolic costs and heart rate responses to treadmill walking in water at different depths and temperatures. Am J Sports Med 17:248–252, 1989.
20. Tajima F, et al: Renal and endocrine responses in the elderly during head-out water immersion. Am J Physiol 254(6 Pt 2): R977–R983, 1988.
21. Claybaugh JR, et al: Fluid conservation in athletes: responses to water intake, supine posture, and immersion. J Appl Physiol 61:7–15, 1986.
22. Epstein M: Cardiovascular and renal effects of head-out water immersion in man: application of the model in the assessment of volume homeostasis. Circ Res 39:619–628, 1976.
23. Coruzzi P, et al: Renin-aldosterone system suppression during water immersion in renovascular hypertension. Clin Sci (Colch) 68:609–612, 1985.
24. Tei C, et al: Acute hemodynamic improvement by thermal vasodilation in congestive heart failure. Circulation 91:2582–2590, 1995.
25. Tei C, Tanaka N: Treatment of chronic congestive heart failure to improve their quality of life—clinical study of thermal vasodilation therapy [in Japanese]. Nippon Naika Gakkai Zasshi 84:1475–1482, 1995.
26. Borg G: Perceived exertion as an indicator of somatic stress. Scand J Rehabil Med 2:92–98, 1970.
27. Borg GA: Perceived exertion. Exerc Sport Sci Rev 2:131–153, 1974.
28. Borg GA: Psychophysical bases of perceived exertion. Med Sci Sports Exerc 14:377–381, 1982.
29. Bishop PA, Frazier S, Smith J, Jacobs D: Physiological responses to treadmill and water running. Phys Sports Med 17:87, 1989.
30. Wilder RP, Brennan DK: Physiological responses to deep water running in athletes. Sports Med 16:374–380, 1993.
31. Hong SK, et al: Mechanics of respiration during submersion in water. J Appl Physiol 27:535–538, 1969.
32. Agostoni E, et al: Respiratory mechanics during submersion and negative-pressure breathing. J Appl Physiol 21:251–258, 1966.
33. Choukroun ML, Kays C, Varene P: Effects of water temperature on pulmonary volumes in immersed human subjects. Respir Physiol 75:255–265, 1989.
34. Choukroun ML, Varene P: Adjustments in oxygen transport during head-out immersion in water at different temperatures. J Appl Physiol 68:1475–1480, 1990.
35. Craig AB Jr, Ware DE: Effect of immersion in water on vital capacity and residual volume of the lungs. J Appl Physiol 23:423–425, 1967.
36. Taylor NA, Morrison JB: Pulmonary flow-resistive work during hydrostatic loading. Acta Physiol Scand 142:307–312, 1991.
37. Taylor NA, Morrison JB: Static and dynamic pulmonary compliance during upright immersion. Acta Physiol Scand 149:413–417, 1993.
38. Taylor NA, Morrison JB: Static respiratory muscle work during immersion with positive and negative respiratory loading. J Appl Physiol 87:1397–1403, 1999.
39. Mangelsdorff G, et al: Strength of inspiratory muscles in chronic heart failure and chronic pulmonary obstructive disease [in Spanish]. Rev Med Chile 129:51–59, 2001.
40. Romer LM, McConnell AK, Jones DA: Inspiratory muscle fatigue in trained cyclists: effects of inspiratory muscle training. Med Sci Sports Exerc 34:785–792, 2002.
41. Romer LM, McConnell AK, Jones DA: Effects of inspiratory muscle training upon recovery time during high intensity, repetitive sprint activity. Int J Sports Med 23:353–360, 2002.
42. Nishimura Y, et al: Respiratory muscle strength and hemodynamics in chronic heart failure. Chest 105:355–359, 1994.
43. Adams MA, Chandler LS: Effects of physical therapy program on vital capacity of patients with muscular dystrophy. Phys Ther 54:494–496, 1974.
44. Pachalski A, Mekarski T: Effect of swimming on increasing of cardio-respiratory capacity in paraplegics. Paraplegia 18:190–196, 1980.

45. Epstein M: Renal effects of head-out water immersion in humans: a 15-year update. Physiol Rev 72:563–621, 1992.
46. Balldin UI, et al: Changes in the elimination of 133 xenon from the anterior tibial muscle in man induced by immersion in water and by shifts in body position. Aerosp Med 42:489–493, 1971.
47. Ernst E, Saradeth T, Resch KL: A single blind randomized, controlled trial of hydrotherapy for varicose veins. Vasa 20:147–152, 1991.
48. Elmstahl S, et al: Hydrotherapy of patients with intermittent claudication: a novel approach to improve systolic ankle pressure and reduce symptoms. Int Angiol 14:389–394, 1995.
49. Gatti CJ, Young RJ, Glad HL: Effect of water-training in the maintenance of cardiorespiratory endurance of athletes. Br J Sports Med 13:161–164, 1979.
50. Avellini BA, Shapiro Y, Pandolf KB: Cardio-respiratory physical training in water and on land. Eur J Appl Physiol Occup Physiol 50:255–263, 1983.
51. Svedenhag J, Seger J: Running on land and in water: comparative exercise physiology. Med Sci Sports Exerc 24:1155–1160, 1992.
52. Hamer TW, Morton A: Water-running: training effects and specificity of aerobic, anaerobic and muscular parameters following an eight-week interval training programme. Aust J Sci Med Sport 22:13, 1990.
53. Poyhonen T, et al: Electromyographic and kinematic analysis of therapeutic knee exercises under water. Clin Biomech (Bristol, Avon) 16:496–504, 2001.
54. Harrison RA, Hillman M, Bulstrode S: Loading of the lower limb when walking partially immersed. Physiotherapy 78:165, 1992.
55. Nakazawa K, Yano H, Miyashita M: Ground reaction forces during walking in water. In Miyashita MY, Richardson AB (eds): Medicine and Science in Aquatic Sports. Basel: Karger AG, 1994, p 28.
56. Krishna GG, Danovitch GM: Renal response to central volume expansion in humans is attenuated at night. Am J Physiol 244:R481–R486, 1983.
57. Epstein M, Levinson R, Loutzenhiser R: Effects of water immersion on renal hemodynamics in normal man. J Appl Physiol 41:230–233, 1976.
58. Larsen AS, et al: Volume-homeostatic mechanisms in humans during graded water immersion. J Appl Physiol 77:2832–2839, 1994.
59. Epstein M, et al: Relationship between renal prostaglandin E and renal sodium handling during water immersion in normal man. Circ Res 45:71–80, 1979.
60. Sagawa S, et al: Effect of dehydration on thirst and drinking during immersion in men. J Appl Physiol 72:128–134, 1992.
61. Grossman E, et al: Effects of water immersion on sympathoadrenal and dopa-dopamine systems in humans. Am J Physiol 262(6 Pt 2): R993–R999, 1992.
62. Krishna GG, Danovitch GM, Sowers JR: Catecholamine responses to central volume expansion produced by head-out water immersion and saline infusion. J Clin Endocrinol Metab 56:998–1002, 1983.
63. Miller NC, Seagrave RC: A model of human thermoregulation during water immersion. Comput Biol Med 4:165–182, 1974.
64. Downey JA, Darling RC, Miller JM: The effects, of heat, cold, and exercise on the peripheral circulation. Arch Phys Med Rehabil 49:308–314, 1968.
65. Bonde-Petersen F, Schultz-Pedersen L, Dragsted N: Peripheral and central blood flow in man during cold, thermoneutral, and hot water immersion. Aviat Space Environ Med 63:346–350, 1992.
66. Craig AB Jr, Dvorak M: Thermal regulation during water immersion. J Appl Physiol 21:1577–1585, 1966.
67. Craig AB Jr, Dvorak M: Thermal regulation of man exercising during water immersion. J Appl Physiol 25:28–35, 1968.
68. Vogelaere P, Deklunder G, Lecroart J: Cardiac output variations in supine resting subjects during head-out cold water immersion. Int J Biometeorol 39:40–45, 1995.
69. Allison TG, Reger WE: Comparison of responses of men to immersion in circulating water at 40.0 and 41.5 degrees C. Aviat Space Environ Med 69:845–850, 1998.
70. Boone T, Westendorf T, Ayres P: Cardiovascular responses to a hot tub bath. J Altern Complement Med 5:301–304, 1999.

71. Toner MM, Drolet LL, Pandolf KB: Perceptual and physiological responses during exercise in cool and cold water. Percept Mot Skills 62:211–220, 1986.
72. Nelson M: Pool temperature and high level training. Personal correspondence 12/09/01.
73. Smith DW, Clarren SK, Harvey MA: Hyperthermia as a possible teratogenic agent. J Pediatr 92:878–883, 1978.
74. Harvey MA, McRorie MM, Smith DW: Suggested limits to the use of the hot tub and sauna by pregnant women. Can Med Assoc J 125:50–53, 1981.
75. McMurray RG, et al: The thermoregulation of pregnant women during aerobic exercise in the water: a longitudinal approach. Eur J Appl Physiol Occup Physiol 61:119–123, 1990.
76. McMurray RG, Katz VL: Thermoregulation in pregnancy: implications for exercise. Sports Med 10:146–158, 1990.
77. McMurray RG, et al: Cardiovascular responses of pregnant women during aerobic exercise in water: a longitudinal study. Int J Sports Med 9:443–447, 1988.
78. McMurray RG, et al: Thermoregulation of pregnant women during aerobic exercise on land and in the water. Am J Perinatol 10:178–182, 1993.
79. Gunther V, et al: Fibromyalgia—the effect of relaxation and hydrogalvanic bath therapy on the subjective pain experience. Clin Rheumatol 13:573–578, 1994.
80. Mano T, et al: Sympathetic nervous adjustments in man to simulated weightlessness induced by water immersion. J UOEH 7(Suppl):215–227, 1985.
81. Joyce PR, et al: Urinary catecholamines and plasma hormones predict mood state in rapid cycling bipolar affective disorder. J Affect Disord 33:233–243, 1995.
82. Brown AS, Gershon S: Dopamine and depression. J Neural Transm Gen Sect 91:75–109, 1993.
83. Robiner WN: Psychological and physical reactions to whirlpool baths. J Behav Med 13:157–173, 1990.
84. Watanabe E, et al: Comparison of water- and land-based exercise in the reduction of state anxiety among older adults. Percept Mot Skills 91:97–104, 2000.
85. Perini R, et al: Heart rate variability in exercising humans: effect of water immersion. Eur J Appl Physiol 77:326–332, 1998.
86. Sheldahl LM: Special ergometric techniques and weight reduction. Med Sci Sports Exerc 18:25–30, 1986.
87. Gwinup G: Weight loss without dietary restriction: efficacy of different forms of aerobic exercise. Am J Sports Med 15:275–279, 1987.
88. Kieres J, Plowman S: Effects of swimming and land exercises versus swimming and water exercises on body composition of college students. J Sports Med Phys Fitness 31:189–195, 1991.
89. Tajima F, et al: Cardiovascular, renal, and endocrine responses in male quadriplegics during head-out water immersion. Am J Physiol 258(6 Pt 2):R1424–R1230, 1990.

Chapter 3
Facility Design and Water Management

Alison Osinski, PhD

DESIGN PROCESS

Before embarking on a major facility design project, an aquatic therapist should learn the basics of how to design a patient- and therapist-friendly warm water pool and have the knowledge necessary to select appropriate equipment and features to complement the programming and therapy goals. The therapist should be able to make informed decisions as to which products, chemicals, pieces of equipment, and surface and construction materials are best suited for use in warm water therapy pool environments. He or she should have a basic understanding of the therapy pool design process, know the advantages and disadvantages of constructing a pool versus purchasing and installing a prefabricated pool, have an understanding of space requirements, and be able to estimate costs of building a therapy pool.

POOL DESIGN TRENDS

Today, the trend in the United States is to build multiple pool facilities that include leisure concept pools and special-use pools designed specifically for a single purpose such as fitness, competition, diving, recreational swimming, or therapy rather than single, multipurpose pools.

In general, pools are becoming shallower overall. They often incorporate water features that involve moving water. Incorporation of a theme is a widespread trend and, in addition, the environment is made more aesthetically pleasing through the use of natural and artificial light, plants, and graphics. The facilities are designed to be accessible to disabled users and incorporate multiple means of ingress and egress to accommodate user preferences and needs. Many aspects of the operation and maintenance of pools are becoming automated.

Special-use pools serve a broader community base than traditional swimming pools. They are often used by individuals with little or no swimming ability. Usually they are designed to be financially self-supporting, and, if they are managed efficiently, capital costs as well as operating expenses will be covered, and profits will be generated soon after the initial start-up.

POOL DESIGN PROJECT PHASES

Following a logical sequence of planning stages will allow the design process to progress smoothly. The project should be analyzed thoroughly, and objectives and goals should be set before the design process actually begins. The design process consists of nine phases:

- Site analysis
- Determination of programming requirements
- Preliminary design and project feasibility
- Selection of a project design team
- Production of construction documents
- Obtaining of permits and plan check
- Bidding and awarding of contracts
- Construction phase
- Turnover and acceptance of the completed facility

Pool Site Analysis

The first phase of the project, pool site analysis, includes determining whether a particular site is an appropriate location for building a therapy pool facility. During this phase, marketing and demographic surveys should be conducted. The therapist should visit similar nearby facilities to check on the competition and identify design features he or she would like to incorporate, eliminate, or improve upon. Zoning regulations should be investigated thoroughly to make sure there are no prohibitions or restrictions to building the desired facility at a particular location. An environmental impact study may be required. The availability of utilities and access to the site from major roads should be verified. Otherwise, the cost of building access roads or bringing natural gas pipelines or electrical lines to the site may make the project cost prohibitive.

A geotechnical engineer or soil specialist should be hired before the land is purchased to conduct topographical and soil surveys, evaluate ground water table conditions, and identify earthquake potential and seismic zone restrictions to determine whether the proposed site is an appropriate location for pool construction. Although a pool can be built almost anywhere, costs will be substantially higher in some locations. The geotechnical engineer or soil specialist should do test borings to determine soil stability. Inappropriate soil conditions or unstable ground can lead to settling, sinking, cracking, or floating of the pool; heave from freezing or wet, expanding soil; hillside erosion and landslides; and ground creep from seismic activity. The engineer will identify ground conditions and load-bearing capacity and determine whether there is suitable drainage and whether installation of hydrostatic relief valves or drain tile or the use of sump pumps may be necessary. He or she will analyze soil samples for moisture content and composition and differentiate soil by particle size into four categories (gravel, sand, silt, or clay) to determine whether the soil will need to be modified or stabilized by compacting or dewatering. Groundwater or water table level conditions, along with springs, flood plains, and tidal variations will be identified. He or she will look for underground hazards or unexpected obstacles such as large buried rocks that may need to be blasted away or for subterranean cavities that will have to be filled before construction. Retaining wall construction or major changes in the topography or earthwork before construction may be necessary.

Demographic Survey

A demographic study should be undertaken to determine whether there is interest in the project or a real need for the facility. Who will use the facility, and why will they select your facility over other existing therapy facilities? Will there be competition from other nearby aquatic facilities that provide similar programs and services or cater to the same clientele? Are the existing aquatic facilities overcrowded, unsafe, aging, or obsolete? What impact will your facility have on the neighborhood? Will nearby residents object to the facility based on the impact on the environment, traffic congestion, availability of parking, or noise or light pollution?

Programming Requirements

Pool design should be program driven if the goal is to generate profits while serving the aquatic therapy needs of the community. When designing the facility, determine how much space is needed to accommodate both current and future programming needs. Prioritize your areas of programming. Which programs are most important and will generate the most revenue? Who is your patient population? What type of patients will you see—general population, older adults, pediatric population, or athletes with sports-related injuries? What treatments or techniques will you provide? How long will treatment sessions be? What are the space and depth requirements for particular therapies? Ranking program importance helps ensure that the aquatic facility will be designed to meet program needs, that certain pieces of equipment and materials will be specified, and that design or operational conflicts will be solved logically.

Preliminary Design and Project Feasibility

List and prioritize desired equipment and design requirements based on an awareness of activities and programs that are planned for the pool. With your consultant, fill out an aquatic facility design checklist and prepare a "design program" to help prioritize program offerings and determine pool and equipment requirements to meet anticipated needs. The design program will specify the number, size, dimensions, tolerances, type, brand names, markings, location, color, technical data, and performance standards for all pool components and equipment.

When initially planning the size of the facility, determine in-water space needs for various therapies and programs and the maximum number of patients who would be in the water at the same time if your facility is successful beyond your wildest dreams. Depending on the activity, space needs per individual range from 60 square feet for stationary activities to more than 500 square feet for activities that involve swimming, water walking, or moving up and down the length of the pool. For instance, if you wanted to run a small group wellness activity that involved no more than 20 participants standing vertically in the water and not moving more than one step in any direction, each participant would need a minimum of 64 square feet of space in the pool. The minimum amount of usable space (not counting steps, ramps, seating tiers, etc.) would be 1280 square feet. Assume that the actual pool size is 30 by 50 feet or 1500 square feet. Suppose that at the same time, one-on-one therapy is taking place in an adjacent 12 foot by 15 foot, 180 square foot prefabricated therapy pool. Decks area is usually 1.5 times the size of the pool area. The space needed for men's, women's, staff's, and families' locker rooms is at least equal to the size of the pools. Auxiliary spaces needed to run the pool, which include pump rooms, chemical rooms, storage rooms for therapy devices and equipment used in the pool, a first aid room, and maintenance closets, are at least equal to the size of the pools. The minimum size of the building that will accommodate the pool, decks, locker rooms, and auxiliary spaces can be estimated by taking the area of the pool, in this example 1680 square feet, and multiplying by a factor of 4.5 for a minimum building size of a little over 7500 square feet. Space for offices, reception areas, meeting rooms, saunas and steam rooms, waiting rooms, patient screening rooms, and therapy treatment rooms may also be needed.

Review all applicable health and safety, building, fire, electrical, and plumbing codes; state and local statutes and regulations; federal regulations; and industry standards and guidelines to make sure your facility design complies with all of these.

Develop a financing plan that identifies funding sources and includes cost projections and a budget. Determine costs of construction, and review the financial viability of the project based on available resources. Costs of building a therapy pool facility range from a low of about $85.00 per square foot for outdoor facilities to more than $400.00 per square foot for high-end, indoor facilities. Develop a contingency plan for cost overruns. Refer to industry cost books that can be purchased at technical bookstores or may be available at your local library. Apply geographic cost modifiers to help determine actual construction costs in your region of the country. You may want to hire an economic research consultant to conduct studies and prepare projections for costs and income potential.

Design Team

Assemble your design team. An aquatic facility design team should consist of the facility owners and their representatives, including aquatic programming, maintenance, and management staff who will be working in the facility; your architect, engineers, and builders/contractors; your aquatic consultant; and local regulatory or health department officials.

The architect is the individual who prepares the specifications and drawings from which the contractors work. The architect estimates project costs, supervises the construction, inspects the completed project, and certifies that the work was completed in compliance with the specifications. The architect must be licensed in the state in which the facility is constructed.

The engineer designs the operation and layout of the mechanical equipment, machinery, and building systems. He or she makes sure systems work in compliance with performance standards. An engineer who is competent to work on an aquatic facility design project should have knowledge and experience in designing hydraulic, heating, ventilating, and air conditioning (HVAC), electrical, plumbing, and mechanical systems.

The builders and licensed contractors purchase building supplies, materials, and equipment that conform to the specifications. A general contractor and several subcontractors are likely to be involved with a complex project such as a therapy pool facility. It is unusual to find one company that specializes in construction of both buildings and pools and employs all the various tradesmen needed to complete the project. The contractors construct the facility, install the equipment, provide the tools and construction equipment, schedule workers and jobs to be done, obtain building permits and schedule inspections, and guarantee that the facility is built to specifications.

The aquatic consultant is the specialist familiar with pool design trends, equipment, and codes. He or she helps establish priorities and goals based on your program needs. The consultant assists the architect in writing or revising specifications and is responsible for educating the design team about equipment options and comparing the costs and effectiveness of various products, materials, and systems. The aquatic consultant reviews and critiques the construction documents for common design errors, safety hazards, code compliance, appropriateness to stated goals and primary facility usage, and compliance with common and acceptable practices of the aquatic industry, manufacturers' recommendations, and design guidelines.

State or county health officials who have jurisdiction over the facility should be invited to participate in the design process so that plans and specifications move smoothly through the plan check process and gain swift approval. This is especially important if the facility or specified equipment is of an unusual, innovative, or controversial design or if code variances are being requested.

When selecting members of your facility design team, make sure the firms or individuals have experience working on comparable projects. Find out if they are open to input from consultants, consulting architects, and other design team members. Are they willing to try innovative design ideas, or do they basically build the same facility project after project? Do all their projects look the same? Make sure that they capable of discussing and providing advice on the advantages and disadvantages of various pool systems and equipment. Have they had problems obtaining approval for past aquatic projects? Ask if they are independent, or if they are affiliated with a specific aquatic product, retailer, builder, or design group. Ask about the number of current projects the firm is involved in and plans to work on simultaneously. Make sure they have the time and staff necessary to devote to your project. Request references and a client list.

Construction Documents

Construction documents that must be prepared include construction diagrams or drawings (commonly, but incorrectly, referred to as blueprints), "as built" plans, specifications, change requests, and change orders. They may also include models and aerial photographs.

Drawings or construction diagrams graphically depict the work to be done. They include floor or site plans that depict the building itself, structural details, elevations, grading, pool orientation, water supply, sewer, and utility connections. Detailed construction plans show the location of inlets, drains, hydrostatic relief valves, perimeter overflow systems, surge chambers, piping, decks, drains, hose bibbs, water fountains, walls, ladders, stairs, rails, ramps, lights, diving boards, starting blocks, bulkheads, filtration and circulation equipment, and locker rooms. Landscape drawings show trees, plants, and irrigation systems. Other schematic diagrams include those that show pool piping; electrical, mechanical, and plumbing details; and cross-sectional and longitudinal views of the pool.

Specifications are the written instructions for the contractor that provide technical information for the various building tradesmen and subcontractors on the work to be completed. Specifications describe materials, size, and type of equipment; standards of workmanship; the quality of materials, options, alternatives, or acceptable substitutions; installation methods or procedures; and inspection and testing requirements. Specifications usually include details that are not found or duplicated on the drawings. If there is a discrepancy, specifications take precedence over the drawings.

The contractor is responsible for ensuring compliance with design specifications, drawings, and codes. Selected equipment must meet the performance requirements specified or the contractor must replace the defective materials.

Today, specification writing and the arrangement of technical information for the trades are computerized using the industry standard CSI MasterFormat system. The CSI Format for Building Specifications has 16 basic divisions, with each division representing several trades. It is used to provide a better and faster method of construction estimating. The 16 divisions include the following:

1. General requirements: Permits, fees, liability bond, insurance, supervision, clean-up, temporary facilities, security, tax, plan check, general contractor, summary of work, responsibilities, items furnished by owner, work to be performed at a later time, applicable codes, abbreviations or symbols, reports, storage and protection of materials and equipment
2. Site work: Clearing, grading, excavating, drainage, utilities, roads, landscaping, demolition, earthwork
3. Concrete: Formwork, reinforcing, material, finish, deck, grout
4. Masonry: Material, reinforcing, grouting, placement of rigs, mortar, and stone
5. Metals: Structural, steel, metal, joists, ornamental iron
6. Carpentry: Millwork, casework, walls, framing, rough carpentry, finish carpentry, adhesives, wood, and plastics
7. Moisture protection: Roofing, weatherproofing, insulation
8. Doors, windows, glass: Doors, windows, skylights
9. Finishes: Drywall, tile, flooring, interior and exterior painting, plaster, tile, carpeting, acoustic ceilings, wall coverings
10. Specialties: Toilet accessories, chalkboards, lockers, signs, clocks, fire-fighting equipment, prefabricated products, pest control, fireplaces, flagpoles, telephones
11. Equipment: Athletic or recreational equipment, theater equipment, spas, saunas, snack bars, cabinets, kitchen and office equipment
12. Furnishings: Seating, artwork, drapery, blinds, shades, carpeting, furniture, plants
13. Special construction: Swimming pools, filtration equipment, wave generators, courts, special purpose rooms
14. Conveying systems: Elevators, escalators, lifts, hoists
15. Mechanical systems: Water supply, fixtures, sprinklers, heating and air conditioning, waste water, fountains, plumbing, air handling systems
16. Electrical systems: Lighting fixtures, communications systems, controls

As the project progresses, the specifications will be appended with addenda and change orders to clarify procedures, correct errors or omissions, and change the scope or quality of work. Upon completion of the project, the owner should request at least two sets of as-built plans. As-built plans reflect changes that occurred during construction and show the work that was actually done. One set of as-built plans should be kept on site and available for frequent reference. The other set of as-built plans should be stored in a safe location for future retrieval when necessary.

Obtaining Permits

An application for construction of a new swimming pool, drawings, and specifications must be submitted to the appropriate authorities for review and approval before construction is begun. The plans must be prepared by and bear the seal of a registered professional engineer or architect licensed to practice in the state. Plans must be accompanied by the required fee. Fees may or may not be waived for nonprofit agencies.

Each state has specific requirements for how applications for construction will be processed and what materials must be submitted for review. Usually though, the person planning to construct, alter, or modify a pool, except for routine maintenance, must submit plans to the county health officer for review and approval. Occasionally, plans must be submitted to other regulatory agencies such as the department of water quality, department of agriculture, or state department of health and rehabilitative services.

Typically, a completed construction permit application form and three sets of plans and specifications prepared and signed by an engineer or architect must be submitted. The package usually includes construction plans (blueprints) drawn to scale and in sufficient detail to completely illustrate the proposed construction, including plan views, cross-sectional views, plans showing the pool in relation to other facilities in the area, dimensional drawings, a detailed view of the equipment layout, a piping schematic showing piping configuration, pipe size, valves, inlets, drains, outlets, water flow pattern, make-up water, and water disposal. Decks, fences, barriers and alarm systems, pool components, pool appurtenances, steps, ladders, rails, ramps and handicap accessibility equipment, bottom markings, depth markings, signage, equipment rooms, chemical rooms, first aid treatment rooms, lifeguard stands and location of rescue equipment, food and beverage service facilities, heating and heat retention, air distribution, ventilation, and dehumidification system components, locker rooms and sanitary facilities, and lighting and plumbing fixtures must be shown. Information on the approved source of potable water that will be used to fill the pools and the method of chemical neutralization and water disposal must be submitted. Information must be provided to show that there are no cross connections between the domestic water supply, the pool recirculation system, and the sewer system and that appropriate backflow prevention and air gaps have been provided.

Detailed written specifications must be submitted to permit a comprehensive engineering review. The name of the manufacturer and model number of all equipment must be provided, along with proof of NSF International listing or approved equivalent for filters, pumps, pipes, valves, disinfection, and other listed equipment. The volume, water surface area, and linear footage/perimeter, construction and surface materials, and color of the pool must be provided. The filter type, filter media, filter surface area, design flow rate, recirculation pump capacity, velocities, turnover time and flow rate, and total dynamic head and pump curves for the filtration and circulation system components must be provided. Detailed descriptions of treatment chemicals and systems and of chemical feeders, controllers, and related equipment that will be used must be provided.

The application, plans, and specifications will be reviewed by the regulatory agent, and at the completion of plan check, the agent will forward written approval or rejection or may require modifications or additional information to be submitted. When all conditions are met, the regulatory agent will issue a construction permit.

The construction permit must be posted in a conspicuous place on the construction site. The permit is typically valid for a period of time of between 12 and 18 months. Changes in plans or specifications during construction require that the documents be resubmitted for approval. The facility owner must ensure that any modification or alteration is completed according to approved plans and specifications.

Bidding and Awarding of Contracts

Advertise the opportunity to bid on the project. Construction documents, including the schedule of drawings and specifications, should be made available to prospective bidders. The bid package should also include an invitation to bid, instructions explaining how the bid is to be submitted, how the contract will be awarded, conditions for which bids will be rejected, sample proposal forms so all bids are submitted in a similar fashion, conditions of the contract, and the agreement. Identify a time frame for project completion and specify a penalty if work is not completed within the scheduled time. Allow a reasonable amount of time for contractors to prepare their bids and hold a pre-bid meeting at the site to answer questions potential contractors might have. Review and accept or reject the bids, negotiate fees, and award the contract.

Construction Phase

During the actual construction phase, a construction manager will supervise the subcontractors, tradesmen, and laborers. The architect or engineer should be on-site as often as necessary but at least once per week to make sure that the facility is being built in compliance with the approved plans. If possible, the owners or their representatives should visit the site regularly to observe and photograph or videotape the progress of the project.

Turnover and Acceptance of the Completed Facility

When construction is completed, conduct a pre-opening walk-through and inspection of the facility. Thoroughly inspect the pool and all of its equipment before it is put into use, and either accept, reject, or conditionally accept the project. Obtain an operating permit from the regulatory agency. Make sure that all operations manuals, instructions for proper preventative maintenance of all equipment, as-built drawings, and warrantees are turned over to the owner. Train the aquatic facility staff in the proper operation and maintenance of the facility and equipment.

Inspect the facility again approximately 120 days after the initial start-up to determine if the equipment is operating as specified and whether systems are performing to expectations. Be sure to conduct a final inspection within 1 year after start-up, and make sure all defects have been corrected or have been identified and are in the process of being fixed before taking final control of the facility. When everything is working properly and the owner is satisfied that the work has been completed, the architect or registered professional engineer certifies that construction was completed in compliance with the approved drawings and specifications.

PREFABRICATED THERAPY POOLS

Very early in the design process, a decision should be made as to whether the therapy pools are going to be designed and constructed from scratch or whether prefabricated pools are going to be purchased and installed. There are, of course, advantages to each.

Constructed pools are permanent and long lasting. They can be custom designed to meet your unique programming needs and can be built to fit specific size and space requirements. By designing and building a pool, you can select from a wide variety of equipment and material options not available when buying a prepackaged system.

Prefabricated therapy pools have the advantage of portability. You can take the pool with you when you move to a new location or a larger facility. There is less of a financial commitment if you are just entering the field or expanding your rapidly growing aquatic therapy practice. The speed of installation allows you to be up and running very quickly. A therapy pool design and construction project often takes 2 to 5 years from the time of the first design meetings to actual occupancy. A prefabricated pool facility can be in operation in less than 1 year. Most prefabricated therapy pools have been classified as Food and Drug Administration–approved class II medical devices. There is a tax advantage with installation of a prefabricated pool. A prefabricated pool is usually considered a piece of equipment rather than part of the building, and, like any other piece of business equipment, it can be depreciated over 5 to 7 years.

Remember though, when comparing prefabricated pools to constructed pools, not to just compare the stated cost of the pool to construction costs. Work typically not contained in the base price stated by manufacturers of prefabricated pools includes site preparation and excavation, electrical or plumbing hook-ups requiring work by licensed professionals, finish work, decking and floor drains, sump pumps for pools without plumbed suction outlets, and HVAC units. Payments for permits and inspections, taxes, and the cost of shipment and delivery of the prefabricated pool to your location will probably be your responsibility. Travel and lodging expenses for the manufacturer's installation crew may or may not be included in the quoted price.

Do not forget the weight-load on the floor. Floors other than ground floors may not be able to support the weight of the pool. Water weighs 8.33 pounds/gallon or 62.4 pounds/cubic foot. Your floor will need to safely support from 200 to 500 pounds/square foot. Floors will probably have to be reinforced to support even a small prefabricated pool.

If you are seriously considering the purchase of a prefabricated therapy pool, be sure to compare features of several pools that are on the market today so that you can make an informed purchase. Each manufacturer includes special or unique features. Features may include movable floors, treadmills, lifts, handrails, exercise bars, parallel bars, seating tiers, underwater windows, hydrotherapy jets, countercurrent jets to provide laminar resistance, built-in work stations, underwater cameras, current resistance gauges, treadmill speed gauges, angled plyometric boards, and attachment points for stabilization and support devices. Some manufacturers provide access to all pool functions through waterproof hand-held remote control devices. Some models include computer monitoring, tracking, and documentation of patient treatment, which allow you to repeat treatment protocols, demonstrate progress toward achieving functional goals and outcomes, and show that skilled intervention is taking place and functional gains are being achieved. Some provide printed progress reports for your records and third party reimbursement.

Factory response time to repair equipment breakdowns, the availability of service contracts, and limited warranties should also be considered.

COMMON DESIGN ERRORS

Design errors that are overlooked in the early stages of the design and planning process can cause astronomical cost overruns and may influence the expense and time involved in maintaining and operating the facility for years to come. To avoid typical pool design errors, examine common mistakes made by other therapists when designing their aquatic facilities.

The biggest mistake many therapists make is designing an aquatic therapy facility that is not program driven. One size does not fit all. Know how you plan to use the facility before you design it and prioritize your programming needs. Do not try to make a single, traditional, multiuse pool fit your needs. Make sure you include necessary features in the original design of the pools. If the feature or piece of equipment does not appear on the construction drawings or in the specifications, it will not be part of your facility. Know which items you are not willing to compromise on when a budget crunch occurs and cuts have to be made.

Do not undersize the facility. No one ever complains that their facility is too big. The facility is undersized if it is at maximum capacity within 1 year of opening and the therapist is turning away patients. Common sizing errors include not enough shallow (or deep) water, crowded pump rooms that do not allow proper air circulation around components or provide easy access for maintenance and repair, no provision of off-deck viewing rooms, inadequate storage space, limited convenient parking, and small, poorly laid out locker rooms, which lack amenities and privacy, are inaccessible, and do not accommodate caregivers of the opposite sex.

Just because a therapy pool is relatively small does not mean that only design professionals familiar with small, residential pool construction are qualified to work on your facility. Do not hire local pool contractors, architects, or engineers who have no commercial pool design/building experience, are unfamiliar with therapy programming needs, and have little familiarity with the demands placed on the facility by a successful aquatic therapy practice.

Pay attention to the work environment and the comfort and health of your employees. Poor design of the HVAC and air handling systems, inadequate illumination, and poor acoustical quality will make the facility an unpleasant and unhealthy place of business. Employees will develop health problems related to sick building syndrome and the facility and equipment will rapidly deteriorate.

Hire a qualified, experienced, certified, and/or licensed pool operator to run the facility. Someone must take care of the ongoing day-to-day routine operation and maintenance of the facility. You need a trained operator on site. Having a pool service firm come in once or twice a week to perform minor maintenance is not adequate. Depending on the size of the facility, this may be a full-time job. Do not expect to take care of daily and preventative maintenance on the pools during the hour before you see your first patients of the day.

Do not select and purchase inexpensive residential quality equipment and components just because the pool is small in size. Install commercial grade equipment. The heavy use of warm water therapy pools puts extreme demands on materials and equipment. Frequent breakdowns and repairs can be costly to a business in which therapy cannot be provided when the pool is out of service.

Size equipment and circulation system components to accommodate peak bather loads. Many therapy pools have insufficient water turnover times and flow rates, even though the equipment may comply with minimum code requirements. Chronic water clarity and water quality problems develop as a result of improper filter sizing, media selection, and filter maintenance.

A good rule of thumb is to keep the bather load to total filtered water (in gallons per day) ratio at 1 bather to 1400 gallons or less. The onset of turbidity is constant and related to the number of bathers, not just to turnover time. If debris, including airborne dirt, dust, plant matter, pollen, rain water, and bather waste, is added to the pool water faster than the filter can remove it, turbidity will increase. Here is an example of the calculation of bather load and clarity:

24,000 gallon therapy pool (20 feet wide × 40 feet long × 4 feet deep)

250 actual bathers per day × 1400
= 350,000 gallons/day ÷ 24 (hours/day) ÷ 60 (min/hr)
= 243 gallons/min (flow rate needed to maintain clarity)

24,000 gallons ÷ 243 gallons/min
= 98 min ÷ 60
= 1.64 hours (required turnover time)

Oversized, commercial-quality filter tanks should be installed to remove particles, to keep the nephelometric turbidity unit value below 0.25, and to help keep the water crystal clear. A particular type or brand of filter should be selected based on several considerations, such as the type of filter media used, the cost of purchase, operation, and replacement; the pool size and required flow rates; filter surface area and space requirements in the pump room; ability to get the filter into an existing room; plumbing requirements; filtering capability (size of particle the filter is able to remove from the water) and clarity achieved; the availability of water for backwashing; water disposal restrictions; and the time requirements and ease of maintenance. In addition to filtration, knowledgeable use of flocculents and clarifiers, sequestering and chelating agents, enzymes and absorbent foam products, and secondary nanofiltration or granulated activated carbon filtration systems will help maintain proper water clarity.

Because of lack of education and experience in the area of water chemistry, many therapy pool designers inadvertently install inadequate and unsafe water treatment systems. Stand-alone halogen systems with no auxiliary or supplemental treatment systems are likely to be inadequate. Minimal automation of the chemical treatment process, improper dispensing methods including hand feeding of chemicals directly into the pool, undersized chemical feed pumps, ignoring water balance, unsafe chemical storage practices, poor choice of chemicals for use in warm water, high bather-load-to-water-volume-ratio pools with heavy organic loading, and estimating rather than calculating precise chemical adjustments all contribute to the water quality problems experienced by many therapy facilities. Many therapy pool operators are not familiar with appropriate chemical ranges or routine or preventative maintenance practices and do not know how to deal with common pool problems such as algae, mineral staining, excessive chloramine buildup, or fecal contamination.

Select appropriate chemicals after a review of your source water chemistry, costs of purchasing bulk chemicals from local distributors, dispensing methods, storage capacity, and safety considerations. Purchase properly sized chemical feeders and top-quality pH/oxidation-reduction potential controllers, and maintain the oxidation-reduction potential at greater than 750 mV at all times to assure proper sanitation and oxidation of pool water. Monitor mineral saturation and keep the water balanced at all times. Purchase good field-quality water testing instruments, test kits and reagents, and air monitoring equipment; test water regularly and record all results. Send samples regularly to the laboratory for microbial testing and analysis to prevent disease transmission through pool water. Learn proper disinfection and decontamination procedures. Use the flowmeters, influent and effluent pressure, and vacuum gauges installed on the circulation system to provide information on the system status. Learn to read a chemical log, to identify common water problems before they get out of control, and to make adjustments as necessary.

Design a facility that is accessible to all patients. The building itself, the therapy pools and services provided, and auxiliary facilities such as locker rooms must be accessible to all users. Many therapy facilities are designed with unintentional barriers. Often decks are too narrow to accommodate users and their conveyances. The need for off-deck space for stowing wheelchairs and walkers and securing guide animals is overlooked.

The purchase and installation of specialized pieces of access equipment may be needed to accommodate participants covered under the Americans with Disabilities Act. Disabled individuals should be able to enter, use, and exit a pool with little or no assistance and without drawing undue or unwanted attention to themselves. Various means or methods of providing safe, comfortable, and dignified ingress and egress for all pool patrons are available. Because of individual differences, more than one modification or piece of equipment may be needed to make aquatic facilities accessible to the entire population.

Follow the swimming pool accessibility guidelines developed by the U.S. Architectural and Transportation Barriers Compliance Board. When only one means of accessibility to the pool is provided, it must be a swimming pool lift, wet ramp, or zero depth entry. Swimming pools with more than 300 linear feet of pool wall should have at least two accessible means of water entry and exit located on accessible routes. The second access method should not be the same as the first method and may include lifts, movable floors, wet or dry ramps, transfer tiers, zero depth entry, or accessible steps.

Many therapy pool designers make poor choices when selecting materials for surfacing pools, decks, locker room floors, and adjacent hallways. Slip-and-fall accidents are the most common reasons for lawsuits being filed in the aquatic environment. It makes sense to install slip-resistance surfaces and provide sturdy handrails in all wet areas of the facility. The coefficient of dynamic friction when wet should not be less than 0.6, regardless of materials chosen. All walking surfaces should slope $\frac{1}{4}$ inch/foot toward drains and should be designed to prevent water accumulation or puddling. To prevent biofilm growth and the resulting slipperiness, surfaces should be both cleaned and disinfected daily or as needed, using either steam or pool water–compatible cleaning and disinfecting products.

With the rising cost of energy, designing an energy-efficient aquatic facility should be a priority. After staffing costs, energy will be your largest operating expense. Design errors and energy-wasteful choices in the selection of equipment have made the difference between profit and loss for many therapy facilities. Design the layout of the pump room for energy efficiency. Locate the pump room near the pools. Provide space inside the pump room to allow straight pipe runs whenever possible and to eliminate the need for installation of many 90-degree elbows. Oversize the filters. Size the circulation pipe to prevent extreme velocities greater than 7 feet/sec. Reduce head loss and resistance to flow, and select a pump that operates at peak efficiency on its pump performance curve. Install high-efficiency pool water heaters. Natural gas heaters with thermal efficiency ratings of more than 90% are available. Replace energy-wasting, 500-watt incandescent, underwater pool lights with efficient, long-life fluorescent bulbs. Provide windbreaks, and use thermal insulating pool covers or monomolecular film products to substantially reduce energy loss due to evaporation off the water surface.

ESSENTIAL DOCUMENTATION AND OTHER CONSIDERATIONS

Before the facility is opened, staff must be hired and trained, standard operating procedures must be established, and operations manuals must be developed.

In addition to therapists and therapy assistants, other instructors, lifeguards, a pool operator, housekeeping staff, an office manager, and receptionists must be employed. All employees should have training in basic water rescue, cardiopulmonary resuscitation, and first aid; should participate in rescue drills; and should be familiar with the emergency communication system and how to obtain assistance in an emergency. Employees should have the appropriate prerequisite current certification or licensing, attend pre-employment training sessions specific to the facility, and participate in regular in-service training.

A comprehensive policies and procedures manual should be developed for the facility. It should include general information such as the mission statement, a map and directions to the facility, phone listings, general program information and a menu of services, customer service principles, hours of operation, admissions requirements, facility rental information, facility description, facility diagram, and a list of employees.

Employee policies and procedures should be clearly defined. Written job descriptions for each position, an explanation of employee responsibilities, and a list of required certifications and licenses should be included. Pre-service and in-service training requirements, testing procedures, in-house and independent staff auditing, uniform guidelines, staff use of facilities, and employee performance evaluation procedures should be explained. Information on employee benefits, resources and equipment support, absence, vacation, employee substitution, rotation and breaks, and payroll information and procedures should be provided. Employee protection policies dealing with employee accidents and on-the-job injuries, universal precautions, use of personal protective gear, skin and eye protection, and critical incident stress assistance should be described.

Chemical, biohazard, and electrical safety guidelines and procedures for injury prevention should be explained in detail. Closure procedures for inclement weather and weather-related emergencies, natural disasters, fire, chemical spills, and electrical power outages should be outlined.

Explain all therapy practices and protocol. Include lesson plans and details concerning each therapy, program, or procedure provided. List the required qualifications of therapists or employees providing each therapy or type of instruction. Explain patient contact procedures, and list contraindications and prohibited practices.

Maintenance practices and standard operating procedures for each pool and piece of equipment should be enumerated.

Patron surveillance procedures for each area of programming should be spelled out. Include information on scanning and surveillance techniques, surveillance during special activities, guarding zones, the 10/20 supervision rule, rotation procedures, victim recognition, and a drowning overview and timeline. Explain how patients will be supervised, how capacity limits will be enforced, how established facility rules will be enforced, how more serious incidents or undesirable behavior will be dealt with, what circumstances will bring about expulsion from the pool, and when security or police will be contacted for assistance in diffusing an explosive, dangerous, or out-of-control situation. If surveillance of the pool area includes use of electronic or remote devices (alarms, video cameras, closed circuit TV monitors, drowning detection systems, or other security system components) in addition to that provided by personnel, the equipment and its operation should be described.

A list of all facility use rules should be included along with the rationale for each rule.

Emergency procedures and emergency action plans for life-threatening and non–life-threatening emergencies should be explained in detail. Describe your communication system, how to call for help in an emergency, and how to activate the emergency medical system. Provide information on filling out accident report forms, notifying relatives of an injured patient, providing information to the media after an emergency, and emergency follow-up procedures.

Accountability, cash register controls, and loss prevention procedures should be explained. Copies of revenue receipts, deposit slips, fee schedules and waivers, billing codes, and claim forms should be provided.

The final section of the policies and procedures manual should include copies of all forms used at the facility. Numerous records and reports must be kept to provide data for making decisions regarding equipment, personnel, and procedures; to provide data used to determine costs of operation, patron satisfaction, causes and prevention of injuries; as a basis for budget recommendations and justification for future expenditures; to ensure the proper operation of the facility; and to comply with state, federal, and local ordinances. Employees should be familiar with all forms used at the facility and should know how to properly fill them out. Employees should be reminded that records should be completed accurately and on time and never forged or filled out in advance. Records should be stored for an extended period of time in case documentation or retrieval of information is necessary as part of a legal defense if an accident results in litigation.

Examples of the following forms should be included in the policies and procedures manual:

- Employee procedures
- Operating manuals and procedures

- Chemical safety procedures
- Evacuation procedures and emergency plans
- Safety literature and posters
- Model release form
- Request for leave of absence
- Work schedule sheet
- Daily cash receipt
- Pool rental agreements
- Fee waiver forms and log
- Accident report form
- Victim and witness statement forms
- Minor injury report form
- Incident report form
- Agreement to participate
- Liability release forms and waivers
- Patient assessment
- Refusal of emergency medical treatment form
- Blood/bodily fluids contact report
- Notice to our guests
- Verification of employee certification and licenses
- Employee training log
- Staff audit forms
- Employee substitution form
- Daily pool log
- Chemical additions log
- Daily maintenance checklists
- Preventative maintenance checklists
- Seasonal maintenance checklists
- Facility safety inspection checklist
- Swimming pool inventory form
- Equipment disposal form
- Maintenance request form
- Code compliance checklists
- Marketing brochures, advertisements
- Phone call log

CONCLUSION

Aquatic therapy has become a mainstream component of rehabilitation. It is now being used extensively in sports and orthopedic rehabilitation, as well as in the management of many neurologic disorders. The establishment of an aquatics program can be a therapeutically beneficial addition to a continuum of patient care. It can also be economically beneficial to a clinical practice.

As seen from the preceding chapter content, these benefits do not come without effort. The planning and development of an aquatics facility requires foresight, diligence, and care. The maintenance of such a program requires continuous oversight, careful documentation, and meticulous discipline on all matters of safety and hygiene. The rewards are high in terms of patient satisfaction and clinical benefit, but such a project should not be undertaken lightly. An inadequately constructed pool can be an economic disaster, requiring constant cash infusions and frequent downtime. A poorly managed maintenance program can put patients, staff, and the facility at risk. But with an understanding of the tasks needed to build a successful aquatic therapy program, and consistent attention to the details of program and facility management, the rewards are great.

Chapter 4
The Halliwick Concept

Johan Lambeck, BPT, Fran Coffey Stanat, PhD, and Douglas W. Kinnaird, BA, NCTMB, ATRIC

INTRODUCTION

Halliwick began as a sequential method, known as the Ten-Point Program, for teaching children with disabilities to swim. When the therapeutic benefits of Halliwick became apparent, the program was extended and described as Water Specific Therapy.

The Halliwick Concept,* as it is used today, retains both elements: a sequential instructional strategy (Ten-Point Program) and its application as a rehabilitation technique (Water Specific Therapy). Because the instructional and therapeutic components are interrelated, both are described in this chapter. The theoretical framework of the Halliwick Concept precedes a description of the possibilities in therapeutic practice. Explanations of the terminology of fluid mechanics can be found in Chapter 2.

DEVELOPMENT

The Halliwick Concept was developed by James McMillan (1913-1994), a fluid mechanics engineer. Returning to London after service in World War II, McMillan pursued his enjoyment of water sports by teaching swimming to children with disabilities. In 1950, he started a swimming program at London's Halliwick School for Crippled Girls.

Until then, few attempts had been made to teach swimming to children with physical or mental impairments. Trial and error led McMillan to the realization that a lack of stability in the water was the major impediment to progress. So, using principles of fluid mechanics, he developed techniques to coach a person toward attaining stability in the water.[1,2] Children taught with his method showed improvements in disassociated head activity, trunk stability, mouth control, and self-esteem within a few weeks.

---

*References to Halliwick use both *Concept* and *Method*. We use the word *Concept,* according to the official subheading of the International Halliwick Association: "promoting the Halliwick Concept of Swimming and Rehabilitation in Water."

This was the origin of both adapted aquatics programs and programs to train lay helpers in teaching swimming skills to people with disabilities. The first swimming club, The Halliwick Penguin Swimming Club, was founded in 1951, and in 1952, several similar clubs for swimmers with disabilities joined in the Association of Swimming Therapy.[3]

McMillan's goals were both recreational and educational, with the aim of helping swimmers achieve independence in the pool. It was quickly apparent that the therapeutic outcomes in water carried over to similar effects on land.

In 1963, McMillan was asked to teach his method in Bad Ragaz, Switzerland, first annually, then from 1974 through 1979, as a permanent instructor at the Medical and Postgraduate Center. During that time, McMillan headed a project group on aquatic therapy, working with a group of physical therapists to develop Water Specific Therapy.

Today, the Halliwick Concept is used around the globe, especially in neurology and pediatrics.[4-8] Further development of the Halliwick Concept is a task of both the International Halliwick Association and the International Halliwick Foundation.

THE LEARNING PROCESS

Several aspects of the Halliwick Concept are critical to the success of the Ten-Point Program (Table 4-1). First, McMillan considered everyone to be a swimmer. With proper adaptations, he maintained, anyone could become proficient and comfortable in the water. The ultimate goal is enabling the swimmer to be as independent as possible, both in water and on land.

McMillan considered swimming a means to independence, not a goal in itself, so he never used flotation devices as stabilizing equipment. He demonstrated that balance depends on body shape and density and that flotation devices compromise one's independence and stability in the water.

Learning to manage the body in water using McMillan's approach requires one-to-one support in the form of a helper. Teaching strategies incorporate music, games, and group activities in which all participants are required to actively engage.

McMillan developed the Ten-Point Program, using General System Theory (GST), a holistic management approach developed in the 1930s. GST suggests that knowledge is not acquired in a vacuum but grows as learning from one area of study influences and informs other areas of study. Applying many rules of evidence-based practice, McMillan used GST to bring together knowledge from physiology, psychology, learning theory, medicine, therapies, and education to establish the practical framework of his Ten-Point Program.

Table 4-1. Key Concepts of the Ten-Point Program

Everyone is a swimmer!
Swimming is a means to independence, not a goal in itself.
Balance depends mainly on body shape and density.
Proper supports are essential.
Most activities require a one-to-one attendance/support.
Flotation aids are never used.
The student participates actively in all activities.
Most activities take place in groups.

For example, using GST in establishing the Halliwick Concept, the client learns specific skills to become independent in the pool, combining principles from motor learning with those of the mechanics of stability. Adaptations in communication and didactics are incorporated for clients with limited learning abilities.

Moving in water requires knowledge of the fluid mechanical features of water. A body will react to the effects of fluid mechanics, and controlled movement requires stability and security, cued by proper manual handling by the therapist. The situation must be "physically controlled and mentally desired." The therapist's skills are of utmost importance, especially when a client is unable to learn automatically, due to incapacity in coordination, perception, comprehension, or pain. Learning of postures (equilibrium and trunk control) and movements will commence with a limited coordination as discussed in the following:

> It is well known that encountering the unfamiliar physical properties of a change in environment can affect balance and coordination. A client, for example, may utilize adaptive motor behavior such as widening the base of support, using hands for support, and stiffening the body to stabilize the center of gravity.[9] This is especially true in the aquatic environment.
>
> Buoyancy or relative weightlessness is an important constraint in water, affecting coordination, especially when the client begins to float. In general this happens with the lower part of the lungs immersed, approximately to the level of the xyphisternum of T11 in an upright position. Walking from the shallow part to the deep end of a pool, a client loses contact with the floor rather suddenly, so normal ankle strategy in postural control must be compensated for with more cranial strategies. In the Halliwick Concept, this is called head balancing. When the client cannot react quickly and appropriately, the result is stress behavior: muscular tone increases, disassociation decreases, the client looks for fixed points (absolute: a landing, or relative: swimming movements), physiologic extension decreases, the base of support is increased, and walking may change from crosslateral to ipsilateral. This behavior may coincide with associated reactions or even tonic reflexes in persons with neurologic incapacities. McMillan allowed these "primitive reflexes" as a kinesiologic adaptation due to the mechanical changes that water provides. Providing stability and then reducing support are some of the most important activities of the therapist. The Halliwick Concept can be regarded as "a struggle to change closed kinetic chains into open ones."
>
> Based on our understanding these primitive reflexes, the Halliwick Concept is regarded by some as a neurotherapeutic facilitation rehabilitation technique.[10] This is not entirely accurate. McMillan allowed the "primitive reflexes" to some extent, at a time when these reflexes were discouraged in other methods, such as Bobath. McMillan developed his view independent of contemporary neurologic developments, basing it instead on his knowledge of (fluid) mechanics and an excellent power of observation. Later, neurophysiologic research supported his ideas on using exteroceptive cues (plasticity), primitive reflexes and reducing of stiffening (degrees of freedom/using coordinated structures), and achieving movement instead of inhibiting postures (task-oriented activities).[11]
>
> Looking at the nature of many Halliwick activities and games, the Ten-Point Program can be regarded as a task-type training approach utilizing the variations that water offers to enhance dry land skills. Recent studies show that being in and moving in water indeed vary the practice of balancing skills and have transfer effects to dry land.[12]

THE TEN-POINT PROGRAM

McMillan organized the instructional application of the Halliwick Concept as a program of ten steps, or points, eventually evolving to a swimming stroke, the Halliwick Movement. These ten points are arranged into three phases of a sensory/psychologic learning process incorporating (1) mental adjustment, (2) balance control, and (3) movement.

Table 4-2. The Ten-Point Program and the Three Phases of the Halliwick Concept

Ten Points	Phases
1. Mental adjustment and disengagement	Mental adaptation/adjustment (point 1)
2. Sagittal rotation (control)	
3. Transverse rotation (control)	
4. Longitudinal rotation (control)	
5. Combined rotation (control)	Balance control (points 2–8)
6. Upthrust/mental inversion	
7. Balance in stillness	
8. Turbulent gliding	
9. Simple progression	
10. Basic Halliwick Movement	Movement (points 9, 10)

The three phases of the Ten-Point Program are delivered in order, and although points can overlap, new phases are not introduced until all previous points have been accomplished (Table 4-2).

Mental Adjustment and Disengagement—Phase One and Point One

The purpose of mental adjustment is to enable the client to react automatically, independently, and appropriately during upright activities in water. Acquisition of breath control is a key issue (Fig. 4-1).

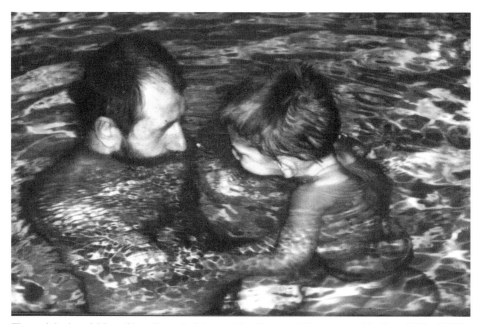

Figure 4-1. Acquisition of breath control in mental adjustment. Treatment objectives (TO)—FBPR or keeping symmetry and alignment of the head over the trunk; rotational axis (RA)—transversal and sagittal; working positions (WP)—sitting; water depth (WD)—N+; treatment techniques (TT)— providing closed chains to facilitate head and mouth activity; exercise patterns (XP)—asymmetrical, focused on alignment; mode of treatment (MT)—pretraining (breath control) and inhibition.

To produce a desired movement in the water, one must be comfortable in an altered mechanical environment. This requires learning adaptations for dealing with buoyancy, hydrostatic pressure, flow, and wave action.

Point one addresses this adaptation. The client experiences and becomes comfortable with altered balance, helped by a therapist who introduces a variety of vertical movement patterns (Figs. 4-2, 4-3, and 4-4). The client experiences mechanical stimuli resulting from buoyancy and impedance. Feedback to the client is focused on instructions to use the head to steer the trunk and the lower extremities.

The instructor also uses verbal cues: "Water is heavy, you can push against it"; "Water provides direction of movement, you can feel it"; and "Water has depth, you can float." These cues are used to enable body awareness and space relationship.

Mastering breath control, especially exhalation, is of utmost importance. The client is instructed to "blow" whenever his or her mouth gets close to the water, so "blowing" becomes automatic when the mouth touches water. This prevents swallowing and chocking. It also facilitates head control, because the head comes forward when one blows, reducing the risk of a loss of balance. The therapist may cue manually by bringing the head into good alignment and/or the cheeks into good position.

Breath control can be regarded as a part of orofacial therapy and an extension of techniques from speech therapy. Blowing, humming, singing, and talking are variations of breath control. Rhythm is used to facilitate movement. Speed of singing can be adapted to change velocity of movement in water.

Breath, head, and trunk control must be considered simultaneously. The therapist must use support properly to ensure control in all three areas. Support should provide stability without providing too much comfort. The client should be out of

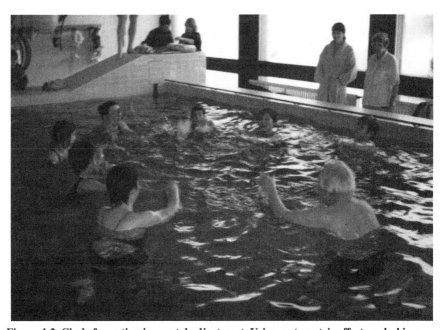

Figure 4-2. Circle formation in mental adjustment. Using metacentric effects, splashing, changing the direction of walking, singing, and changing distance as principles of disengagement. The objectives are independence and automatic balance control with elements of distraction.

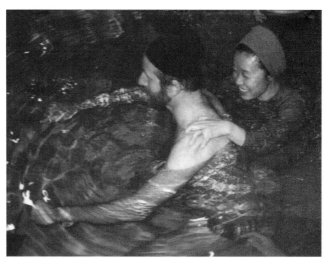

Figure 4-3. Space ships. An activity in mental adjustment. The client is asked to walk around the therapist and just hold when necessary. Treatment objectives (TO)—FBPR/upright postural control; rotational axis (RA)—combined rotation; working positions (WP)—stand (in fact, here motion rather than a position is practiced); water depth (WD)—N+ to N– can be chosen, depending on weight-bearing, treatment techniques (TT)—turbulence resisted and waves; exercise patterns (XP)—both symmetrical and asymmetrical; modes of treatment (MT)—facilitation (using turbulence and waves).

balance enough to be challenged, but not enough to lose balance and become panicky (or anxious). McMillan maintained that the client should always be in a situation that is "physically controlled and mentally desired."

Disengagement—the gradual process of increasing the difficulty of the tasks or movement to be accomplished—is an important part of mental adjustment, and a part of every point in the program. Because the purpose is to enable the client to balance in open kinetic chains, most of the disengagement principles address the change from closed (absolute/relative) to open chain postural control. The quality of this postural control will change during the course of therapy and can be operationalized in the change of variables listed in Table 4-3.

There are many possible methods to increase difficulty by changing variables of disengagement (Table 4-4). Placement of hand supports, depth of the water, radius of the body, turbulence, metacentric forces, and range of motion are a few of the variables that can be introduced to accomplish disengagement.

Suggested therapeutic possibilities in this phase include exercising orofacial control (lip closure, vocalization, breathing through the nose, desensitization, and contraction of the diaphragm) and exercising head/trunk control (normalizing muscular tone, disassociation of patterns, facilitation of righting reactions, and midline symmetry). This phase is also used for getting to know the effects of water, so more functional goals—walking, jumping, turning around, and reaching—are possible as well. These possibilities have been described in numerous typical Halliwick games and activities.[8]

Balance Control—Phase Two and Points Two through Eight

Balance control—phase two of the Ten-Point Program—is the ability to change a position slowly or to keep a position without support. As discussed for the mental

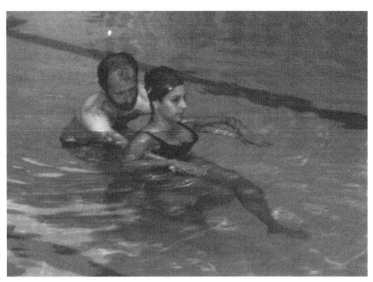

Figure 4-4. Bicycling or suspended sitting with fixation at the upper extremities. This is an activity in mental adjustment, reducing eye contact. Treatment objectives can be static stabilization of the shoulder girdle, dynamic stabilization of the pelvic girdle, and increased range of motion (ROM) of hip and knee joints. Treatment objectives (TO)—strengthening (stabilization)/ROM hips and knees; rotational axis (RA)—transverse rotation; working positions (WP)—suspended sitting with fixation at the upper extremities; water depth (WD)—N+; treatment techniques (TT)—turbulence resisted (because of client's leg movements); exercise patterns (XP)—asymmetric (alternating leg movements); modes of treatment (MT)—facilitation (use of turbulence).

adjustment point, a client's control is challenged in the water by the altered mechanical environment. Initially, control is inefficient, with the client relying extensively on peripheral movements or fixed points.

In the balance control phase, the client learns to centralize balance control and demonstrate effective postural control. Seven points comprise this phase, including control of four types of rotation, upthrust, stillness, and gliding.

Sagittal Rotation Control—Point Two

Sagittal rotations are movements around sagittal axes. These movements include lateral flexion of every part of the spine and abduction/adduction of the extremities.

Table 4-3. Effect of Feedback and Experience on Changes in Motor Behavior

Novel Skill	Controlled Skill
Variable execution	Consistent execution
Inaccurate, clumsy	Precise
Slow	Fast
Much co-contraction	Smooth
Visual control needed	No visual control necessary
Visible postural adaptations	Invisible postural adaptations
Stiff in performance	Flexible in performance

Adapted from Smits-Engelsman BCM, van Tuijl ALT: Toepassing van cognitieve motorische controle-theorie van in de kinderfysiotherapie: het controleren van vrijheidsgraden en beperkingen. In: Syllabus 'Leren en herleren van motorische vaardigheden bij pati enten met chronische benigne pijn.' Amersfoort, Nederlands Paramedisch Instituut, 1999.

Table 4-4. Possibilities to Make Balancing More Difficult, Using Principles of Disengagement

Simple Equilibrium	Progression or Disengagement Principles
Support at the shoulder girdle	Change supports caudally
Support at the hands or forearms	Change supports centrally
Applying many points of support	Few or no points of support
Water depth around T11/xyphisternum	Depth above T11/xyphisternum
Large radius	Decrease the radius
Wide basis of support	Small basis of support
With compensating arm movements	No arm movements
No turbulence around the body	Turbulence around the body
No waves	Waves
No metacentric torque effects	Metacentric torque effects
Small range of motion	Large range of motion

This point contains movements not only in place but also in walking sideways and changing direction. Sagittal rotations are most functional in upright positions (Fig. 4-5), but also are seen in supine position as lateral flexion of the trunk in seaweeding activities or in swimming a crawl stroke.

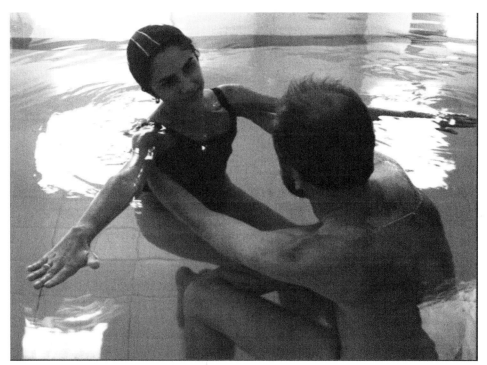

Figure 4-5. Suspended sitting. By tilting the client in the lateral direction (sagittal rotation), automatic equilibrium reactions can be facilitated. This support enables stability of the trunk and therefore a muscular release of head and cervical spine. Voluntary head movements occur when the client is asked to keep the head upright when being tilted. This could be used for a gentle mobilization of the cervical spine. Treatment objective (TO)—FBPR/ROM cervical spine/activation of the deltoids; rotational axis (RA)—sagittal rotation; working positions (WP)—suspended sitting; water depth (WD)—N+; treatment techniques (TT)—metacentric assisted (the head is used to counterbalance); exercise patterns (XP)—asymmetrical; modes of treatment (MT)—facilitation (metacentric effects are used).

Sagittal rotation can be used therapeutically to mobilize or stabilize the spine with lateral flexion movements to lengthen the trunk, to facilitate optical righting reactions and equilibrium reactions (reaching out), to stimulate abduction of arms or legs, or to shift weight from left to right.

Transverse Rotation Control—Point Three

Transverse rotations are movements around *any* transverse axis in the body. The end form is the rotation from a standing/sitting position to supine lying and vice versa. Forward and backward somersaults are an example from swimming.

Transverse rotation control is generally introduced with a supine position. The supine position is favored for safety reasons, because the nose and mouth are free of the water. Later, the prone position (a very stable position) is introduced as a challenge. Rolling out of the prone position is quite difficult.

In the supine position, the body behaves like a canoe. The main and fastest rotation takes place around the longitudinal axis. Loss of balance/midline symmetry or even the feeling of loss of balance may result in massive (pathologic) equilibrium reactions, combined with increased extension and/or flexion of the spine. The reasons are obvious: fixed points between feet and floor have disappeared, normal visual input has changed, communication is more difficult (ears under water), fear of swallowing water arises, and the body rotates quickly around the longitudinal axis.

Therefore, transverse rotation must be taught slowly by gradually increasing the client's range of motion toward the supine position in small, manageable stages. It is equally important to teach the client how to stand independently, because inability to achieve a stable vertical position is a major source of fear.

Cues for transverse rotation are to move the head forward, reach forward with the arms, catch an object above the water, blow out, tuck in head/hips/knees, and try to sit on the floor of the pool.

Therapeutically, transverse rotation is a kind of selective extension. All elements of this selective extension can be used therapeutically: positioning of the head on the trunk, alignment of the spine, extension of the dorsal spine, achievement of appropriate scapular depression, control of pelvic tilt, eccentric contraction of the abdominal muscles, inhibition of associated reactions, and development of symmetry of movement (Fig. 4-6*A* and *B*).

Longitudinal Rotation Control—Point Four

Longitudinal rotation takes place around the longitudinal axis or midline of the body. This rotation is most important in the supine position. Preparations can begin in upright positions.

The first movements are symmetrical with a gradually decreasing radius (arms at the body and legs together). Support is provided at the center of balance (at the second sacral segment). Balance control is focused on (contra)rotational head activities of the client. Next, the client actively rotates by using the head in rotation and crossing the midline of the body with the arm and leg. Ultimately, the goal is to roll 360 degrees, back to the supine position. Basically this is a safety skill, because the supine position is considered a safe position for breathing.

Each of these skills is taught separately; then all are executed together to accomplish the full rotational pattern. This analytical approach is necessary, because longitudinal rotation requires maximal disassociation between head, shoulder girdle, and pelvic girdle during a fast movement that also involves a breath skill (Figs. 4-7 and 4-8).

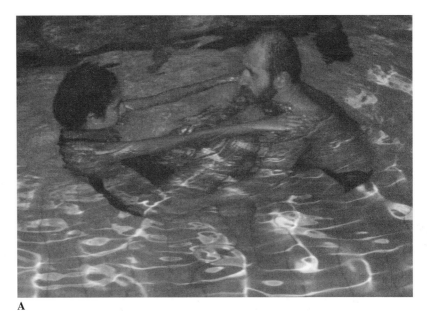

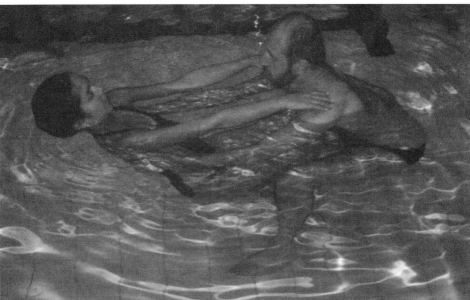

Figure 4-6. Transverse rotation control. This change of position can be used for training the lower abdominal muscles, especially when during the movement the client is asked to keep a certain position for a while (and move other parts of the body). Other objectives are to increase ROM or to work on symmetry. *A*, transverse rotation control, still in a flexed position. *B*, transverse rotation control, changing to extension.

The therapeutic application of longitudinal rotation is facilitation of the head-to-trunk righting reactions. The abdominal muscles, which are active during this rotation, are important rotators; increasing their selective and stabilizing function is one of the major therapeutic objectives in longitudinal rotation, important for both swimming and walking. This rotation may also be used to reduce muscular tone of spastic trunk muscles, such as the quadratus lumborum and the latissimus dorsi.

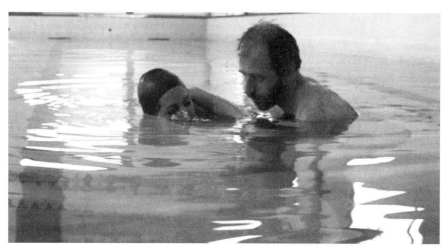

Figure 4-7. Supine lying. Teaching breath control in longitudinal rotation. The objective is disassociated head over trunk activity.

Combined Rotation Control—Point Five

Combined rotation control includes (1) *transverse* and *longitudinal* rotations during a forward roll and (2) *sagittal* and *longitudinal* rotations during a sideways roll (Fig. 4-9). Combined rotation might seem more difficult to accomplish than the

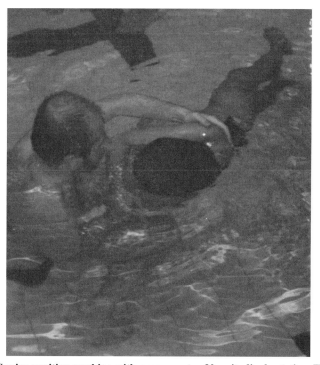

Figure 4-8. Supine position working with components of longitudinal rotation. The objectives are mobilization of the glenohumeral joint and facilitation of the scapulothoracal rhythm.

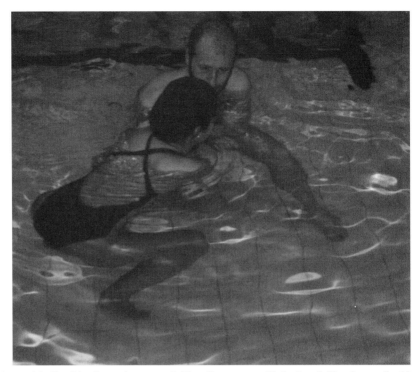

Figure 4-9. Combined rotation control. The clients are guided when falling forward with a rotation around the longitudinal axis at the same time.

individual rotation patterns, but actually it is rather easy because it combines previously mastered patterns. The goal is to roll out of trouble when one loses balance and end in a supine position.

In fact, all rotations in water have a combined character. Bodies move three dimensionally, so they must have control in three dimensions. Moreover, clients with impairments usually have asymmetric distributions of shape and/or density (specific gravity). This increases the need to teach combined rotation control by putting separate rotations together.

The most important therapeutic use of combined rotation is teaching clients how to fall and stand up again. Water allows one to "dare to make errors"—losing balance without the risk of pain or injury. Begin in deep water and work progressively to shallow water.

Upthrust or Mental Inversion—Point Six

Understanding the concept of upthrust—that one cannot sink, but always will rise to the surface again—is fundamental to comfort and safety in the water. Many people are afraid to sink or of being unable to inhale air when they need to do so.

With simple activities, a client can learn that it is nearly impossible to sink to the bottom of the pool and stay there. When a swimmer understands—and can demonstrate—this concept, he or she is considered to be waterfree. *Waterfree* means that the client is unsinkable, controls all rotations, can fall and stand up again, has good breath control, and can walk to the side of the pool.

This point concludes the first part of the Ten-Point Program that is focused on rotational control with positional changes. Although this phase has important therapeutic potentials in itself, it is the foundation for the more advanced work of Water Specific Therapy.

Balance in Stillness—Point Seven

Balance in stillness is a static point in the Ten-Point Program, the point at which the client begins to perfect rotational control. Focus is on posture: equilibrium and stability in various positions—standing, sitting, kneeling, oblique, and supine. The client must react with "central motor activity" of the axial structures such as head and trunk. Compensating is not allowed—no hand movements, no widening of the stance, no stiffening of muscles, etc. The therapist disturbs balance with manual turbulence around the swimmer, asking for metacentric effects or using a wave during step-stop activities. Because this is preparation for swimming, positions progress from upright to supine. In the supine position, the client might be supported, a departure from the disengagement the therapist maintains when the client is in other positions.

Balance in stillness can be used therapeutically when stability (co-contraction, and isometric activity) is needed. The most important regions to work on are the shoulder girdle, the trunk, the pelvic girdle, and the hip region. This point is the same as the phase of inhibition in Water Specific Therapy.

Turbulent Gliding—Point Eight

Turbulent gliding is a dynamic follow up to balance in stillness. The client is supine and controls all rotations (good alignment of the spine, hips extended, and trunk symmetrical, with no lateral flexion or abduction). The therapist tows the client in a wake of turbulence, which challenges balance.

Therapeutic options are restricted and are mainly focused on facilitation of dynamic trunk control during this specific activity.

Movement—Phase Three and Points Nine and Ten

In the movement phase, the client learns to propel effectively in the water, usually swimming. Other methods of moving, such as walking or jogging, are also acceptable.

Simple Progression—Point Nine

When the client can control his or her position during turbulent gliding, the therapist introduces propulsion. Initially this involves a symmetrical motion of the hands, under water and close to the pelvis. Although the movement is not particularly effective for propulsion, the goal is to introduce (effective) peripheral movements while maintaining adequate control of the trunk and head.

Therapeutic possibilities are similar to those for turbulent gliding. The difference is that the client now has to control both central stability and propelling movements. This double task is more difficult than the previous skill.

Basic Halliwick Movement—Point Ten

The basic Halliwick swimming stroke uses only the arms for propulsion. Features are symmetry, ROM for the recovery movement from 0 to 120 degrees abduction, and only hands taken out during the recovery.

These symmetrical movements with the arms are easier to control than alternating arm-crawl movements (affecting midline symmetry) or leg movements (affecting pelvic stability). This is the first attempt to really move efficiently and effectively.

At this point, the swimming stroke may have to be adapted to the individual abilities of the client. Development of swimming strokes will include alternating strokes, side-lying positions, prone positions, and use of fins and other equipment.

Large arm movements influence trunk and head control more than simple progression does. Therapeutically, swimming can be used to work on local and general aerobic endurance.

As stated previously, the movement phase can also focus on walking, jumping, and other dynamic activities in upright positions. Therapeutic goals are the same as those for the swimming sequence: controlling posture in a dynamic way, while using arms and legs functionally, in closed or open chain activities.

WATER SPECIFIC THERAPY (WST)

As discussed earlier in this chapter, the therapeutic effects of the Halliwick Ten-Point Program were immediately apparent. McMillan and the physical therapists in Bad Ragaz began exploring both the therapeutic outcomes of the Halliwick Concept and methods for applying the concept as WST.

WST also is based on application of fluid mechanics, reactions of the body in water, and application of aspects of the Ten-Point Program as therapeutic interventions.[2,5,14,15] It is a decision-making system containing elements needed to prepare, perform, and assess aquatic therapy. This decision-making system will be described (Table 4-5), with examples of interventions that arise from the WST system.

Assessment

Before actual treatment starts, a dry land assessment is carried out according to the system required for that particular client. Regular tests and questionnaires are used before a more water-specific assessment takes place.

Water-specific skills are assessed sequentially and include: (1) water adjustment, especially breath control, (2) positional changes or rotations, (3) movement through the pool—walking and swimming, and (4) positions—standing, sitting, oblique, supine, and prone.

This sequence of assessment follows the Ten-Point Program. In each activity or position, the therapist identifies the quality of the motor performance, the problems that exist, and the reasons for the problems. In most cases, this will be a qualitative interpretation of factors such as symmetry or tonus. Quantification during a water-based assessment is difficult, but simple measurements like time and distance will give an indication of changes.

Both during assessment and treatment, some golden rules apply:

- Do not touch the client too much or too quickly ("put your hands in your pockets").
- Do not say "stop" too often—give the client time to correct.*

---

*Especially when working on facilitation of posture and balance reactions (see treatment objectives), water offers great possibilities to work with "trial and error," allowing the client to make mistakes and learn from them. On dry land, guidance of movements is used much more often with voluntary motor activity work.

Table 4-5. Elements of Water Specific Therapy

Treatment Objectives (TO)	Rotational Axis (RA)	Working Positions (WP)	Treatment Techniques (TT)	Exercise Patterns (XP)	Mode of Treatment (MT)
1. Strengthen weak muscle groups (+WMG)	1. Sagittal rotation control (SR)	1. Standing • N± = Water at T11 • N+ = Water above T11 • N− = Water below T11	1. Turbulence assisted	1. Symmetric	1. Pretraining • Mental adjustment • Rotational controls • Upthrust
2. Increase range of motion (+RM)	2. Transverse rotation control (TR)	2. Sitting	2. Turbulence resisted	2. Asymmetric	2. Inhibition—posture control • Balance in stillness
3. Facilitate posture and balance reactions (FPBR)	3. Longitudinal rotation control (LR)	3. Suspended sit	3. Metacentric assisted		3. Facilitation—change of posture, shape, or base • Controlled movement, e.g., turbulent gliding on simple progression
4. Improve physical condition (+GPC)	4. Combined rotation control (CR)	4. Kneeling	4. Metacentric resisted		4. Dynamic—change of posture, shape, and base • Challenging controlled movement, e.g., basic Halliwick Movement
5. Reduce pain (−P)		5. Supine	5. Wave of transmission		
6. Reduce spasticity (−Sp)		6. Prone	6. Non-fluid mechanic techniques • Working in open chains • Working in closed chains • Transference		
7. Improve mental adaptability (IMA)		7. Oblique			

- Get water between you and your client to ensure disengagement.
- Be dynamic, give clients movement experience.
- Do not assess or treat the things one can do on land.

Another way to facilitate motor activity is to work on automatic reactions for righting, protection, and equilibrium. In both assessment and treatment, differences in feedback cues will be seen between these approaches.

Treatment Objectives (TO)

The purpose of WST is to enable a client to improve functional abilities on land. So, if aquatic therapy can enhance a client's functional abilities, treatment in the water should be used as an introduction, complement, or extension to land therapy.

WST includes seven treatment objectives:

1. Strengthen weak muscle groups (+WMG)
2. Increase range of motion/stretching (+RM)
3. Facilitate posture and balance reactions (FPBR)
4. Increase general physical condition (+GPC)
5. Reduce pain (–P)
6. Reduce spasticity (–Sp)
7. Increase mental adaptability (+IMA)

(The use of abbreviations to develop short, succinct treatment plans will be demonstrated later.)

These objectives have been described at the level of impairment (World Health Organization, International Classification of Impairment, Activity/Disability, Participation/Handicap [ICIDH 2]). More functional goals—walking, reaching, sitting down, and rolling over—are part of the program. These are hidden in the facilitation of balance and posture reactions and in the increase in mental adaptability, using the activities of the Ten-Point Program (Table 4-6).

Facilitation of posture and balance reactions is a very broad objective and applicable to most clients with neurologic impairments. Currently, therapists using WST have narrowed the FPBR objective to include intents such as symmetry, disassociation, centralization, and reciprocal motion. Physiologic rules of muscle strengthening, cardiovascular training, and stretching of connective tissue must be included in these objectives.

When assessment has been completed and treatment objectives identified, the therapist selects the appropriate rotational plane, starting position, exercise patterns, treatment techniques, and mode of treatment.

Rotational Axis (RA)

Selection of the best rotational axis is based on the effect of impairment on the client's body shape and density. A hemiplegic client will have to be taught

Table 4-6. Focus of the Two Halliwick Systems

	Impairment	Activity	Participation
Ten-Point Program	+	++	++
Water Specific Therapy	++	+	+/–

lengthening activities of the trunk, or sagittal rotation, to assist with learning righting reactions for work in the vertical position.

The same client might begin work in longitudinal rotation, along the longitudinal axis, to facilitate posture and balance reactions in the supine position. A client with ankylosing spondylitis would need extension exercises of the trunk, using transverse rotation movements. A person with athetosis might work in combined rotation, along the combined axis, to normalize tonus, increase ROM, and enhance symmetry and extension.

Including a rotational axis is important, because this includes the most prevalent rotational control activities needed by the client.

Working Positions (WP)

As previously stated, many of the activities in the Halliwick Concept are dynamic, asking for movement or positional changes. Working positions provide another important aspect, utilized for treatment objectives such as increased ROM, joint stabilization, and inhibition of hypertonicity.

These working positions are standing, sitting in a cube, suspended sitting, kneeling, oblique lying, supine, and adapted prone. Figures 4-4, 4-5, 4-10, 4-11, and 4-12 show each of these positions and an analysis of their possibilities.

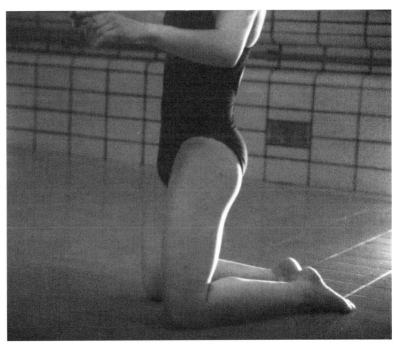

Figure 4-10. Kneeling. The client is asked to gently lean forward, lift the toes off the floor, and keep balance. This results in an increased activity of the gluteal muscles. The therapist may have to correct a wrong pelvic tilt. Objectives are to increase of ROM of the hips, lengthen the rectus femoris, and balance around the transversal axis. Treatment objectives (TO)—ROM of the hips/strengthen gluteal muscles; rotational axis (RA)—transverse rotation; working positions (WP)—kneeling; water depth (WD)—N+ to N–, depending on the weight-bearing component; treatment techniques (TT)—metacentric resisted (when the hands are out of the water); exercise patterns (XP)—symmetrical; modes of treatment (MT)—facilitation (using metacentric effects).

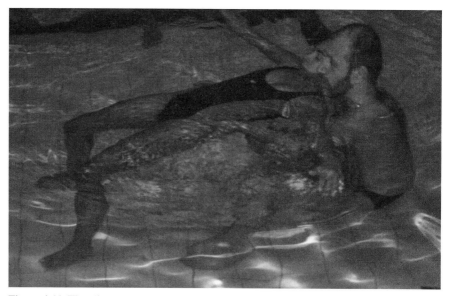

Figure 4-11. The client should keep her feet on the floor (as a cue the therapist may put his foot on the client's feet). In this position any small flexion/extension activity can be asked in one single joint while holding a certain position in the other joints. (Note: The water should not be too deep to prevent lumbar hyperlordosis.) Treatment objectives (TO)—gluteal strength/coordination (without extension of the knees as a disassociated extension); rotational axis (RA)—transverse rotation; working positions (WP)—oblique position; water depth (WD)—N+; treatment techniques (TT)—open chain extension (metacentric when hands are lifted); exercise patterns (XP)—symmetrical; modes of treatment (MT)—inhibition (facilitation when metacentric effects are used).

Water Depth (WD)

Water depth is an important factor[16,17] for weight-bearing purposes, but also for determining the contribution of the lower extremities to total postural control.

As soon as the client loses friction between feet and floor, a transition occurs, leading to a greater contribution from more cranial parts of the body. This brings an increase of head activities or of arm movements when head and trunk control has not been sufficiently developed. This shift occurs with the body immersed to approximately T11, the exact level depending on the specific gravity of the client.

The choice of water depth is important because it will determine whether a treatment technique is upthrust (buoyancy) dominant or gravity dominant. Water depths above T11 (N+) are used for facilitation of head balance in relatively open chains. As the water level drops below T11 (N−), the client experiences increased weight-bearing and more proprioceptive (weight-bearing) input, so more closed chain activities of the lower extremities are possible. Generally, a client standing in water at T11 is neutral (N±), and many clients will use this depth automatically to ambulate (an important consideration, incidentally, in the design of therapy pools).

Depth is equally important for therapists, who also start to float in depths above T11. For their own stability, therapists must to be able to work in water of proper depth.

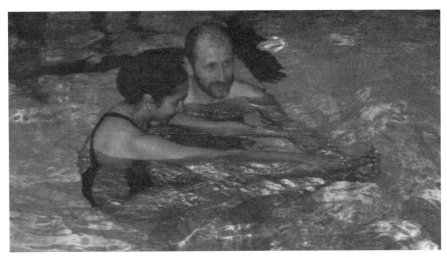

Figure 4-12. This position can be used to stretch the dorsal connective tissue structures (slump), but also to facilitate activity around the sagittal axis as, e.g., lengthening/shortening of the trunk when the client is tilted laterally. Treatment objectives (TO)—ROM; rotational axis (RA)—transverse rotation; working positions (WP)—suspended sitting with extended knees; water depth (WD)—N+; treatment techniques (TT)—metacentric resisted in a closed chain; exercise patterns (XP)—transverse rotation; modes of treatment (MT)—facilitation (client is tilted backward; this provides a metacentric torque which activates flexors).

Treatment Techniques (TT)

WST uses five treatment techniques to challenge balance, with the intention of stimulating use of inertia patterns to develop postural control and movement. Although each of these techniques will be discussed individually, one should understand that each technique can be used for multiple objectives and should consider the broader impact on the client.

For example, a client who is challenged to regain posture and balance will perform isometric and dynamic activity, with variable resistance that aids in the strengthening of weak muscle groups. Buoyancy and the concomitant weightlessness will naturally cause a reduction in muscle stiffness. The reduction in stiffness, coupled with increased movement and strength of weak antagonists, will enable a greater ROM. The combination of all the activities and hydrodynamic forces will create a favorable environment for a reduction in pain.

The first and second treatment techniques are turbulence assisted and turbulence resisted. In the first, the therapist manually produces turbulence to assist the client, to maintain postural control and balance, and to achieve movement. The turbulence-resisted technique is used to advance the difficulty of exercises. By producing turbulence, the therapist can work without touching the client, preventing compensatory activity.

The third treatment technique utilizes metacentric effects, which are effects created by the force-couple gravity and buoyancy. Both forces are of almost equal magnitude, so any small change will produce torque and large rotational destabilizing effects.[2] Examples are lifting a hand out of water, changing head position, or putting a floating object under water.

The therapeutic impact is that the client must resist rotation to maintain balance (see Fig. 4-3). Maintaining balance requires the client to work with rhythmic, stabilizing, isometric activities in the joints of the spine and lower extremities, while changing hand positions regularly. Metacentric effects normally are used in a resistive way to challenge balance but may also be used to assist a client's balance when trunk control is insufficient.

The fourth technique is the wave of transmission, which is used for stabilizing. The client walks through the water one step forward and stops. Water rushing into the area of low pressure created by the preceding movement creates a wave from behind, challenging the client to hold a balanced position until the wave has passed.

Two non-fluid mechanical techniques are also used in WST. The first uses supports to enable clients to work in closed chains, providing at least two points of support to allow work with leverage. This can produce various (stable) postures, balance, and movements, depending on the extent of stability provided. When support is put at the center of balance, the client must balance in open chains all over the body.

Supports in the Halliwick Concept are subtle. When one is working in an open chain fashion, a support is a reference point for proprioceptive cueing, rather than a real fixed point as in the Bad Ragaz Ring Method (Figs. 4-13 and 4-14).

The second non-fluid mechanical treatment technique is transference. The client first engages in movement in the unaffected region of the body, perceiving the muscular activity required for the movement, and then attempts to duplicate the action in the affected region. This technique is predicated on the idea that the client will transfer learning into the affected region, because even small contractions (changes in body shape) will facilitate movement and proprioceptive feedback.

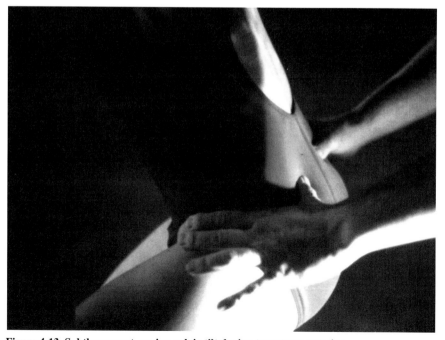

Figure 4-13. Subtle support, cueing pelvic tilt during transverse rotation.

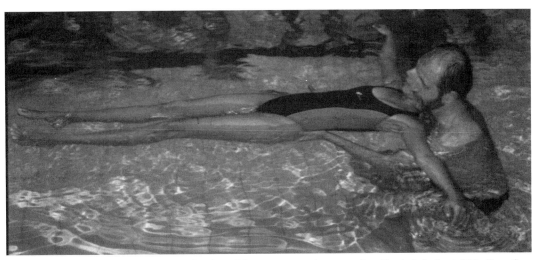

Figure 4-14. Supine position, allowing abduction of the arms as an increase of radius to help in stabilization of midline symmetry. Support at the center of gravity, working in an open chain to facilitate righting or equilibrium reactions when starting to rotate around the longitudinal axis.

EXERCISE PATTERNS (XP)

The type of exercise pattern—symmetrical or asymmetrical—used in a treatment technique determines the kind of action in which a client will engage.

In a symmetrical pattern, both sides of the body perform simultaneously. This can be seen when the therapist applies a centered manual turbulence or when metacentric effects are applied symmetrically.

Only one side of the body is performing in an asymmetrical pattern, such as walking-stopping-standing in a stride. The destabilizing effect of the wave hitting the body from behind must be controlled with predominantly asymmetric (rotational) activity by the client.

MODES OF TREATMENT (MT)

The final aspect of the Halliwick Concept as an aquatic therapy technique is the mode of treatment, which considers the phase and elements of treatment delivery. Phases in the WST (pretraining, inhibition, facilitation, and dynamic) are similar, but not identical, to the phases (mental adaptation, balance control, and movement) of the Ten-Point Program.

The elements of treatment delivery include the selection of appropriate interventions from the first five aspects (treatment objective, rotational patterns, starting positions, exercise patterns, and treatment techniques) of WST and the intensity of the chosen activities.

Intensity encompasses many factors, including, but not limited to, amount of weight-bearing, velocity, change of radius and levers, length of time, visual control, and position during movement. Decisions regarding which aspects and intensities to use are based on the phase of the program in which the client is participating. Explanations of each phase, point, and element of WST follow.

Pretraining

Client comfort and independence in the water are prerequisites for WST. The client should be adjusted to water on the face and in the ears and must have adequate breath control. The client also must have mastered a rough sense of sagittal, transverse, longitudinal, and combined rotation. The client moves to one of the WST phases (inhibition, facilitation, on dynamic) when he or she is able to submerge, rise to the surface, and use a rotational pattern to achieve a comfortable breathing position.

Therapists must also be certain that the client can tolerate the physiologic response to immersion (see Chapter 2).

Inhibition

Inhibition is basic posture control. In this phase, there is no motion through the pool. The client's posture, position, shape, and base remain the same. The posture may be sitting ("cube" position), kneeling, standing, supine, prone, or oblique.

Postural control is challenged with the use of buoyancy only (gravity and upthrust dominant, N+, N−, N±), the easiest form of posture control, because the client is not subjected to any change of forces.

The inhibition phase also can be used for the reduction of pain or spasticity.

Facilitation

Facilitation is posture control with changes occurring in the client's position, posture, and/or shape or with changes in the base. Examples of changing posture are moving from sitting to standing and supine to oblique. During this activity, the relationship between buoyancy and gravity changes. Thus, torque affects postural control more than inhibition does.

Examples of changing the base are walking (step/stop) and bicycling (see Fig. 4-2). In these cases, postural control is challenged by reaction forces in the body, which are generated by turbulence and waves. Thus, postural control is challenged with metacentric effects and turbulence assisted/resisted with waves of transmission.

Dynamic

The dynamic phase is postural control with changes occurring in the client's position, posture, and/or shape and the base.

An example of changing posture is jumping. Postural control is challenged with metacentric effects and turbulence assisted/resisted with waves of transmission. This is the most difficult form of postural control because all fluid mechanical factors influencing posture are incorporated.

Table 4-7 shows how modes of treatment can be developed with respect to the treatment objectives.

Table 4-7. Development of the Mode of Treatment with Respect to the Treatment

Treatment Objectives	Modes of Treatment		
+WMG: strengthen weak muscle groups		Facilitation	Dynamic
+ROM: increase range of motion		Facilitation	Dynamic
FPBR: facilitate posture and balance reactions	Inhibition	Facilitation	Dynamic
+GPC: increase general physical condition		Facilitation	Dynamic
–P: reduce pain	Inhibition	Facilitation	
–Sp: reduce spasticity	Inhibition	Facilitation	Dynamic
+IMA: increase mental adaptability	Inhibition	Facilitation	Dynamic

Questions

1. What are some of the ways a therapist can disengage from the client to promote independent activity (Table 4-4)?
2. How can a client slow down the transverse rotation from sitting to supine?
3. What is the rationale for the use of the Halliwick Concept for a client with a hemiplegia after a stroke?

Answers

1. Possibilities for disengagement include the following:
   1. Supports: from firm to loose
   2. Eye contact: present at first, later none
   3. Changes in rhythm: first with, later without
   4. Inclusion of doubletasks
   5. Increase in the amount of repetitions
   6. Increase in leverage when using metacentric effects
   7. Fast changes of direction when moving through the pool

2. Slowing down transverse rotation can be done by:
   1. Bringing the arms forward
   2. Taking the hands out of the water
   3. Providing fixed points, e.g., standing on client's feet
   4. Blowing out to contract the abdominal muscles
   5. Keeping the head forward as long as possible

3. The rationale for using the Halliwick Concept with a hemiplegic stroke client include the following:
   1. The Halliwick Concept facilitates automatic/involuntary motor control in an environment in which the effects of gravity and pathologic reactions against gravity are decreased.
   2. Walking aids do not have to be used, so independent gait is stimulated. Assisted turbulence and metacentric effects can be used to help balancing.
   3. Loss of balance is a relatively slow process, due to turbulence resistance effects, so the client has time to correct this loss of balance.
   4. The client is unstable and has to balance constantly. This stimulates physical and mental activity.

5. Input changes: skin stimulation from friction between water and the skin provides massive exteroceptive and proprioceptive information. This change of information can be important as a feedback source in motor learning.
6. Many clients like to be in water and are willing to (re)learn to swim; this is important as a motivator for movement and as an activity in secondary prevention.

CASE HISTORY

History and Current State

A 63-year-old truck-driver had a CVA (stroke or apoplexia) 2 months ago, resulting in a right-sided hemiplegia with minor problems with dysphasia. After a short period in acute care, he was referred to a center for clinical rehabilitation. The rehabilitation method used by all disciplines is Bobath/NDT (neurodevelopmental therapy).

Currently, the patient can ambulate slowly with manual facilitation by a therapist. He needs an ankle-foot orthosis to hold the right foot in dorsal flexion. Both physical therapy and occupational therapy focus on posture training, because the affected side of the trunk shows a marked tendency to shorten.

The patient still needs a wheelchair for daily activities, but transfers are independent, as is personal care. The right hand is spastic. The arm shows some signs of recovery, but even with a sling, the patient experiences shoulder pain.

Before his stroke, the patient enjoyed recreational swimming.

Treatment Plan in Water

The physical therapist suggested hydrotherapy to support sensorimotor rehabilitation. The objectives are to:

1. Facilitate independent head to shoulder movements, i.e., to facilitate righting reactions
2. Relax the right shoulder and arm for decreased tone and reduction of pain
3. Work on trunk symmetry and to train the affected (hypotonic) abdominal muscles
4. Disassociate hip-pelvis-thorax-head activity
5. Reinforce sensory input and vary experience for enhanced motor learning
6. Increase aerobic capacity and stamina
7. Work on independent ambulation
8. Teach the patient to swim again
9. Present an enjoyable activity that distracts from dry land rehabilitation and encourages movement

Considerations

1. Immersion in water prevents mechanisms that can occur to compensate for the normal physiologic extension against gravity.

2. Immersion in warm water, coupled with slow movements, promotes relaxation in preparation for stretching (neurodynamic) techniques.
3. Relative instability of the body in water (fixed points fail) forces the body to actively balance, especially around its symmetry axis.
4. Lack of fixed points facilitates use of the head during balancing activities.
5. The tactile input of water provides a different source of feedback, compared with dry land, and is important in motor learning.
6. Without exercise, the patient risks having a sedentary lifestyle. There is a clear need for a familiar physical activity that he enjoys, such as swimming.

Important Considerations

The following program requires a pool with sufficient space for ambulation and swimming. The water depth should enable the patient to swim, including a safe way to stand up (make a transverse rotation). It also must be deep enough for the patient to ambulate so the advantages of buoyancy (weight reduction) and gravity (working in a relatively closed kinetic walking chain) can be combined.

Methods to Choose

1. Relaxation (e.g., using the rhythmic initiation technique of the Bad Ragaz Ring Method) of the right arm and shoulder. The therapist gently moves the patient through the warm water and asks for a guided active motion within the limits of pain. Flotation aids are used to enable the therapist to localize stretching and mobilization.
2. Halliwick Concept for all other objectives.
3. Adapted swimming, e.g., according to Halliwick.

Program

Start with relaxation and the Halliwick Concept, continue with Halliwick techniques, and finally proceed to swimming. At least two sessions per week, lasting from 30 to 45 minutes each, are necessary to establish proper progress. Upon release, the patient should continue swimming in a swimming club or community program for people with special needs.

REFERENCES

1. Nicol K, Schmidt-Hansberg M, McMillan J: Biomechanical principles applied to the Halliwick Method of teaching swimming to physically handicapped individuals. In Terauds J, Bedingfield EW (eds): Swimming III. Champaign, Ill: Human Kinetics, 1979, pp 173–181.
2. McMillan J: The role of water in rehabilitation. Fysioterapeuten 45:43–46, 87–90, 236–240, 1977.
3. McKinnon K: An evaluation of the benefits of Halliwick swimming on a child with mild spastic diplegia. A.P.C.P. J. Dec. 30–39, 1997.
4. Dorpmans J, Lambeck J: Zwemmen met gehandicapten. Haarlem, The Netherlands: De Vrieseborch, 1992.

5. Gamper UN: Wasserspezifische Bewegungstherapie und Training. Stuttgart: Gustav Fischer Verlag, 1995.
6. Lambeck J: De Halliwick methode, oefentherapie in water en zwemmen voor gehandicapten. Kwartaaluitgave NVOM 2:53–57, 1997.
7. Martin J: The Halliwick Method. Physiotherapy 67:288–291, 1981.
8. Reid-Campion M: Hydrotherapy: Principles and Practice. Oxford, UK: Butterworth-Heinemann, 1997.
9. Carr J, Shepered R: Neurological Rehabilitation, Optimizing Motor Performance. Oxford, UK: Butterworth-Heinemann, 1998.
10. Morris DM: Aquatic rehabilitation of the neurologically impaired client. In Ruoti RG, Morris DM, Cole AJ (eds): Aquatic Rehabilitation, Philadelphia: Lippincott, 1997, Chap. 7.
11. Lambeck J (ed): Neurophysiological Basis for Aquatic Therapy: Theoretical Topics. Spokane, Wash: Constellate, 1996.
12. Poteat-Salzman A: Justifiable aquatic therapy: scientific support for intervention, neurological and neurosurgical population. In Lambeck J, Bult H (eds): Congresboek: Hydrotherapie "van practice based naar evidence based." Amersfoort: Nederlands Paramedisch Instituut, 1999.
13. Smits-Engelsman BCM, van Tuijl AL T: Toepassing van cognitieve motorische controletheorien in de kinderfysiotherapie: het controleren van vrijheidsgraden en beperkingen. In Syllabus 'Leren en herleren van motorische vaardigheden bij patinten met chronische benigne pijn.' Amersfoort: Nederlands Paramedisch Istituut, 1999.
14. Cunningham J: Halliwick Method. In Ruoti RG, Morris DM, Cole AJ (eds): Aquatic Rehabilitation. Philadelphia: Lippincott, 1997.
15. Paeth B: Schwimmtherapie 'Halliwick-Methode' nach James McMillan bei erwachsenen Clienten mit neurologischen Erkrankungen. Z Krankengymnastick 36:100–112, 1984.
16. Becker BE: Biophysiologic aspects of hydrotherapy. In Becker BE, Cole AJ (eds): Comprehensive Aquatic Therapy. Boston: Butterworth-Heinemann, 1997, Chap. 2.
17. Harrison RA, Hilman M, Bulstrode S: Loading of the lower limb when walking partially immersed: implications for clinical practice. Physiotherapy 78:164–166, 1992.

Chapter 5
Watsu

Harold Dull, MA and Peggy Schoedinger, PT

INTRODUCTION

It is uncommon to be a witness at the birth of a new therapeutic technique. Although rehabilitative technology is constantly developing, most of the changes are evolutionary rather than revolutionary. Watsu is revolutionary, a significant departure from previous aquatic treatment methods. To observe the emergence of Watsu in the early 1980s and its development over the 20+ years since its inception has been fascinating. As editors of this book, we felt strongly that Watsu needed representation within its covers. Harold Dull's interest has not been in investigating the physiologic effects of the technique, but in a more Eastern view of the methods. Peggy Schoedinger added a careful exposition of some of the clinical applications of the technique and is a practitioner who has extensively used and studied the method.

This chapter does not give the reader the knowledge to perform Watsu. It is a technique that must be experienced and learned in the water. In the same way that an inward dive cannot be skillfully or even safely performed through textbook reading, Watsu should be learned at the side of a skilled instructor. It is not a simple technique, although many of the moves are not complex and the mind-body interaction is more integrated than in most other techniques. The flow of movements becomes a potential dance of healing and of sharing between giver and receiver in a way that alters both. We have had patients show major clinical breakthroughs with the use of the technique, but always with skilled therapists assisting them. It is perhaps more demanding than any other common aquatic methodology, but with its use clinical gains that would otherwise have been unimaginable have been achieved.

PRINCIPLES UNDERLYING WATSU'S EFFECTIVENESS IN THERAPY

The way a person is held while being floated in a Watsu move facilitates a level of presence, a physical empathy, that amplifies the therapeutic effects of Watsu's moves and stretches. Watsu's inception in 1980 opened up a new field, aquatic bodywork, that, being distinct from purely therapeutic modalities, has a value to the general public in its potential for stress reduction and personal growth. Almost immediately, therapeutic communities around the world began adopting Watsu because of the unique benefits it offers the populations they serve. The benefits of touch have long been acknowledged. The idea that the advantages of being held can even be greater can be seen in the response of infants. When a child falls and cries, having a parent reach down and touch him or her does not have the same effect as being picked up and held. What parents instinctively provide by holding a child close to their heart is the greatest presence they can give. Their physical empathy calms and allows healing to proceed. By moving bodywork into water, where being held is accepted as essential, the primary contact has moved from being touched to being held. Being floated in warm water, with all its benefits, adds the sensation of being held by the water itself. This helps to depersonalize the experience and to avoid transference or attachment, as does the way Watsu practitioners are trained to communicate to receivers that the water is doing everything. Every session begins with practitioners encouraging receivers to stand in front of them and experience the water lifting and lowering them with each breath, to surrender to the water and let the water do everything. Then after practitioners have seen receivers enough times to sense their surrender, they lift and float them close to their hearts. Each time practitioners feel the person become lighter in their arms, they too breathe in and the water effortlessly lifts them both. And when they both breathe out, the water accepts them back in. For practitioners, this Water Breathe Dance becomes a powerful shared meditation. It establishes a common breathing pattern to which all of Watsu's subsequent moves and stretches are executed. This connected breath adds greatly to the receiver's sense of connection and physical empathy during a session. This connection, with the trust it creates, and the continuum of a Watsu, with the relief from pain it often provides, helps receivers access levels of their being that can aid in their recovery. This includes levels implicated in the initiation or perpetuation of their condition, as well as those that may hold resources for self-healing. One level often implicated is that on which we judge our own worth, a judgment that the care experienced during a Watsu may help correct. The continuum of Watsu may allow material suppressed in emotional levels to arise and be released during the continual flow of the Watsu. Transpersonal levels may be accessed. Many identify the connection they feel during a Watsu as a connection to everything. Experiencing that oneness may free some from identification with their condition and may provide a perspective from which they can more easily cope. There seems to be no level of our being that has not been reported to be accessed during a Watsu. There is no way of knowing just what level persons floating in our arms with their eyes closed are on. If we see tears coming from their eyes, we do not know if it is sadness at not being held this way before, or joy, or both, or something else. We do not ask. A Watsu practitioner's primary training is in non-interference, in being present without trying to do something to someone. We do not try to direct anyone into any particular level. We do not try to re-parent, re-birth, use psychotherapy, transfer energy, or heal. The receiver's experience of having someone just being with them, without trying to do something to them, is integral to Watsu's therapeutic effectiveness. Feeling someone trying to do something to you arouses resistance, even if it is just the reverse resistance of trying to help. An example of this on a physical level was documented at the Timpany Center in California when a greater range of motion in a limb was achieved through Watsu than with traditional exercises. In traditional exercise, the focus on moving the limb elicited the client's assistance. In Watsu, with the whole body being moved, there was no focus to arouse that assistance. In Watsu when a receiver feels free to explore whatever level of his or her being opens to him or her, that freedom itself is healing.

One level of our being that may be directly affected by Watsu's kind of presence is a level being researched at the Heart-Math Institute. These researchers found that certain irregularities in the heart's rhythms that are chaotic in conditions of stress convert to regular waveforms when a person enters the kind of state commonly encountered in a Watsu. When that happens, the rhythms of the brain, the breathing, and other rhythms of the body take on the same waveform. They posit that it is in this state that the heart-mind can fulfill its function of managing the emotions. This may be what is happening when we see tears coming into someone's eyes during a Watsu. The researchers have also found that when someone who has entered this level of "heart coherence" touches another, his or her coherent rhythms can be measured in the brain waves of the receiver. I often feel a connection on this level when I float someone next to my heart—what I have called a "heart wrap." The coherence of these rhythms may extend throughout the body and show up in the spontaneous vibrations we occasionally see in a Watsu. It was my own experience of this "body wave" while someone was floating me in the warm pool at Harbin Hot Springs and the desire to share it with others that started the development of Watsu.

On the Development of Watsu

When I look back on Watsu's development I see how much it depended on being the right person in the right place at the right time. I do not believe Watsu as we know it could have been developed in any other place at any other time. In 1980 the warm pool at Harbin Hot Springs was frequented by body workers and yoginis who readily volunteered to be guinea pigs for the development of this new form. Our bodywork school there was not as closely regulated by the state as it is today. Today, a new form cannot be introduced into a school's program until it is demonstrated there are employment opportunities for those who study it. I was a relative newcomer to bodywork. I had not experienced any kind of bodywork until I was 40 years old. My background was in creative arts, poetry, and teaching English as a second language, not in medicine or therapy. I had little discipline and few inhibitions. Being so far outside the mainstream, I was not aware of any potential for malpractice suits or other problems. But most importantly I found in Watsu something I greatly enjoyed, something that connected me to others and became an arena for creativity. I had been studying Zen Shiatsu for 5 years and had started teaching it at our School of Shiatsu and Message at Harbin.

Zen Shiatsu was developed in the middle of the last century by Masunaga, who combined many different oriental modalities with the point work of Shiatsu. He considered stretching an even older form of activation and balancing meridians (the flows of energy through our body) than acupuncture. He emphasized the importance of connecting to the breath and establishing a meditative presence. In Zen Shiatsu each stretch is seen as bringing a particular meridian closer to the surface where its energy can be balanced. Each meridian represents one of the functions of our life force. Where it flows on our body is related to that function; e.g., the stomach meridian flows down the front. We go out in front of ourselves to get the food our body needs. Imbalances in this meridian of the front can be related to going too much out in front of ourselves, in worrying, in obsessions, etc. A session of Shiatsu is usually preceded by a diagnosis to determine which meridians are out of balance. Many of the principles of Zen Shiatsu continue to underlie our work in Watsu, but no attempt has been made to bring oriental diagnosis into the water. All the meridians are naturally stretched and mobilized, and hopefully balanced, during a session. Practitioners are encouraged to spontaneously respond to what they feel is needed at each moment. This can be a response to what is happening on levels beyond those focused on in Shiatsu. The word *Watsu* itself came from combining Water and Shiatsu, but over the years Watsu has evolved beyond those origins. In water, practitioners learn to move from a base similar to that established in Tai Chi. Their training culminates in the creative freedom of Free Flow. Those who work in a clinical setting learn to adapt their sessions to the growing number of populations Watsu is being found to benefit. In addition, the benefits that learning to share the simpler forms of Watsu can provide for the nonprofessional are being explored.

THE USES AND MODIFICATIONS OF WATSU IN REHABILITATION

In rehabilitation, we know the importance of looking at each patient as an individual. We strive to consider the needs of the entire person, including physical, cognitive, and psychosocial aspects. At the same time, we are under tighter and tighter pressure to improve each patient's functional status as quickly as possible. Watsu is a passive form of aquatic therapy, and yet when used as a part of a patient's rehabilitation program, it can help address many different needs. It can help improve both the functional status and the quality of life for many of our patients.

Physiologic Effects

First, let us consider the physiologic effects of Watsu. During a session, the client's heart and respiration rates decrease, the depth of respiration increases, and muscle tone decreases. Clients report a deep and profound state of relaxation. Scaer[1,2] has seen these effects in his patients time after time. Scaer is a neurologist who utilizes Watsu in treatment programs for his patients with chronic pain and posttraumatic stress disorder. He suggests that Watsu has a balancing effect on the autonomic nervous system (ANS), causing a quieting of the sympathetic nervous system and an enhancement of the parasympathetic nervous system.

These seemingly simple effects lead to far-reaching benefits, especially for the musculoskeletal and neuromuscular systems. For patients with edema, Watsu aids in the resolution of swelling via the compressive forces of hydrostatic pressure and the deep relaxation that enhances the functioning of the lymphatic system.[3] For patients with orthopedic impairments, there is a decrease in muscle spasm, which provides pain relief. The warmth of the water, coupled with Watsu's gentle stretches into all ranges for the spine and extremities, amplifies these benefits and leads to improvements in soft tissue mobility and range of motion. Patients with neurologic impairments experience improvements in soft tissue mobility and a decrease in muscle tone, which leads to a decrease in hypertonicity. Watsu's rhythmical, gentle rocking motions combined with repeated trunk rotation and trunk elongation further help to decrease muscle tone and improve range of motion.[4]

Although there has been little research done directly with Watsu, it is reasonable to extrapolate from work done in other established areas of therapy. Virtually all areas of neurorehabilitation, including neurodevelopmental treatment and Brunnstrom, recognize the value of trunk rotation in decreasing excessive muscle tone in the trunk, shoulders, hips, and also the extremities. Proprioceptive neuromuscular facilitation also incorporates rotation into all activities as the key element

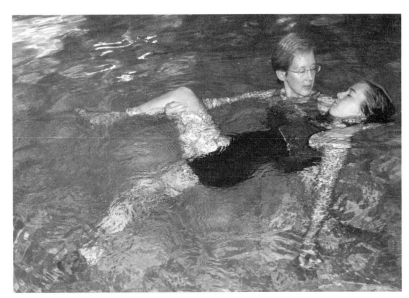

Figure 5-1. This movement is called far leg rotation. It is one of the frequently used movements in Watsu. With the weight bearing joints unloaded, this gentle rotational stretch for the hips and spine benefits many patients (Courtesy Peggy Schoedinger).

in facilitating normal patterns of movement.[5] Watsu utilizes both static rotational stretches for the trunk, and rhythmical, repeated trunk rotation in many of its commonly used movements. These include the most basic Watsu movements of rotating accordion, and near and far leg rotation (Fig. 5-1). Farber[6] and others working in the field of sensory integration have noted the benefits of neutral warmth, as provided by the temperature of most Watsu and therapy pools, in decreasing muscle tone. Work done in sensory integration also supports the muscle-tone–reducing benefits of the slow, rhythmical repeated movements used throughout a Watsu session.[7] These movements gently stimulate the vestibular system, causing a dampening effect on muscle tone. However, overstimulation of the vestibular system may have the opposite effect, and care must be taken during a Watsu session to monitor the system.[5]

In discussing the physiologic benefits of Watsu, it is important to remember that for expediency, clinical impairments are often referred to as either orthopedic or neurologic. However, the body functions as an endlessly interconnected whole. An injury to or impairment of either the musculoskeletal system or the neuromuscular system will have an influence on the other system. If a joint loses mobility for whatever reason, the functional consequences will be similar. With a decrease in joint mobility, the peripheral nerve begins to lose its ability to change in the length of the nerve bed. This loss of elasticity causes problems in connective tissue function, which then affects the function of the motor system's control over the musculoskeletal component.[8] A patient who has had a stroke and has hemiparesis with hypertonicity may initially have limited mobility caused by damage to the central nervous system. This immobility will lead to a loss of elasticity of the peripheral nerves and to myofascial restrictions. These limitations will then further affect motor control.[9] Watsu influences both the neuromuscular and musculoskeletal systems, allowing patients to experience movement with less pain and greater freedom of mobility.

Watsu's influence on the ANS may reach even farther in helping our patients. As more is learned about the adverse effects of ANS imbalance, many propose that ANS imbalance is the basis for disease processes and impairments.[1] These impairments range from fibromyalgia to reflex sympathetic dystrophy to post-traumatic stress disorder and many other conditions.[10] Patients experiencing ANS imbalance may be trapped in their fight/flight/freeze response, which creates a physiologic imbalance similar to that of pushing on the accelerator and the brake simultaneously.[11] Watsu has been used to help patients move beyond the fight/flight/freeze response and onto a healthier life by helping to rebalance the ANS.[1]

Psychological Effects

In addition to Watsu's physiologic effects, many patients and clinicians report psychological benefits in resolving past traumas as well as stress related to daily life. Watsu often affects receivers deeply and profoundly, sometimes to the point of laughter or tears. The graceful movements through warm water, the calming tactile, auditory and vestibular input, and, perhaps most importantly, the nurturing touch and unconditional acceptance of the practitioner all combine to create an extraordinary environment for healing. Many patients report feeling safe for the first time since the time of their trauma. It is this safe environment that provides the foundation for the healing process. By touching both the physical and the psychological aspects of patients, Watsu has enormous potential to move patients forward on their path to improved function and improved quality of life.

Watsu in Acute Rehabilitation Treatment Programs

During the acute rehabilitation phase, the emphasis of therapy programs is on restoring functional abilities as quickly as possible. Although Watsu might benefit nearly every patient, consideration must be given to the most efficient use of the patient's rehabilitation dollars. If the patient can be treated effectively on land, that is where he or she should be treated. If the patient is unable to participate in rehabilitation activities on land because of pain, weight-bearing restrictions, weakness, or other reasons, then the aquatic environment may be selected, and a decision must be made about which techniques to use. Although the focus is on improving functional skills, including walking, dressing, sports, and job-related activities, patients often are unable to practice these skills because of impairments such as those previously mentioned. The therapist must consider what the limiting factors are during each session. Watsu is often the best way to address impairments such as pain, muscle spasm, hypertonicity, and decreased range of motion, at the beginning of the treatment session. When used in this way, the Watsu session is relatively short, generally 10 to 30 minutes, depending on the needs and the response of the patient. The remainder of the session then addresses functional skills and exercises (Fig. 5-2).

Consider two patient scenarios.

1. A patient is experiencing pain and muscle spasm at levels that make it extremely difficult for him to work on stretching and strengthening. Watsu would be an excellent choice for beginning the treatment session. Using Watsu would help decrease the patient's pain and muscle spasms and increase both soft tissue and

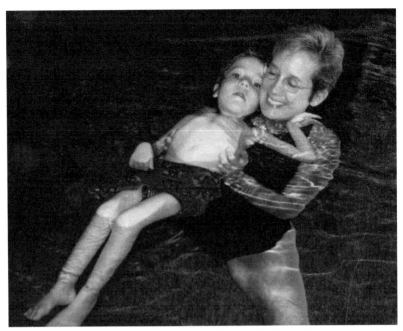

Figure 5-2. This child with spinal muscular atrophy benefits from alternating short periods of active movements with short periods of passive movements. This program has helped him improve his strength, mobility, and functional skills without excessive fatigue. This child has been free of hospitalization for the past year. Previously, he was hospitalized several times each year for respiratory infections (Courtesy Peggy Schoedinger).

joint mobility, thereby allowing the patient to participate more fully in therapeutic exercises and functional activities.
2. A patient has hypertonicity that limits her movements and her ability to practice functional activities. The patient also has limited range of motion because of soft tissue restrictions caused by the neurologic impairment. Using Watsu at the beginning of the session would help decrease the muscle tone and improve the soft tissue mobility, enabling the patient to perform functional activities with greater ease.

Watsu in Postrehabilitation Treatment Programs

After discharge from acute rehabilitation programs, many patients benefit from Watsu sessions to help manage their symptoms. Keeping symptoms under control allows patients to continue to advance or at least maintain their functional skills. This allows many patients to continue working at their jobs or to continue living independently. Watsu sessions at this stage tend to be longer and comprise most or all of the treatment session.

Consider three patient scenarios.

1. A patient with Parkinson's disease may choose to receive Watsu sessions to help him maintain mobility. The mobility gained in these sessions often has multiple beneficial effects, including improvements in walking, balance, posture, respiration, and daily life skills such as dressing and bathing.

2. A patient with fibromyalgia may seek Watsu to assist in modulating symptoms so she can remain more active in daily life. For this patient, Watsu may be beneficial in decreasing her pain and allowing her to relax and sleep more deeply at night. She can then participate more fully in life, including her family, job, hobbies, and a consistent exercise program.
3. A patient with late-stage metastatic cancer may find that Watsu decreases pain, improves relaxation, and assists him in finding peace within himself.

Essentials in Every Watsu Session

The foundation for every Watsu session is unconditional acceptance. In rehabilitation there is generally a sense of needing to "do" something to or for someone to rehabilitate and therefore change the person. In Watsu, awareness is maintained of the specific needs of the individual while openly and completely accepting the person "as is." This translates into the session as quiet listening with responsiveness to all aspects of the individual. It becomes a dance of sometimes leading and frequently following the patient's movements. Therapists are also sensitive to subtle physiologic changes such as changes in muscle tension and respiration. Although the therapist is mindful of the patient's needs, movements are not imposed to achieve specific goals. Instead, some movements may be invited or encouraged while therapists remain sensitive to and accepting of rejection of any of those movements. The session may evolve in completely unexpected ways. Although there may be few words exchanged during the session, the first words from patients at the end are often, "Thank you for listening."

Therapists learn a wide variety of Watsu moves that form a Watsu vocabulary. However, because each patient is unique and each session develops differently, there is an infinite variety in the sequence of the movements as well as in the movements themselves. Subtle variations in the movements occur with every patient, and sometimes entirely new movements develop spontaneously while therapists are following the needs of the individual. With each movement, part of the body is moved through the water. Turbulence causes drag on other parts of the body, which move and stretch freely in the aquatic environment. Although the movements are generally slow and rhythmical, they may be interspersed with bolder, stronger movements or stillness. Various types of soft tissue mobilization techniques are also easily incorporated into sessions (Figs. 5-3 and 5-4).

Before beginning Watsu with a patient, the therapist needs to explain the technique to the patient. Patients are instructed to notify their therapists immediately if a movement causes discomfort or motion sickness. Patients are encouraged to adjust their heads and necks as needed for comfort, although therapists strive to maintain optimal cervical alignment with elongation throughout the session.

Watsu Sessions for Patients with Neurologic Impairments

Patients with upper motor neuron impairments often exhibit limitations in range of motion resulting from soft tissue restrictions.[12,13] These restrictions, combined with hypertonicity, can impede functional recovery. Watsu is generally used at the beginning of a treatment session to improve soft tissue mobility and decrease hypertonicity so the patient can work on functional activities more successfully. Short

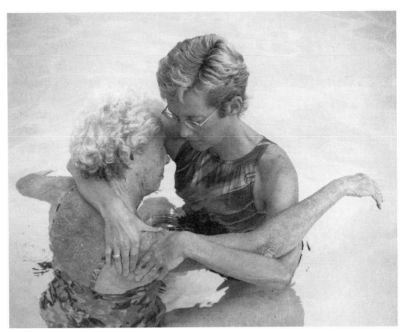

Figure 5-3. This position with the patient resting on the therapist's lap is often used in rehabilitation. The patient and therapist are both comfortable and relaxed, and various types of soft tissue and joint mobilization techniques are easy to incorporate. Many areas of the spine and extremities are accessible in this position (Courtesy Peggy Schoedinger).

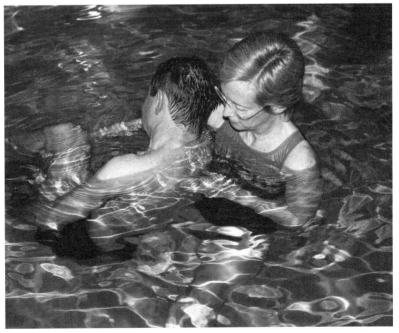

Figure 5-4. This is one of many different Watsu positions that allows the therapist to incorporate different forms of bodywork from both eastern and western medicine (Courtesy Peggy Schoedinger).

periods of Watsu may also be alternated with short periods of functional activities if the patient's activity tolerance is very low or the level of hypertonicity is very high.

Watsu dramatically changes the sensory input for the patient. The eyes are usually closed and the ears are under water most of the time. Combined with these quieting sensations is the calming tactile and gentle vestibular stimulation resulting from the movements through the water. In particular, the rhythmical, repeated rotational movements through the water gently stimulate the vestibular system and thus aid in quieting the patient's tone.

Water temperature is crucial, with neutral warmth being the goal with most patients, so they do not become chilled or overheated. A water temperature of 94 to 95°F (34.4 to 35°C) is generally considered ideal. However, the patient's condition or the external environment may necessitate a different temperature. For example, a patient with multiple sclerosis may respond better to a cooler temperature. In other situations, very dry or very cool air temperatures in the pool environment may dictate a slightly higher water temperature. Most therapy pools where Watsu is used have water temperatures between 92 and 95°F (33.3 to 35°C); however, patients have responded favorably in cooler or warmer water. Wastu done in water that is too cool generally does not decrease the patient's tone as much as Watsu done in neutrally warm water. Patients must also be kept warm when they exit the pool and when they are in the changing area to maintain the benefits gained during the session.[14]

Most Watsu sessions begin with movements of the trunk; however, for patients with neurologic impairments, the trunk becomes the primary focus. The emphasis is on encouraging trunk rotation, flexion, and elongation through a variety of positions

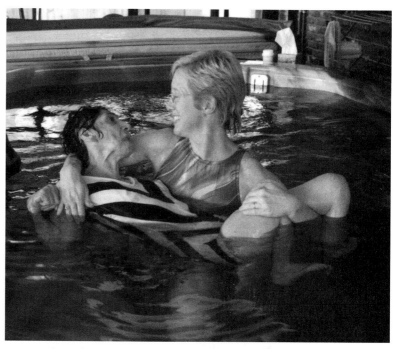

Figure 5-5. For patients with more severe spasticity, typical Watsu movements that utilize turbulent drag are generally not effective for stretching the body. Manual pressure is needed to sustain gentle, prolonged stretches. In this photo, the patient's right shoulder is being pressed while her knees are being pulled toward the therapist, allowing the therapist to maintain a trunk rotation stretch (Courtesy Peggy Schoedinger).

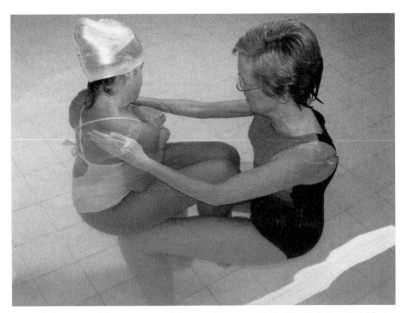

Figure 5-6. Patients with severe spasticity can be supported with their legs held between the legs of the therapist. This helps to stabilize the patient's lower trunk and allows the therapist to use both hands to turn the upper portion of the trunk. This rotation of the trunk helps to decrease hypertonicity (Courtesy Peggy Schoedinger).

and movements. With a more able-bodied patient, the turbulent drag of the water is usually adequate for causing the trunk, and therefore the spine, to rotate, flex, and elongate. However, for patients with hypertonicity, turbulent drag alone may not be enough. Gently maintained manual pressure may be needed to sustain a slow stretch to give the body time to respond (Figs. 5-5 and 5-6). As the patient's hypertonicity begins to diminish, movements may progress from proximal, shoulder, and hip joints, to distal extremity joints.[14] This movement sequence is similar to that used in many other areas of neurorehabilitation, including neurodevelopmental treatment.[13]

Watsu Sessions for Patients with Orthopedic Impairments

For patients with orthopedic impairments, Watsu may be used at the beginning of the session if their pain, muscle spasms, or range of motion restrictions make it difficult for them to work on exercises and functional activities. The Watsu session begins with movements that decrease the patient's symptoms. These movements will be different for each patient and are determined in the initial evaluation on land. Some patients will need more emphasis on flexion, whereas others may need more on extension or rotation (Fig. 5-7 A, B, C). These movements form a starting point from which other movements are free to develop. Therapists maintain their awareness of movement precautions for each patient as well as range of motion medical restrictions that may suggest movements to be avoided. Awareness of the patient's physiologic needs may also suggest movements to be encouraged. At the same time, therapists remain open, allowing the session to evolve in sometimes unexpected ways.

As the patient begins to relax, pain and muscle spasms decrease and movement ranges can be increased to permit more stretching and elongation (Fig. 5-8). Floating supine in the water with the gentle support of the therapist and buoyancy, the patient's body is free to move in a multitude of ways, including movements not possible on land. With the joints unloaded, joint compression forces, especially through the spine, are greatly reduced, allowing for greater range of motion and more pain-free movement (Fig. 5-9). Soft tissue mobilization techniques can also be incorporated into the session to augment Watsu's benefits. Stretching is enhanced by increasing the speed, and therefore the turbulent drag, of some movements and by using a manual stretch for others.

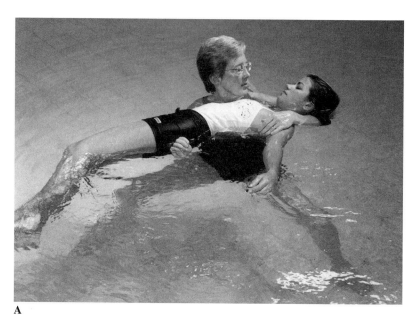

A

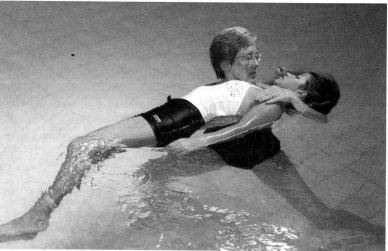

B

Figure 5-7. For patients with orthopedic impairments, Watsu sessions begin with movements that help alleviate symptoms. Therapists carefully select the initial movements based on the results of the evaluation on land. Initial movements will vary with each patient, but may include one of the options demonstrated in these photos. *A,* Hip extension and gentle extension of the spine. *B,* Gentle extension focused in the thoracic spine. *C,* Trunk, hip, and knee flexion (Courtesy Peggy Schoedinger).

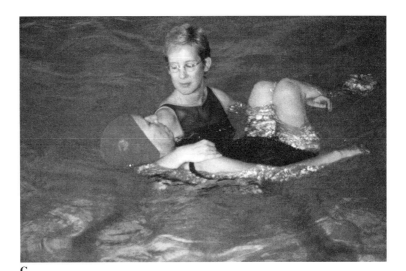

C

Figure 5-7. cont'd

Precautions for Watsu

With all aquatic therapy techniques, therapists must first consider the safety and inherent risks of having each patient in the water. All general precautions for aquatic therapy must be taken into consideration. Safety is always the top priority. Each therapist must also consider his or her professional background and knowledge base, and treat patients only within this framework. If a patient comes to a therapist with a condition about which he or she is unsure, it is critical for the therapist to seek further medical advice first.

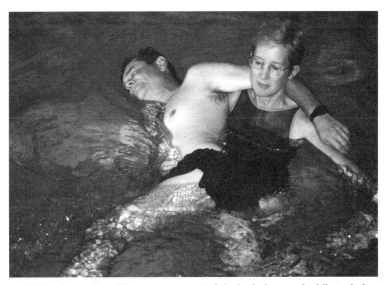

Figure 5-8. During various Watsu moves, part of the body is moved while turbulent drag causes movement in other parts of the body. In this photo, one leg is being pulled backward into hip extension while turbulent drag causes the other leg to move into hip flexion. This allows the hip flexors of one leg to be gently stretched while the opposite hip is flexed. This helps to protect the lumbar spine by preventing hypertension (Courtesy Peggy Schoedinger).

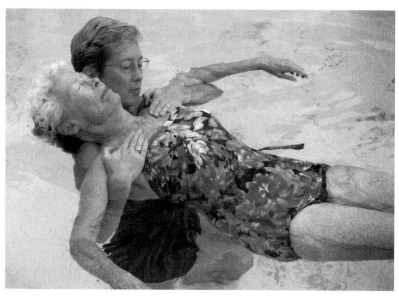

Figure 5-9. Watsu is helpful in improving thoracic mobility in patients such as this woman who has osteoporosis and who has had coronary artery bypass surgery. The improved mobility decreased her pain, improved her posture, and enabled her to participate in a strengthening and aerobic exercise program (Courtesy Peggy Schoedinger).

In addition to general precautions for the aquatic environment, there are some precautions specific to Watsu. It is essential to remember that Watsu movements affect the entire body. While floating supine in the water, the body is free to move. Although this is an overwhelming benefit, therapists must also be aware of how each motion is influencing other areas of the body. For example, many movements focus on the spine,

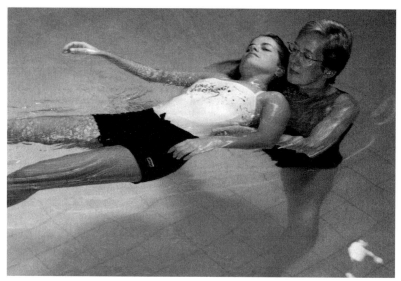

Figure 5-10. With the patient's head resting on the therapist's shoulder, the spine and extremities are free to move. Although this is an advantage for most patients, care must be taken if there are medical reasons to limit movement. This patient has back pain, but if she had additionally had a recent total hip replacement, this movement would be contraindicated because it causes adduction of the hip past midline (Courtesy Peggy Schoedinger).

but the extremities are also moving in the water at the same time. If a particular patient has range of motion precautions due to injury, disease, or surgery, the therapist must constantly be observing and analyzing each movement for safety (Fig. 5-10).

Patients with conditions in which movement could potentially cause harm must also receive special care and attention (Fig. 5-11 A, B). These might include patients with osteoporosis, an acute flare of rheumatoid arthritis, or ligamentous instability. With patients such as these, it is important to keep the movements slow and smooth to avoid any sudden loading of joints. If the condition at a particular joint is severe, Watsu must be significantly modified, or an external splint may be needed to protect the joint.[14]

It has been noted previously that Watsu causes an increase in vestibular stimulation. Although gentle stimulation has a dampening effect on muscle tone, overstimulation may have the opposite effect and cause physiologic distress. Each patient has

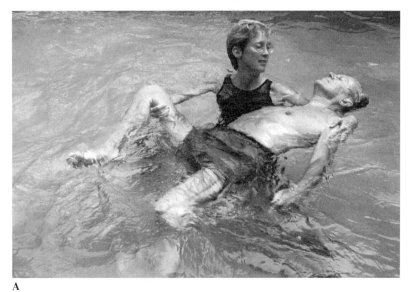

A

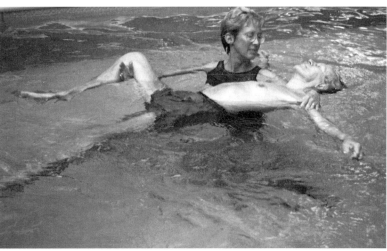

B

Figure 5-11. Watsu encourages gentle stretching of most joints during a session. However, care may need to be taken to support and protect a painful joint such as the shoulder of the patient in photo *A*. As the joint improves, turbulence can be used to gently stretch the joint as shown in photo *B* (Courtesy Peggy Schoedinger).

a different tolerance to vestibular stimulation, and therapists must use caution, particularly with patients who are susceptible to overstimulation. These may include people who report motion sickness in cars or on boats, and patients with traumatic brain injuries or some other type of injury to the central nervous system that causes them to be easily overstimulated by various types of sensory stimuli. Therapists must watch carefully for any physical signs of overstimulation, especially with patients who are unable to communicate verbally. Signs of overstimulation in patients may include reported dizziness or nausea, sudden facial pallor, facial sweating, increased rate of respiration, or nystagmus. However, symptoms may vary from person to person. In some patients, these symptoms, except for nystagmus, may signal other physiologic responses or emotional release. Therapists need to gain skill in differentiating the cause of the symptoms. For patients who are sensitive to vestibular stimulation, it may be necessary to focus on *slow*, linear movements and avoid rotational movements in which the head rolls from side to side.[14]

Summary

From its development for able-bodied clients, Watsu has grown into a useful tool in rehabilitation. Through its wide range of effects on patients, both physical and emotional, Watsu has far-reaching benefits. Although Watsu is a passive aquatic therapy technique, it has the potential to help many patients with both neurologic and orthopedic impairments, especially when used in conjunction with treatments focusing on functional activities and exercises.

REFERENCES

1. Scaer R: The Body Bears the Burden: Trauma, Dissociation, and Disease. Binghamton, NY: Haworth Medical, 2001.
2. Kauder C: Healing waters. Boulder Daily Camera 1B–5B, Sept. 27, 1999.
3. Jamison L: The therapeutic value of aquatic therapy in treating lymphedema. Rehab Manage: Interdisciplinary J Rehabil Aug–Sept, 2000.
4. Dougherty L, Dunlap E, Mehler S: The rehabilitative benefits of Watsu. In Dull H (ed): Watsu: Freeing the Body in Water. Middletown, Calif: Harbin Springs Publishing, 1997.
5. Umphred DA: Classification of treatment techniques based on primary input systems. In Neurological Rehabilitation, 3rd ed. St. Louis: Mosby-Year Book, 1995.
6. Farber S: Sensorimotor Evaluation and Treatment Procedures, 2nd ed. Indianapolis: Indiana University–Purdue University at Indianapolis Medical Center, 1974.
7. Huss J: Sensorimotor Treatment Approaches in Occupational Therapy. Philadelphia: Lippincott, 1971.
8. Butler DS: Mobilization of the Nervous System. New York: Churchill Livingstone, 1991.
9. Morris DM: Aquatic rehabilitation of the neurologically impaired client. In Routi RG, Morris DM, Cole AJ (eds): Aquatic Rehabilitation. Philadelphia: Lippincott, 1997.
10. Greenman PE: Principles of Manual Medicine, 2nd ed. Baltimore: Williams & Wilkins, 1996.
11. Levine P: Waking the Tiger. Berkeley, Calif: North Atlantic Books, 1997.
12. Ballantyne B: Factors contributing to voluntary movement deficits and spasticity following cerebral vascular accidents. Neurology Rep 15(1):15–18, 1991.
13. Craik RI: Abnormalities of motor behavior. In Lister MJ (ed): Contemporary Management of Motor Control Problems. Alexandria, Va: Foundation for Physical Therapy, 1990, pp 155–164.
14. Schoedinger P: Adapting Watsu for people with special needs. In Dull H (ed): Watsu: Freeing the Body in Water. Middletown, Calif: Harbin Springs, 1997.

Chapter 6
Equipment Options and Uses for the Aquatic Therapy Pool

Marilou Moschetti, BSc, PTA

There is a wide variety of equipment available for use during aquatic physical therapy. The equipment may include either built-in apparatus such as treadmills, massage hoses, or swim jets or be hand-held, slip-on, lightweight foam, expandable resistance, or contoured systems to provide impact-free exercise. All pieces of pool equipment are designed to take advantage of the properties of water and at the end of physical therapy treatment to help facilitate improvement of a patient's function on dry land.[1]

Each piece of aquatic equipment has a special shape, style, and features, allowing the therapist to select multiple products for multiple uses. Individual patients' needs dictate which equipment the therapist will utilize.

PATIENT POPULATIONS

Common ailments treated in the pool include (1) prepartum or postpartum pelvic and low back pain,[2,3] (2) lower or upper extremity edema,[4] (3) joint replacement,[5] (4) arthritis,[6] (5) spine dysfunction,[7–9] (6) cerebral palsy,[10] (7) neurologic disorders including Parkinson's disease,[11] (8) decreased balance or fear of falling in older adults for initiation of an early balance retraining program,[12,13] (9) connective tissue disorders,[14] (10) multiple fractures,[15] (11) heart disease, (12) breast cancer, and (13) spinal cord injuries[16–22] (Figs. 6-1 and 6-2).

Often referrals come from medical specialists such as physiatrists and orthopedic surgeons. However, primary care physicians, rheumatologists, obstetrician/gynecologists, cardiologists, and neurologists are also important referral sources.[23] After the doctor's diagnosis and the physical therapist's evaluation are completed, an individualized program for the patient is designed. The patient's pool exercise or rehabilitation program will most probably use a wide array of equipment, and the therapist has many such types of equipment to choose from.

116 COMPREHENSIVE AQUATIC THERAPY

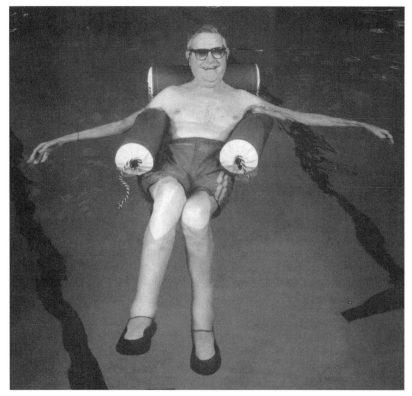

Figure 6-1. For patients who need lower extremity strengthening and have balance deficits, a float chair may be used as a supplemental device in the pool. (Courtesy of Aqua S.E.A.T.S., Birmingham, AL, 2001.)

THE BASIC PRINCIPLES OF CHOOSING AQUATIC THERAPY EQUIPMENT

With such a wide variety of equipment available, choosing the appropriate pieces for use in an aquatic therapy practice can often become confusing and/or expensive. Before equipment is purchased, specific criteria should be met, including the product's (1) safety, (2) durability, (3) reliability, (4) effectiveness, (5) utility, and (6) potential liability.

The element of safety in the aquatic environment should be the foremost criterion, because drowning is still the major risk management concern for aquatic therapists, even when supports or other devices are used in the pool.[24] Products must be safe for both the patient and therapist. Many patients may be nonswimmers and/or be deconditioned. Products should feature quick-release clips if they are going to be attached to the body. During the first treatment session, the therapist should discuss the appropriate use of the specific piece of equipment, assure a proper fit, and be sure there are no protruding pieces that could get caught on a bathing suit or injure the patient's skin.

The equipment, regardless of the size or probable use, must be durable and be able to withstand the harsh, corrosive chemical actions of the pool environment. The presence of atmospheric chlorides can lead to corrosion of materials such as stainless steel, with either pitting or eating away of metal products. Hand rails,

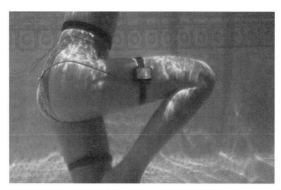

Figure 6-2. Specific muscle strengthening data can be collected with the use of surface electromyograph biofeedback devices such as the Aquanex. (Courtesy of Swimming Technology Research, Tallahassee, FL, 2001.)

poles, door jams, ceiling materials, or other metal products may be affected. Cosmetic corrosion may affect the structural integrity of stainless steel with a wall thickness of 0.145 inch, and may also affect the material's safety.[25] Not only do chemical reactions and water temperature affect stainless steel, but most foam and polyvinyl chloride (PVC) piping break down over time, even when coated with liquid vinyl. Before purchasing the equipment, the therapist should look for a manufacturer's guarantee or return policy.[26]

Watch Your Step
People do occasionally get injured through no fault of the facility, owner, or staff. A frequently litigated class of accidents results from defective or unreasonably dangerous products and equipment.

There are three basic theories of recovery available under product-liability law: (1) strict liability, (2) negligence, and (3) breach of warranty. Strict liability, which is also referred to as liability without fault, holds that a manufacturer or supplier is liable for personal injuries or property damage if the product they supply is "unreasonably dangerous." The reason typically is that the manufacturer and supplier are in the best position to bear the expenses associated with defective products.

As a general rule, the courts will impose strict liability if the product in question subjects a person to an unreasonable risk of harm and it was feasible to design the product in a safer manner. To defeat a strict liability claim, the manufacturer or supplier must demonstrate that the product's utility outweighs the risk of injury to the consumer and that the product has been designed so that the risks are reduced to the greatest extent possible, while the product's inherent usefulness is retained at an acceptable cost. A risk utility test is used for such claims.

The risk utility test identifies seven factors for consideration:

1. The magnitude and seriousness of the danger in using the product
2. The likelihood of injury
3. The obviousness of the danger
4. The product's utility to the public and the individual user
5. The technologic and economic feasibility of a safer design
6. The ability to avoid injury by use of instructions or warnings
7. The ability to have avoided injury by careful use of the product

Negligence requires that the manufacturer and supplier of products exercise reasonable care in preparing, designing, and selling the product. Failure to inspect or test the product, improper design or construction of the product, or failure to warn of product defects or dangers associated with the product may lead to a lawsuit.

Breach of warranty is based on contract law and can be either an express or implied warranty. When a manufacturer or supplier makes specific statements about the quality and characteristics of the product and the product does not meet minimum industry standards, that is a breach of an *express warranty*. An *implied warranty* results simply from selling of the product, and the assumption is made that when a manufacturer sells a product, that product is fit for the ordinary purpose for which it is intended. (Reprinted with permission of the author and *Athletic Business*, © 2001.)

If the equipment is too expensive to purchase, the clinic or hospital may want to consider renting or leasing. Therapists should preview or test the device before the purchase is made. Customization of pieces of equipment to meet specialized patient needs may be arranged with the manufacturer. The manufacturer may have produced a video showing the possible uses of the equipment or device. Information concerning the proper assembly, maintenance, and storage of the equipment should also be provided.[27] Lastly, the product should be visible to both patient and therapist. Bright colors in yellow, black, red, green, or dark blue make the object easily identifiable to lifeguards on deck or retrievable from the pool floor.

The product must be comfortable to touch, because many patients undergoing rehabilitation suffer from sensitive skin or painful joint ailments. The equipment must be versatile and adjustable to fit a variety of body sizes and types (Fig. 6-3). The pool size and patient load must be considered when certain pieces of equipment are used, and the equipment should not interfere with the treatment of other patients. A variety of products should be available for program progression, categorized by buoyancy assist, super assisted, buoyancy resist, or super resist, depending on their construction and design by the manufacturer (Fig. 6-4).

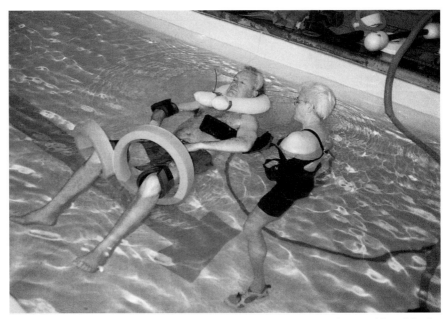

Figure 6-3. Several devices may be used simultaneously for support of extremities while the therapist applies effleurage massage with a water jet. (Courtesy of AquaTechnics Consulting Group, Aptos, CA.)

Equipment Options and Uses for the Aquatic Therapy Pool 119

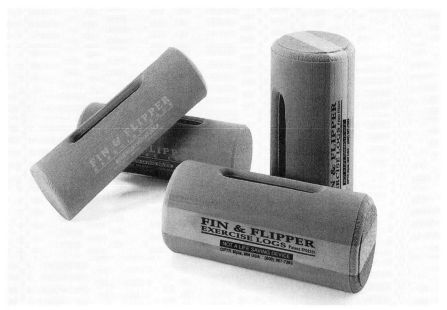

Figure 6-4. Products made from foam provide buoyancy or light resistance. (Courtesy of OPTP, Minneapolis, MN.)

CONSTRUCTION MATERIALS USED IN POOL EQUIPMENT

Standard pool equipment is made from a variety of materials to provide durability. As long as it is properly cared for, the equipment can be used over a long period of time. Product size, quality, strength, absorption, and resistance to chemical breakdown are important considerations for the manufacturer and end user. Certain types of materials conform to a particular shape and are easily constructed. Others require special heating techniques and highly technical methods of blow molding, compression molding, or injection molding by the manufacturer (Fig. 6-5). The materials pool equipment is made from may include one type or a combination of the following:

1. **Polyethylene cross-linked with closed-cell EVA foam** is durable, resistant to chlorine, impervious to rot or sunlight, and able to be molded into many shapes.
2. **Endolite foam** is coated with liquid PVC vinyl.
3. **Neoprene** comes in three grades, has a rubber or Lycra coating, and is used for gloves, outer wear for warmth, or rectangular floats.
4. **Lycra** is a tightly woven nylon fabric that provides light resistance when used in gloves and is commonly combined with nylon in bathing suits.
5. **Polyethylene** is used for contoured buoys or kick boards and is a type of liquid plastic.
6. **Non-latex copolymer** is used for construction of tubing and elastic bands.
7. **Aqua-Cell foam** is a UL-certified product that can be custom molded and is also used by NASA and the U.S. military.

Depending on the manufacturer's product specifications, each piece of equipment is developed specifically for a particular use, be it flotation, resistance, or athletic or therapeutic performance.

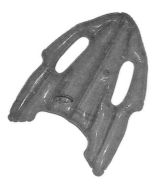

Figure 6-5. Blow molding or injection molding allows special contours for product manufacturing and use in the therapy pool. (Courtesy of Zura, Inc., Westerville, OH.)

Proper care consists of rinsing the product with clean water and drying the product by hand or hanging the item to maximize air circulation. Belts made with vinyl outer coverings should be washed with a pH-neutral soap and rinsed thoroughly. They should be hung to dry away from other wet surfaces and unclipped to help prolong their lifespan. All equipment should be allowed to dry thoroughly before the next day's use and should be replaced at the first sign of cracking, dryness, or other damage.[28]

W.A.T.E.R. SCALE AND EQUIPMENT OPTIONS

For the licensed professional to maximize the limited time available to treat patients in the therapy pool, equipment, mode of treatment, and other options need to be chosen when the plan of care is created. The W.A.T.E.R. Scale Classification System describes and defines equipment choices and the necessary elements of rehabilitation potential, while establishing a standardized system of communication for patient care in the aquatic environment (see Appendix A, Tables A-1, A-2, A-3, and A-4).[29] A partial list of categories that best describes the potential use of equipment during the patient's treatment session includes (1) equipment type, (2) manufacturer, (3) construction materials, (4) patient position, (5) active segment and attachment, (6) movement, (7) variable, and (8) grade of difficulty (see Appendix A).

Functional therapy goals may vary over the course of treatment and program changes may need to be made. Use of a standardized measurement of the patient's functional progress is essential. After the appropriate choice of specialized treatment protocol and equipment is made, direct observation, timed performance, self-administered questionnaires, Subjective Objective Assessment Plan (SOAP) records, and the guidelines within the W.A.T.E.R. Scale can be used to provide information about treatment effectiveness, patient classification, and discharge status to physicians and payers.

EQUIPMENT OPTIONS BY PATIENT TYPE AND SPECIALTY TECHNIQUE

A brief description of pool equipment options is provided in this section. The equipment is categorized by the type of treatment for which it might be most appropriate.

(1) **Watsu** (Water Shiatsu), a form of passive aquatic therapy, is modeled after principles of Zen Shiatsu. The provider always performs Watsu in a hands-on manner. The patient is held or cradled in warm water while being stabilized or moved. The resulting movement is a stretch of another body segment due to the drag effect created by the water. Watsu providers may need equipment such as a **cervical collar, flotation rings**, **Styrofoam bar,** or **ankle floats,** to support patients who are too large to handle. Treatment is possible without using any equipment. **Suggested patient profiles** include chronic pain, acute pain conditions, fibromyalgia, muscle guarding, and decreased range of motion.[30]

(2) The **Bad Ragaz Ring Method,** which has been influenced by proprioceptive neuromuscular facilitation (PNF) and Knupfer exercises, is used mainly for musculoskeletal problems. It was originally developed in Switzerland and is used to guide the patient through specific patterns of movement to increase strength and range of motion. The therapist serves as a point of stability from which the patient moves, generating resistance from turbulent drag of the water. The patient determines the amount of resistance based on the speed of his or her movement. Typical exercise equipment options include a **neck collar, float belt, jacket,** and **float rings**. **Suggested patient profiles** include those requiring strength building, neuromuscular reeducation, and joint rehabilitation.[30, 31]

(3) The **Halliwick Concept,** a method of teaching swimming, is taught on a one-to-one basis, using phases of adjustment, rotations, control of movement, safe breathing, and correct handling until independence is achieved. The method follows a 10-point program, forming a sequence of motor learning patterns. Ideally, there are **no water props** or **equipment** used in this method, because the method relies solely on one-to-one treatment with the aquatic professional. **Suggested patient profiles** include balance disorders; it is often used in training children with disabilities, scoliosis, cerebrovascular accident/hemiparesis, and athetoid cerebral palsy.[30]

(4) **Spine stabilization** is a type of therapeutic exercise that helps patients gain dynamic control of segmental spine forces, eliminate repetitive injury to motion segments, encourage healing of injured motion segments, and possibly alter the degenerative process, while minimizing further spinal injury. Patients may benefit from either prone, supine, or vertical positions in both shallow and deep water and can use **paddles, gloves, collars, float belts or jackets, mask and snorkel, Styrofoam bars, weights, kick boards, balance boards** or a **swim leash** for their progressive therapeutic program. **Suggested patient profiles** include disc disease, pre- and postoperative conditions of the spine, and degenerative disc disease.[32, 33]

(5) **Spinal traction** is a method in which forces are applied to stretch the periarticular tissues and musculature, to separate joint surfaces, and to reduce intradiscal pressure, possibly retracting herniated disc material along the spine. Traction in the aquatic environment can be applied to either the lumbar, thoracic, or cervical spine by the licensed therapist in the prone or supine position, using elastic or nonelastic tethers. Additional hands-on methods can be used when the patient is in traction, including massage, passive movement, tissue mobilization, graded oscillation, and/or progressive stretch mobilization. Types of equipment options include **belts, collars, tethers of nylon cord or elastic tubing, neoprene floats, snorkel and mask, float bars, buoyancy jackets,** or **swim leashes. Suggested patient profiles include** disc herniation, spinal nerve root impingement, degenerative disc disease, zygapophyseal joint pain, and muscle guarding/spasm.[34, 35]

(6) The **Burdenko Method** is the integration and practical application of water and land exercises based on exercise science to maintain health and quality of life and enhance physical performance. Six essential qualities are used: balance, coordination, flexibility, endurance, speed, and strength to achieve goals. Types of equipment options include **barbells, buoyancy vest and cuffs, rings suspended above the water, kick boards,** or **tubing**.[30]

(7) The **Jahara Experiential Method** utilizes the "third arm," offering precise support of the body. A series of gentle stretches are used. Equipment consists of a modified **Styrofoam bar** and one-to-one interaction with an aquatic professional. **Suggested patient profiles** include general relaxation, fibromyalgia, and neuromuscular and musculoskeletal disorders.[30]

(8) **Ai Chi** is a combination of deep breathing and slow broad movements standing in chest-deep water. Tai Chi, Shiatsu, and Qigong concepts are combined with basic movement patterns, and no pool props are used. **Suggested patient profiles** include osteoporosis, balance deficits, and geriatric disorders.[30]

(9) A Russian-born Israeli physicist researched human movement, its relationship to our behavior, and then developed the method of **Feldenkrais,** also known as **Fluid Moves,** in the pool. It is formulated on the basis of the "functional integration" component of the method. A guided exploratory process of sensorimotor learning is used, in which the practitioner works with the patient to reach a level of training or retraining of the brain to control muscles, so the body can move at an optimal level. No equipment is needed in the pool when this technique is used. **Suggested patient profiles** include balance or proprioceptive dysfunction, chronic pain, and restricted extremity range of motion.[36]

(10) The **Task-Type Training Approach** is a set of principles to guide clinicians as they design treatment programs and is best described as a technique emphasizing functional skills performed in functional positions. The patient is encouraged to be an active participant. Equipment includes the **pool wall, functional equipment** specific to the task, i.e., **weighted box, rowing oar, tennis racket, golf club,** and stability provided by the **therapist**.[37] **Suggested patient profiles** include neurologic dysfunctions, cerebrovascular accident, traumatic or anoxic brain injury, spinal cord injury, and functional skill integration.

(11) **Swim Stroke Training and Modification** is used to actively train clients in the horizontal position using verbal, visual, or tactile instruction to modify and execute various swim strokes with the intent to rehabilitate, not teach swim skills. Equipment may include **snorkel/mask, belts, rings, buoys,** or **fins**. **Suggested patient profiles** include both upper and lower extremity amputation, spinal dysfunctions, chronic or acute pain, cerebrovascular accident/hemiparesis, spinal cord injury, and orthopedic or musculoskeletal injuries.[38]

(12) **Aquatic PNF** is an active therapy modeled on the principles and movement patterns of PNF. Patterns can include a series of functional, spiral, diagonal, or mass movements while standing, sitting, kneeling, or lying in the water as the therapist gives verbal, visual, and/or tactile instructions. Equipment may include **collars, belts, rings, jacket,** or the **pool wall,** along with the hands-on approach with the aquatic professional. **Suggested patient profiles** include neurologic deficits, and orthopedic joint rehabilitation.[39]

In addition, **manual therapy** can include soft tissue mobilization, strain-counterstrain, myofascial release, or joint mobilization, and is used for those with orthopedic or neurologic conditions. Support devices are used and can include **Styrofoam bars, support jackets or vests, collars, belts,** or other equipment combinations.

Several underwater techniques have developed from **Watsu** and are called **Wassertanzen**, **Aquadance**, and **Jahara's Unique Underwater Work**. Most use a clip-on type **nose plug** and **earplugs**.

A basic set of equipment is useful for the aquatic professional starting a therapy program (see Appendix B for a listing of equipment and suppliers). The suggested start-up equipment may include flotation rings, flotation belts, long bar buoyancy floats, short fins, kick boards, gloves, Styrofoam bars, inflatable cervical collars, step platforms, tethers, vests, and weights. Accessory items, such as shoes, neoprene wraps, metronomes, surface electromyograph units, heart rate monitors, massage hoses, computerized treadmills, aquatic wheelchairs, and float or sink balls, all add to the flexibility of aquatic therapy programming. A fully equipped first aid kit, automatic external defibrillator (optional except in mandated federal buildings, but may become a standard of care), rescue equipment as required by state bathing code, and a universal precautions spill kit will add to the patient's safety while in the therapy pool.

CONCLUSION

Careful consideration of facility size, budget constraints, patient demographics, and patient safety helps aquatic therapists choose the best equipment to meet the needs of their practices. This will enable them to provide challenging, progressive, and enjoyable therapeutic exercise for their patients.

Acknowledgment

The author thanks Melanie Olson, PT, for her assistance in writing portions of this chapter.

Appendix A
Modified W.A.T.E.R. Scale™ Classification System[29, 40]

I. **Type** category classifies equipment as flotation, resistive, tethered/portable stations, and/or accessory.

II. **Manufacturer** category represents a broad variety of equipment manufacturing companies.

III. **Position** category describes the body during treatment as:

 1. Vertical or upright position
 2. Supine or lying flat on the back face up
 3. Prone or lying flat, face down
 4. Side-lying, on either the right or left side

IV. **Activity/attachment** category refers to the predominant location of the attachment of equipment and function of the body during a particular exercise or specialty technique:

1. Sitting or standing
2. Floating
3. Distance movement or locomotion
4. Foot/feet
5. Hand
6. Watsu
7. Bad Ragaz Ring Method
8. Spine stabilization
9. Spinal traction
10. Burdenko Method
11. Jahara Experiential Method
12. Aquatic PNF
13. Task-Type Training Approach
14. Swim Stroke Training and Modification

V. **Active segment** is used to name the part of the body that is undergoing motion:

1. Upper extremity—hands, arms
2. Lower extremity—legs
3. Both upper and lower extremity
4. Trunk and pelvis
5. Head and neck
6. Thorax or thoracic spine segments

VI. **Movement** category describes motion occurring by the active segments while using equipment:

1. Static
2. Bilateral
3. Reciprocal
4. Unilateral

VII. **Variable** category is used to describe the direction of movement, amount of buoyancy, or water depth while using equipment.

VIII. **Grade** category describes the level of difficulty or intensity while using equipment:

1. Level I—Slow, mild intensity, short duration, 0–30 seconds (50% relative perceived exertion [RPE])
2. Level II—Slow, medium intensity, moderate duration, 30 seconds–1 minute (50%–70% RPE)
3. Level III—Fast, more difficult, long duration, ≥1 minute (80% RPE)
4. Level IV—Difficult, long duration in minutes (90%–100% RPE)
5. Level V—Elite athlete level, very difficult, sustained (100% RPE)

Table A-1. Modified W.A.T.E.R. Scale Classification System Key

Construction Materials	Position	Activity*	Active Segment	Movement	Variable	Grade
Closed-cell EVA = CCEVA	Vertical = V	Sitting = Si	Upper extremity = UE	Static = ST	Buoyancy assist = BA	Level I = I
Endolite = EN	Supine = S	Standing = St	Lower extremity = LE	Bilateral = B	Buoyancy resist = BR	Level II = II
Neoprene = NE	Prone = P	Floating = Fl	Both UE and LE = (B)UE & LE	Reciprocal = R	Water depth = WD	Level III = III
Lycra = LY				Unilateral = Uni	Direction of movement = DM	Level IV = IV
Aqua-Cell UL certified = AC	Side-lying = Sl	Locomotion = Lo	Trunk and pelvis = TP			Level V = V
Blow = Molded		Bad Ragaz Ring Method = BRRM	Head and Neck = HN			
Polyethylene = BMP		Massage = MA				
Compression molded single foam = CMSF		Manual therapy = MT	Thorax = TH			
Injection molded = IM		Spine stabilization = SpSt				
		Spinal traction = SpTr				

*Some techniques are not represented in the key.

Table A-2. Modified W.A.T.E.R. Scale Classification System: Applications for Flotation Devices

Type*	Manufacturer	Construction Materials	Position	Activity	Active Segment	Movement	Variable	Grade
Balls	Variable	Rubber, nylon	V, S, P, Sl	Si, St, Fl, Lo	(B) UE & LE	ST, B, R, Uni	BA, BR, DM, strengthening	I-II
Bar bells	Variable	CCEVA, EN, ET	V, P, St, Sl	Si, St, Fl, Lo, SpSt	(B) UE & LE, TP, HN	ST, B, R, Uni	BA, BR, WD, DM, strengthening	I-IV
Boards	Variable	CCEVA, IM	V, S, P, Sl	Si, St, Fl, Lo, SpST, MT, SpTr	(B) UE & LE, TP, HN, TH	ST, B, R, Uni	BA, BR, strengthening, floating	I-V
Collars	Variable	Rubber, EN	S, Sl	Si, St, Fl, Lo, BRRM, MA, MT, SpSt, SpTr	(B) UE & LE, HN	ST, B, R, Uni	BA, BR, DM, flotation support	I-II
Cuffs	Variable	CCEVA, NE, CMSF, ET, nylon	V, S, P, Sl	Si, St, Fl, Lo, BRRM, MA, MT, SpSt, SpTr	(B) UE & LE, TP	ST, B, R, Uni	BA, BR, WD, DM, strengthening, flotation support	I-V
Float belts	Variety	EN, ET	V, S, P, Sl	St, Fl, Lo, BRRM, MA, MT, SpSt, SpTr	LE, TP, HN, TH	ST, B, Uni	BA, DM, flotation support	I-V
Foam bars	Aqua-Gym, variable	Closed-cell polyurethane foam	V, S, P, Sl	Si, St, Fl, Lo, BRRM, MA, MT, SpSt, SpTr	(B) UE & LE, TP, HN, TH	ST, B, R, Uni	BA, BR, WD, DM, strengthening, flotation support	I-V
Jackets	Bioenergetics, Sterns	NE, Nylon	V, S, P, Sl	Si, Fl, Lo, MT, SpSt, SpTr	(B) UE & LE, TP, TH	ST, B, R, Uni	BA, DM	I-III

*Not all types of equipment are represented.
Adapted from Bedgood D: Comparison of Water Exercise Equipment. Key West, FL: Kona Fitness (now AquaToner), 1982.

Table A-3. Modified W.A.T.E.R. Scale Classification System: Application for Resistive Devices

Type*	Manufacturer	Construction Materials	Position	Activity	Active Segment	Movement	Variable	Grade
Paddles	AquaTherapeutics, AquaToner	Nonimpact plastic	V, P	Si, St, Lo, foot, hand	(B) UE & LE	R, Uni	BR, DM, strengthening	III–V, >250 sq in. surface area
Boots/bells	Hydro-Tone Fitness Systems	High-impact plastic	V, P	Si, St, Lo, SpSt, foot, hand	(B) UE & LE	B, R, Uni	BR, WD, DM, strengthening	II > V
Wheels	Danmar	Nonimpact plastic	V	Si, St, Lo, SpSt, hand	UE	B, Uni	BR, WD, DM, strengthening	III–V
Boards	OTPT	Closed-cell foam	V, S, P, Sl	Si, St, Fl, Lo, SpSt, foot, hand	(B) UE & LE	ST, B, R, Uni	BA, BR, WD, DM, strengthening	I–IV
Fins	Force Fin®	100% durable polyurethane	P, Sl	St, Lo, Fl, SpSt, foot	LE	B, R, Uni	BR DM, strengthening	III–V
Short blade fins	Zoomers	Injected molded rubber	P, S, Sl	Si, St, Fl, Lo, SpSt, foot	LE	B, R, Uni	BR, DM, strengthening	III–V
Single fin	Finis, Inc.	Injection molded rubber	P, S	Fl, Lo, feet	LE	B	BR, DM, strengthening	IV, V
Other types	Aqua-Gym, AquaFlex	Injection molded plastic	V, P, S	Si, St, Lo, hands	UE	B, R, Uni	BR, DM, strengthening	III–V

*Not all types of equipment are represented.
Adapted from Bedgood D: Comparison of Water Exercise Equipment. Key West, FL: Kona Fitness (now AquaToner), 1982.

Table A-4. Modified W.A.T.E.R. Scale Classification System: Applications for Tethers and Portable Stations

Type*	Manufacturer	Construction Materials	Position	Activity	Active Segment	Movement	Variable	Grade
Tethers	Super Swim	Nylon cord, nylon webbing with belt	V, S, P	St, Fl, Lo, MT, SpSt, SpTr	(B) UE & LE, TP, HN, TH	ST, B, R, Uni	BR, DM, strengthening, flotation	I–V
Tethers	Mary Sanders	Rubber tubing	V, S	St, Fl, Lo, MT, SpSt, SpTr	(B) UE, TP, TH	B, R, Uni	BR, strengthening	II–III
Portable Stations	Ferno-Ille, Neptune	Stainless steel, plastic	V, S	Si, St, Fl, SpSt	(B) UE & LE, TP, HN, TH	B, R, Uni	BR, DM, strengthening	II–V

*Not all types of equipment are represented.
Adapted from Bedgood D: Comparison of Water Exercise Equipment. Key West, FL: Kona Fitness (now AquaToner), 1982, 2001.

Appendix B
Where to Buy Accessory Devices and Equipment

AQUATIC EXERCISE TOOL BOX/ BOOKS

Human Kinetics
www.Humankinetics.com
1-800-747-4457

DISPOSABLE SWIM PANTS

Water Safety International
www.swimpants.com
1-800-852-0284
i Play
www.iplaybabywear.com
1-800-876-1574

FIRST AID SUPPLIES

Marine Rescue Products
www.marine-rescue.com
1-800-341-9500

FLOTATION DEVICES AND EQUIPMENT

GyroJoggers with Connector Bar
Aquatic Foam Aids; AFA, Inc.
Rickd@brinet.com
1-828-692-9558

Head floats, sectional raft, Dolphin Float, Swim Rings, Hydro Helpers, Running Water, Tri-Swim support, Stabilizer Bar, Comfort Mat, Flotation Swimsuits, Delta Swim System
Danmar
www.danmarproducts.com
1-800-783-1998

Therapy Collar, Belt, Cuffs, Mat
BlueMoon® Aqua Products
TRMN Enterprises, Inc.
www.bluemoonswim.com
1-800-944-1176

AquaJogger® Float Belt, AquaRunners, DeltaBells®
Excel Sports Science, Inc.
www.aquajogger.com
1-800-922-9544

Wet Vest, II, AT, ATS, Belt, EC, Float-It, Water Weights, Collar, BODYfit Tether
Bioenergetics
www.wetvest.com
1-800-938-8378

Aqua S.E.A.T.S.™ Supportive Exercise & Therapy Seat
Aqua S.E.A.T.S.
www.aquaseats.com
1-205-870-3404

Type III PFD Flotation Jacket
Stearns, Inc. & Mustang Survival Corporation
West Marine Products, Inc.
www.westmarine.com
1-800-BOATING

H2O Aquasizer Gear: Tangles log with seat, belt, dumbbells, boots, boards, mats, Sun Breeze Settee water chair
Fabrionics, Inc.
www.fabrionics.com
1-800-851-2760

Aqua Coach Fitness Trainer Belt
Swimline Intl Leisure Products
www.swimline.com
1-631-254-2155

AquaPower, Hydroflo, Avia, Ear Bandit, Chimal, Wonder Board, Safety Island, Dr. Gordon's Balance Aqua Board, BodyFit Collar®, Saddle Float and Square Float, Burdenko Belt, Rings, Buoyancy Board, Starboard, additional products and educational material
Sprint/Rothhammer
www.sprintaquatics.com
1-800-235-2156

The Sammy, Fillable Dumbbells, Warm Belly Wetsuits, Training Tubes, Aqua Power Bar, Bow Tie Resistance Trainer, The Coil, Wonder Float, additional products, videos, and educational materials
Adolph Kiefer & Associates
www.kiefer.com
1-800-323-4071

LIFTS

Aquatic Access, Inc.
www.aquaticaccess.com
1-800.325-LIFT

Swim-Lift, Econo-Lift®
Spectrum Pool Products
www.spectrumproducts.com
1-800-776-5309
Mengo Industries, Inc.
www.mengo-ind.com
1-800-279-4611

SureHands Wheelchair-to-Water™ Lifts
SureHands Lifts & Care Systems
www.surehands.com
1-800-724-5305

NEOPRENE WRAPS

WetWrap, WetPants, Booties
D. K. Douglas
www.wetwrap.com
1-800-334-9070

RESISTIVE DEVICES AND EQUIPMENT

Aqua-Power Paddle®, AquaToner®
AquaTherapeutics Worldwide
www.AQUATONER.com
1-800-237-0469

GyroJoggers with Connector Bar
Aquatic Foam Aids; AFA, Inc.
Rickd@brinet.com
1-828-692-9558

Th' Horse™, Hand Paddles, Muscle Shells™, Gym Bells™
Aqua-Gym®
www.handsonwounds.com
1-813-960-9040

Foot Floats, Dumbbells, Flotation Belt, Hydro Gloves, Sidekick, Speedray
Zura Sports, Inc.
www.zura.com
1-800-890-3009

Fin & Flipper™ Exercise Logs, AquaPaddle™
OPTP
www.optp.com
1-800-367-7393

LOCH Water Gym Equipment
LOCH Integrated Systems, Inc.
www.lochsystems.com
1-888-887-8853

Professional Aqua Cuff
Water Gear, Inc.
www.watergear.com
1-800-794-6432

Aqua-Cell™ Products—belts, bars, cuffs, boards, buoys
Spongex Corporation
www.spongexcorp.com
1-866-782-7749

Cuffs, gloves, Wave Belt®, Wave Belt® PRO, Hand Buoys™, AQUIS® Micro Fiber Towels, Wet Sack, Water Dogs™, Men's River Trainer™
Hydro-Fit
www.hydrofit.org
1-800-346-7295

Abilitations™ Ring Float, Aquatic Therapy Float, Water Walker, Multi-Sensory Aqua Balls, All Pro™ Aqua Power® Water Weights, Pool Pant Diaper™, Pool Side Therapy Chair, Abilitations™ Aquatic Ball Pack, My Pool Pal® Special Needs Flotation Swimsuit, Wet Vest II® and Wet Vest Collar
Abilitations®
www.Abilitations.com
1-800-850-8602

Swimcizor—The Portable Fitness Machine
Quaker Plastic Corporation
1-888-288-6655

Water Wheel, Aqua Arm
Danmar
www.danmarproducts.com
1-800-783-1998

Speedo Fitness Barbell, Gloves, Elite Fitness Glove, Jog Belt, Surfrunner 2000, Slim Fin® by Force Fin®
Kast-A-Way Swimwear, Inc.
www.kastawayswimwear.com
1-800-543-2763

SHOES, TRAINING TOOLS, VIDEO AND AUDIO TAPES

Aqua Fit™ Ryka Water Fitness Shoes, Polar® Heart Rate Monitors, Karen Westfall's Senior Splash, Aqua Attack, Liquid Toning, Deck Coach by Chatter Vox™, heart rate charts
Hydro-Fit
www.hydrofit.org
1-800-346-7295

SNORKELS

Center Mount Snorkel
Finis, Inc.
www.lane4USA.com
1-888.33.FINIS

SWIM WEAR

Latex Free Swimwear
www.latexfreeswimwear.com
1-352-666-1485
H2O Wear
www.h2owear.com
1-800.321-7848

TETHERS/CORDS

Super Swim-Pro®
Super Swim, Inc.
1-800-848-1222
1-914-275-7600

Tether—3 tensions
Swimcords, Intl.
www.swimcords.com
1-800-482-7946

Mary Sanders Aquatic Tether
Fitness Wholesale®
www.fwonline.com
1-888-396-7337

TREADMILLS

Treadmill, skiing, climbing, cycling, rowing underwater machine
Neptune Aquatic Systems, Inc.
www.pooltherapy.com
1-513-575-2989

AquaGaiter, AquaCiser, Circuit Gym
Ferno-Washington, Inc.
www.ferno.com
1-800-733-3766

WHEEL CHAIRS

Assistive Technology
www.PVCDME.com
1-800-478-2363

Abilitations
www.Abilitations.com
1-800-850-8602

Kiefer
www.kiefer.com
1-800-323-4071

ADDITIONAL BUYER'S GUIDE WEB SITES

www.isoc.net/neptune
www.waterworkout.com
www.splashinternational.com
www.aquastyle.com
www.nzmfg.com
www.spectrumproducts.com
www.flaghouse.com
www.recreonics.com
www.aquaticsintl.com

REFERENCES

1. Hauss D: How to buy aquatic therapy equipment. Rehabil Today Apr 1994:45–49.
2. Aderhold KJ, Perry L: Jet hydrotherapy for labor and postpartum pain relief. Am J Matern Child Nurs 16:97–99, 1991.
3. Katz VL, Rozas L, Ryder R, Cefalo RC: Effect of daily immersion on the edema of pregnancy. Am J Perinatol 9:225–227, 1992.
4. Gehrke A, et al: Hydrotherapy in swellings with special reference to lymphedema. Z Lymphol 5:100–106, 1981.
5. Cirullo JA (ed): Aquatic Physical Therapy (special issue). Orthop Phys Ther Clin North Am 3(2): 1994.
6. McNeal RL: Aquatic therapy for patients with rheumatic disease. Rheum Dis Clin North Am 16:915–929, 1990.
7. Smit TE, Harrison R: Hydrotherapy and chronic lower back pain: a pilot study. Aust J Physiother 37:229–234, 1991.
8. Langridge JC, Phillips D: Group hydrotherapy exercises for chronic back pain sufferers: introduction and monitoring. Physiotherapy 74:269–273, 1988.
9. Cole AJ, Moschetti ML, Eagleston RA: Swimming. In White AH (ed): Spine Care. St Louis: Mosby, 1995, p 727.
10. Prins JH, Merritt DJ, Blancq RJ, et al: Effects of aquatic exercise training on muscle force in sedentary persons with polio disability. Presented at The American College of Sports Medicine Annual Meeting. Dallas, TX, 1992.
11. Morris DM: Aquatic rehabilitation for the treatment of neurologic disorder. J Back Musculoskel Rehabil 4:297–308, 1994.

12. Nashner LM: Sensory, neuromuscular, and biomechanical contributions to human balance. In Proceeding of the APTA Forum. Alexandria, VA: American Physical Therapy Association, 1989, pp 5–12.
13. Heyneman CA, Premo DE: A "water walkers" exercise program for the elderly. Public Health Rep 107:213–217, 1992.
14. Nicholas JJ: Physical modalities in rheumatological rehabilitation. Arch Phys Med Rehabil 75:994–1001, 1994.
15. Revay S, Dahlstrom M, Dalen N: Water exercise versus instruction for self-training following a shoulder fracture. Int J Rehabil Res 15:327–333, 1992.
16. Beasley B: Metabolic and heart rate responses to aquatic exercise [unpublished research]. Tampa, FL: University of Southern Florida, 1986.
17. Prins JH, Havriluk R: Measurement of changes in muscular strength in aquatic rehabilitation. Presented at XIIth International Congress on Biomechanics, University of Western Australia, Perth, Australia, 1991.
18. Lloyd A, Theil J, Holloman P, et al: Water exercise versus land exercise in cardiac patients [abstract]. J Cardiopulm Rehabil 1:10–12, 1986.
19. Cole AJ, Farrell JP, Stratton SA: Cervical spine athletic injuries: a pain in the neck. In Press J (ed): Physical Medicine and Rehabilitation Clinics of North America. Philadelphia: WB Saunders, 1994, p 37.
20. Salzman-Poteat A: Quantifying aquatic exercise with surface electromyography. Adv Phys Therapists PT Assist 6(26):Aug 1998.
21. Fuller R: Aquatic biofeedback treatment of PFPs. Sports Med Update 15(2):27–30, 2001.
22. Olsen P: Gravity-free zone. Phys Ther July/Aug 2000:19–23.
23. Babb B: Personal communication. Centers for Aquatic Rehabilitation, Philadelphia, 2001.
24. Moschetti M: Aquaphysics made simple. AquaTechnics Consulting Group, 1988.
25. Hunsaker J: A stainless reputation? Atmospheric chlorides can lead to corrosion of stainless steel. Aquatics Int May 2001:14–15.
26. Wolohan JT: Watch your step. Athletic Bus 25(12):18–22, Dec 2001.
27. Clement A: Legal responsibilities in aquatics: risk management—equipment. Aurora, OH: Sport and Law Press, 1997, pp 204–205.
28. Clement A: Aquatic therapy: using facilities, equipment and supervision. Adv Phys Therapists PT Assist Oct 2000:12–13.
29. Cole AJ, Moschetti, ML, Eagleston RA: The Water Scale™: a classification system for aquatic exercise. Manuscript in preparation, 1997.
30. Salzman-Poteat A: Aquatic specialty techniques glossary. ARN Newslett 5(1):7, 2000.
31. Boyle AJ: The Bad Ragaz ring method. Physiotherapy 67:265–268, 1981.
32. Cole AJ, Herring, SA: The Low Back Pain Handbook. Philadelphia: Hanley & Belfus, 1996.
33. Ruoti RG, Morris DM, Cole AJ (ed): Aquatic Rehabilitation for Health Professionals. Philadelphia: Lippincott, 1997.
34. Pellecchia GL: Lumbar traction: a review of the literature. J Orthop Sports Phys Ther 20(5):64–69, 1994.
35. Shaffer S: Spinal Traction in the Aquatic Environment. Course Notebook. Watsonville, CA: AquaTechnics Consulting Group, 2000.
36. Salzman-Poteat A: Fluid Moves: the Feldenkrais Method. ARN Newslett 4(2):2, 8, 1999.
37. Salzman-Poteat A: Aquatic task-type training approach. ARN Newslett 4(4):2,12, 2000.
37. Dunlap E: Swim stroke training and modification for rehabilitation. In Ruoti RG, Morris DM, Cole AJ (eds): Aquatic Rehabilitation for Health Professionals. Philadelphia: Lippincott, 1997.
39. Jamison L, Ogden D. Aquatic Therapy: Using PNF Patterns. San Antonio, TX: Therapy Skill Builders, 1994.
40. Bedgood D: Comparison of Water Exercise Equipment. Key West, FL: Kona Fitness (now AquaToner), 1982. Portions adapted and revised in Aquatic Resources Network Newslett 6(1):5, 2001.

Chapter 7
Aqua Running

Robert P. Wilder, MD, FACSM, and
David K. Brennan, MEd

Aqua running is an effective form of cardiovascular conditioning for both injured athletes and those who desire a low-impact aerobic workout. Sufficient cardiovascular responses have been demonstrated to result in a training effect.

Deep-water exercise is thus being used in the treatment and conditioning programs for a number of populations needing rehabilitation. This is especially true in the field of sports medicine, in which aqua running is used as an effective form of cardiovascular conditioning for injured athletes as well as for others who desire a low-impact aerobic workout. Aqua running, or deep-water running, consists of simulated running in the deep end of a pool aided by a flotation device (vest or belt) that maintains the head above water. The participant may be held in one location by a tether cord, thus essentially running in place, or may actually run through the water across the width of the pool. The tether serves to increase resistance, to assist in maintenance of a near vertical posture, and to facilitate monitoring of exercise by a physician, therapist, or coach. No contact is made with the bottom of the pool, thus eliminating impact. The elimination of weight load on joints makes this an ideal method for rehabilitating or conditioning injured athletes, particularly those with foot, ankle, or knee injuries for whom running on land is contraindicated.

Several positive influences of incorporating aqua running into a training program are summarized in the following:

1. Improvement or maintenance of fitness without the associated risk of impact loading
2. Improvement of biomechanics for running (especially upper body mechanics)
3. Decrease in thermal stress
4. Active recovery on days after hard workouts or races
5. Avoidance of training boredom through creative workouts
6. Increase in social component by allowing runners of all ability to train together
7. Improvement in respiratory muscle endurance

Understanding the bioengineering principles of the aquatic environment, proper technique, physiologic response, and methods of prescribing exercise helps practitioners incorporate aqua running into rehabilitation and training programs.

PRINCIPLES OF HYDROTHERAPY

Several properties of water make it an ideal environment for exercise.[1]

Buoyancy

Buoyancy supports a body submerged in water from the downward pull of gravity. The submerged body seems to lose weight equal to the weight of the water displaced, resulting in less stress and pressure on bone, muscle, and connective tissue.

Drag Force

The viscosity and drag force of water provide a resistance that is proportional to the effort exerted, much like running into a stiff wind. This adds to the cardiovascular challenge of aquatic exercise without having impact stress on joints and soft tissue.

Hydrostatic Pressure

Hydrostatic pressure (i.e., pressure exerted by water on a submerged body) is proportional to depth and equal in all directions. It is thought to aid cardiovascular function by promoting venous return.

Specific Heat

Specific heat is the amount of heat needed to raise the temperature of a substance by 1°C. The specific heat of water is several times that of air; therefore, the rate of heat loss in water is much greater than the rate of heat lost to air at the same temperature. This is an especially important consideration in warmer climates, where heat illness is a significant source of morbidity. It is also helpful in training injured athletes who are deconditioned and not acclimated to exercise in warm environments.

Temperature

The aquatic environment allows regulation of the temperature during exercise. An ideal range appears to be 82 to 86°F (28 to 30°C), where little heat is stored and performance is not impaired. In our experience, competitive athletes typically prefer a slightly cooler environment.

BIOMECHANICS OF AQUA RUNNING

The form of running in water is patterned as closely as possible to that used on land (Fig. 7-1). For the runner (or any athlete whose sport requires running), aqua running therefore represents a biomechanically specific means of conditioning

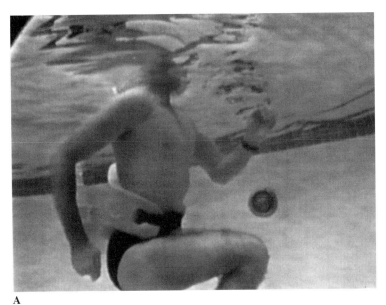 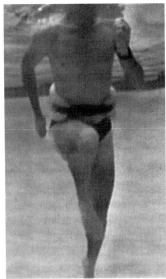

Figure 7-1. The form of running in water closely mimics the form used on land. Notice that the arm carriage is identical to that used with land-based running. *A,* Lateral view. *B,* Frontal view.

during a rehabilitation program or for supplementing regular training. This has special importance because the effects of training include not only improvement in cardiac and pulmonary performance but also improvement in the function of the muscle groups that undergo enzyme, capillary density, and other adaptations to exercise. Compared with land-based running, the elimination of weight bearing and the addition of resistance in aqua running change the relative contribution of each muscle group. Every effort is made, therefore, to reproduce the running form used on land and to ensure the use of the same muscle groups.

The following guidelines will assist the patient in maintaining proper form during aqua running[2]:

1. The water line should be at the shoulder level. The mouth should be comfortably out of the water without cervical spine extension. The head should be looking straight ahead, with the neck unflexed.
2. The body should assume a position slightly forward of the vertical, with the spine maintained in a neutral position.
3. Arm motion is identical to that used on land, with primary motion at the shoulder. Hands are held lightly clenched.
4. Hip flexion should reach 60 to 80 degrees. As the hip is being flexed, the leg is extended at the knee (from the flexed position). When end hip flexion is reached, the lower leg should be perpendicular to the horizontal. The hip and knee are then extended together, the knee reaching full extension when the hip is in a neutral position (0 degrees flexion). As the hip is extended, the leg is flexed at the knee. These movements are repeated, and throughout the cycle the foot undergoes dorsiflexion and plantarflexion at the ankle. The ankle is in a position of dorsiflexion when the hip is in a neutral position, and the leg is extended at the knee. Plantarflexion is assumed as the hip is extended and the leg is flexed.

Dorsiflexion is reassumed as the hip is flexed and the leg is extended. Underwater viewing demonstrates that inversion and eversion accompany dorsiflexion and plantarflexion, similar to land-based running.

EXERCISE RESPONSE TO AQUA RUNNING

The metabolic responses to aqua running and land-based running differ significantly.[3, 4] Nonetheless, aqua running elicits sufficient cardiovascular response to result in a training effect, thus supporting anecdotal evidence of its usefulness in the rehabilitation of the athlete. The American College of Sports Medicine Guidelines for Exercise Prescription state that to obtain a training effect, one must exercise three to five times per week at an intensity level between 40% and 85% of maximum oxygen uptake ($\dot{V}O_{2max}$) or 55% to 90% of maximum heart rate. This level should be maintained for 15 to 60 minutes.[5] Studies have demonstrated that aqua running elicits responses well within these suggested ranges.

Maximal Physiologic Responses

Several studies have compared the maximal physiologic responses to aqua running and land-based running.[6–16] Important measures of response to exercise of maximal intensity include $\dot{V}O_{2max}$ and maximal heart rate. $\dot{V}O_{2max}$ values during supported deep-water running (with a flotation device) are 73% to 92% of those obtained during land-based running. Heart rates during deep-water running range from 86% to 95% of those obtained during land-based running.

Similar relative perceived exertion (RPE) values have been reported for both deep-water running and treadmill running consistent with maximal effort. Cardiorespiratory efficiency as evidenced by O_2 pulse can be calculated as $\dot{V}O_2$/heart rate. Maximal O_2 pulse during deep-water running has been reported to be lower than during treadmill running.[8, 15] Reports have varied regarding lactate and ventilation. Blood lactate concentrations after deep-water running have been reported as higher than,[8] lower than,[9, 14, 15] and similar to[12] those after maximal treadmill running. Ventilation during deep-water running has been reported as both similar to[4, 12] and lower than[4, 6, 13, 14] during treadmill running.

Submaximal Physiologic Responses

Important relationships have also been noted during deep-water running at submaximal intensities. For a given level of RPE, heart rates and oxygen uptake levels tend to be lower during deep-water running than during treadmill running. During graded exercise testing, Svedenhag and Seger[8] noted higher central and peripheral ratings of RPE during deep-water running at any given $\dot{V}O_2$ or heart rate compared with treadmill running at the same intensity. Navia[11] reported a similar relationship between RPE and physiologic responses during graded exercise. Higher RPE values were expressed during deep-water running at any given heart rate than during treadmill running. A similar relationship was noted for RPE and $\dot{V}O_2$. These differences should be noted if perceived exertion is used as the sole measure of exercise intensity.

During submaximal deep-water running for 45 minutes, Bishop and colleagues[17] recorded lower mean $\dot{V}O_2$, ventilation, and respiratory exchange ratio (RER) values than those recorded during a 45-minute treadmill run at a comparable perceived exertion ($\dot{V}O_2$, 29.8 versus 40.6 mL/kg/min; ventilation, 58.1 L/min versus 79.1 L/min). Heart rates were also lower during deep-water running (122 versus 157 beats/min); however, this was not deemed statistically significant with the small sample involved ($n = 7$). Two participants, who were described as the most accomplished and enthusiastic deep-water runners, achieved similar responses during deep-water running and treadmill running, suggesting that motivation or familiarity may play a role in attaining levels of physiologic response.

Ritchie and Hopkins[18] noted that perceived exertion and perceived pain during a 30-minute deep-water run at a "hard" pace were comparable to those ratings obtained during "hard" treadmill running. These ratings were significantly greater than perceived exertions during treadmill running or road running at a "normal" training pace.

Examining the relationship between heart rate and $\dot{V}O_2$ during submaximal graded exercise, Svedenhag and Seger[8] reported lower heart rates during deep-water running than during treadmill running at any given level of oxygen uptake. Oxygen pulse was higher during submaximal exercise in the water. A similar relationship between heart rate and $\dot{V}O_2$ was noted by Navia[11] at higher work loads. These results suggest that an aerobic training effect may occur at lower heart rates during deep-water running than during treadmill running at submaximal levels. Svedenhag and Seger also reported higher RER and similar ventilation during deep-water running at submaximal intensity compared with land running.[8]

Yamaji and associates[19] noted significant interindividual variability in heart rate responses as a function of $\dot{V}O_2$ during unsupported deep-water running. Although group data revealed a similar $\dot{V}O_2$/heart rate relationship for both deep-water running and treadmill running, two of the more skilled participants did have lower heart rate values during deep-water running than during treadmill running at a comparative $\dot{V}O_2$. Ritchie and Hopkins[18] obtained heart rate values during a 30-minute session of hard deep-water running that were lower than those during hard treadmill running (159 versus 176 beats/min). Oxygen uptake values, however, were similar (49 versus 53 mL/kg/min). The heart rate values obtained during hard deep-water running were similar to those obtained during treadmill running at a normal training pace; however, corresponding oxygen uptake was greater during hard deep-water running. This study also supports the contention that deep-water running at submaximal levels may result in greater overall aerobic response if heart rate is used as the measure of exercise intensity.

Frangolias and Rhodes[12] demonstrated lower heart rate and $\dot{V}O_2$ values during aqua running than during treadmill running at the ventilatory threshold. RPE, RER, and ventilation were similar during both aqua running and treadmill running at the ventilatory threshold.

Michaud and colleagues[20] examined eight trained runners completing three separate 15-minute tests as follows: (1) treadmill run at 75% treadmill $\dot{V}O_{2max}$, (2) water run at 75% water run $\dot{V}O_{2max}$, and (3) water run at 75% treadmill $\dot{V}O_{2max}$. Heart rate and $\dot{V}O_2$ were similar during both deep-water running and treadmill running. Blood lactate, RER, and RPE were greater during deep-water running. This study suggests that heart rate may be more reflective of the aerobic demands of deep-water running than RPE.[20, 21]

Gerhing and associates[22] demonstrated that competitive runners were able to maintain similar $\dot{V}O_2$ values during 20-minute submaximal treadmill and water running sessions, whereas noncompetitive runners had lower $\dot{V}O_2$ values in the water compared with those on land. This study suggests that more accomplished runners may be able to utilize aqua running with greater efficiency than noncompetitive runners.

During submaximal running at heart rates equivalent to 60% and 80% of treadmill $\dot{V}O_{2max}$, DeMaere and Ruby[21] demonstrated higher RER and carbohydrate metabolism and lower fat oxidation during deep-water running than during land-based running. Ventilation was higher during deep-water running compared with treadmill running at 80% $\dot{V}O_{2max}$. $\dot{V}O_2$, RPE, and energy expenditure did not differ significantly between trials.

Long-Term Training Effects

Several studies have reported on the long-term effects of a deep-water exercise program. Michaud and associates[10] reported that 10 subjects who underwent an 8-week training program of aqua running showed improvements in $\dot{V}O_2$ during both water-based and land-based graded exercise testing (19.6% and 10.7%, respectively), thus demonstrating a training effect as well as a crossover effect to land-based exercise. Eyestone and colleagues[23] demonstrated that deep-water running was comparable to land-based running and cycling for preserving levels of fitness during a 6-week training period at maintenance duration (20 to 30 minutes) and frequency (three to five times per week). Although a small decrease in $\dot{V}O_{2max}$ was noted for each group, this was much less than the 16% to 17% loss previously reported during a 6-week rest period.

Wilber and colleagues[24] demonstrated no significant differences in treadmill $\dot{V}O_{2max}$, ventilatory threshold, running economy, and blood lactate at $\dot{V}O_{2max}$ after 6 weeks of training in two groups: one training on land and the other training exclusively in water. Additionally, glucose and norepinephrine levels were similar between the two groups. Of note, both groups improved treadmill $\dot{V}O_{2max}$ levels with the land-based training group improving 13.8% and the water training group improving 9.2%. Bushman and associates[25] found no significant differences in a simulated 5-km run time, submaximal and maximal oxygen consumption, or lactate threshold after 4 weeks of deep-water training in recreationally competitive distance runners.

Quinn and colleagues[26] reported a 7% decrease in $\dot{V}O_{2max}$ after a 4-week deep-water training program. Their subjects, however, were previously unfamiliar with deep-water running and exercised at minimum maintenance levels of intensity, duration, and frequency only. Furthermore, the description of the technique as a "high knee bicycle motion" suggests that the less than full range of running motion during aqua running may have influenced results.

These training studies suggest that when performed with proper technique and intensity, deep-water running can provide a stimulus great enough to maintain and even improve running fitness.

Discussion

There are several possible explanations for the differences in metabolic response to deep-water running and land-based running. Differences in muscle use and activation patterns contribute to these differences in exercise response. Furthermore, because weight bearing is eliminated and resistance is increased, the larger muscle groups of the lower extremities do less work, and a comparatively increased proportion of work is done by the upper extremities. This may contribute to the lower maximal oxygen uptakes recorded during deep-water running. Lower perfusion pressures in the legs during immersion, with resultant decreases in total muscle blood flow, also have been proposed to influence a higher anaerobic metabolism during deep-water running.[8]

Hydrostatic pressure is thought to assist in cardiac performance by promoting venous return; thus, the heart does not have to beat as fast to maintain cardiac output. This may contribute to the lower heart rates observed during both submaximal and maximal deep-water running. Temperature also has been demonstrated to have an effect on heart rate during exercise, with higher temperatures correlating with higher heart rates.

Town and Bradley[9] suggested that decreased blood flow to the lower extremities during deep-water running may be responsible in those persons in whom lower blood lactate was measured during deep-water running. Frangolias and Rhodes,[4] however, suggested that level of familiarity with deep-water running may play the most important role in the variability in blood lactate response during deep-water running. It has also been suggested that in those persons in whom ventilation is reduced during deep-water running, an increase in intrathoracic blood volume and hydrostatic chest compression results in an increase in the force required for inspiration by reducing total lung compliance and vital capacity. However, it has also been suggested that a proportionally greater increase in central blood flow during water immersion may compensate for the reduced lung compliance in those persons in whom ventilation is similar.[12]

Familiarity with this form of exercise appears to be an important factor in maximizing the physiologic response to deep-water running when measured at a particular level of perceived exertion. In our experience at The Runner's Clinic at University of Virginia and the Houston International Running Center, strict adherence to proper form and technique ensures a higher physiologic response as measured by $\dot{V}o_2$ and heart rate.

EXERCISE PRESCRIPTION FOR AQUA RUNNING

Three measures are used for grading the intensity of aqua running exercises: (1) heart rate, (2) rating of perceived exertion, and (3) cadence. Workout programs typically are designed to reproduce the work the athlete would do on land and to incorporate both long runs and interval/speed training.

Heart Rate

There is a high correlation between heart rate and oxygen uptake. The American College of Sports Medicine guidelines recommend that for a training effect, one should exercise at a level between 55% and 90% of the maximum heart rate (the target heart rate range).[5] The maximum heart rate can be estimated (220 minus age) or can be based upon heart rate levels attained during exercise of maximum effort. Although heart rate levels in the water tend to be lower than those on land, it is possible to approach land-based values by adherence to proper technique. Heart rate can be monitored by a waterproof heart rate monitor or periodically by palpation.

Rating of Perceived Exertion

Rating of perceived exertion refers to the patient's subjective grading of level of exertion.[27, 28] Perceived exertion for jogging is rated as low, whereas sprinting is rated with a high level of perceived exertion. A high correlation has been identified between perceived exertion and physiologic variables during deep-water running.[2, 29] The most commonly used scale of perceived exertion is the Borg Scale, a 15-point scale with verbal descriptors ranging from very, very light to very, very hard (Table 7-1). For distance runners, we use the Brennan Scale, a 5-point scale designed exclusively for aqua running; verbal descriptors for this scale range from very light to very hard (Table 7-2).[2] We further instruct our athletes that level 1 (very light) corresponds to a recovery jog, level 2 (light) to a long easy run, level 3 (somewhat hard) to a brisk run, level 4 (hard) to 5- to 10-km pace, and level 4.5 to 5 (very hard) to track intervals. The Brennan Scale facilitates the incorporation of both speed and distance work into workouts in a manner easily understood by both coach and athlete. A sample workout protocol is presented in Figure 7-2. A separate perceived exertion scale is used for sprinters (Table 7-3).

Cadence

Wilder and colleagues[30] demonstrated a very high correlation between cadence and heart rate with intraindividual correlations averaging 0.98. Competitive athletes undergo a graded exercise test of aqua running following our standard protocol (Fig. 7-3). Cadence is controlled by an auditory metronome. By recording heart rate

Table 7-1. Borg Scale of Perceived Exertion

Level	RPE
6	
7	Very, very light
8	
9	Very light
10	
11	Light
12	
13	Somewhat hard
14	
15	Hard
16	
17	Very hard
18	
19	Very, very hard

From Borg GV: Psychophysical basis of perceived exertion. Med Sci Sports Exerc 14:377–387, 1982.

Table 7-2. Brennan Scale of Perceived Exertion and Cadence Values for Distance Runners

Level	RPE	CPM*	Land Equivalent
1	Very light		
	1.0	<55	Recovery jog
	1.5	55–59	
2	Light		
	2.0	60–64	Easy run
	2.5	65–69	
3	Somewhat hard		
	3.0	70–74	Brisk run
	3.5	75–79	
4	Hard		
	4.0	80–84	5–10 km pace
	4.5	85–89	Long track intervals
5	Very hard		
	5.0	>90	Short track intervals

*Measured as the number of times each limb moves through a complete cycle per minute (CPM).

From Brennan DK, Wilder RP: Aqua Running: An Instructor's Manual. Houston, TX: Houston International Running Center, 1999. Used with permission.

responses to various levels of cadence, we can anticipate an expected physiologic response to a particular cadence level. Workouts then can be designed that use timed intervals at particular cadence levels.

Studies that have measured leg speed (cadence) as a measured variable of deep-water running intensity reported lower cadences than those during land running at submaximal levels (60% to 70% of peak $\dot{V}O_2$ and heart rate).[2] As subjects in the water approach peak workloads, cadences begin to more closely match those on land. For the elite athlete this may suggest a higher degree of biomechanical

Workout #1

Total Work-out Time	No. of Repetitions	Duration of Repetitions (min)	Exertion Level	Recovery Periods (sec)
37 min	5	× 2	@ SH	30
	8	× 1	@ H	30
	5	× 2	@ SH	30

Figure 7-2. Sample workout protocol. In this case, the workout protocol (#1) would call for 5 repetitions of 2 minutes (2:00) duration each at a perceived exertion level of somewhat hard, followed by 8 repetitions of 1 minute (1:00) duration each at a perceived exertion level of hard, followed by 5 repetitions of 2 minutes (2:00) duration each at a perceived exertion level of somewhat hard, with a 30-second (:30) recovery period consisting of easy jogging after each interval, for a total workout time of 37 minutes (37:00). (From Brennan DK, Wilder RP. Aqua Running: An Instructor's Manual. Houston, TX: Houston International Running Center, 1999.)

Table 7-3. Modified Brennan Scale of Perceived Exertion and Cadence Values for Sprinters

RPE	CPM	Land Equivalent
Very light		
1.0	<74	>800 m
1.5	75–79	
Light		
2.0	80–84	600–800 m
2.5	85–90	
Somewhat hard		
3.0	90–94	400–600 m
3.5	95–99	
Hard		
4.0	100–104	200–400 m
4.5	105–109	
Very hard		
5.0	>110	50–200 m

specificity for deep-water running at intensities that approach 80% to 90% of peak workloads. Additional studies are needed to evaluate and standardize sport-specific biomechanical models for deep-water running.

Measurement of heart rate is used primarily during long runs: prolonged periods of exercise at a specified rate (the target heart rate). RPE and cadence ratings are most often used for interval sessions. RPE is most helpful in group settings, whereas cadence is most appropriate for individual sessions.

PRACTICAL GUIDELINES FOR CLINICIANS

Our athletes typically undergo one or two individual sessions for familiarization and to ensure proper technique. A flotation device is used because it is difficult to adhere to proper technique without support. The athletes then undergo our graded exercise test (GXT), allowing us to correlate cadence and perceived exertion to heart rate responses. Workouts are then designed using perceived exertion and cadence to effect a particular level of physiologic response. Training schedules are designed to follow closely the work that the athlete would do on land. Thus, for example, if an athlete were scheduled to run 6 × 600 m at a pace of 2 minutes each on the track, the athlete would perform six 2-minute intervals in the water at a Brennan RPE level of 4. Longer runs may call for aqua running of up to 1 to 2 hours at a Brennan RPE level of 2.

For nonrunners and athletes seeking general conditioning and fitness maintenance only, three to four sessions per week are performed at maintenance duration (15 to 60 minutes) and intensity (55% to 90% maximal heart rate). Aqua running is also effectively incorporated into cross-training programs involving other forms of exercise such as biking and stair-climbing.

As the athlete gradually returns to land-based running, sessions are tapered; however, many athletes choose to incorporate one or two sessions of aqua running per week into their regular training programs.

Name: _____   Date: _____

Predicted 90% maximum heart rate: _____

Stage	End Point	Cadence (gait cycles/min)	Heart Rate	RPE	Comments
W	at 4 min	48			
1	at 6 min	66			
2	at 8 min	69			
3	at 10 min	72			
4	at 12 min	76			
5	at 14 min	80			
6	at 16 min	84			
7	at 18 min	88			
8	at 20 min	92			
9	at 22 min	96			
10	at 24 min	100			
11	at 26 min	104			
Post	at 27 min	48			
	at 28 min	48			
	at 29 min	48			

Figure 7-3. Houston International Running Center Data Collection Sheet: Modified Wilder Graded Exercise Test for Aqua Running. W, warm-up phase; Post values represent postexercise values during cool down. (Copyright 1990, Houston International Running Center, Houston, TX; used with permission.)

AQUA RUNNING FOR SPECIAL POPULATIONS

We have incorporated aqua running into fitness and rehabilitation programs for nonathletes as well. These include patients with lumbar spine disorders, arthritis, and degenerative joint disease, patients who have undergone orthopedic surgery, lower extremity amputees, and women with uncomplicated pregnancies. We emphasize neutral spine mechanics for patients with lumbar spine disease. These mechanics are then incorporated into land-based exercises. Technique is generally modified in patients with arthritis and degenerative joint disease as well as in patients who have undergone orthopedic surgery so they can exercise within pain-free ranges. In pregnant women who do not have contraindications to exercise during pregnancy, mild to moderate exercise may be performed consistent with fitness level; however, women are counseled not to exercise to exhaustion and to stop exercising if they experience any signs of overexertion, hyperthermia, dehydration, or fetal distress.[31]

CONCLUSION

Despite the differences between deep-water running and land-based running, deep-water running does elicit the physiologic responses necessary to promote a training effect as defined by the American College of Sports Medicine (40% to 85% $\dot{V}O_{2max}$ or 55% to 90% maximum heart rate). These responses can be maximized by adherence to proper technique and by the use of environment-specific means of exercise prescription (established specifically for deep-water exercise). Deep-water running also offers additional benefits, most notably the maintenance of quick turnover (rapid gait cycling) as well as coordinated movements between the arms and legs. These aspects facilitate return to land-based training.

Maintaining conditioning is a challenge for the injured athlete. Aqua running is an effective way to continue training during rehabilitation and can later be incorporated into a regular training program, providing a low-stress form of additional cardiovascular exercise.

Further research will help define the effect of aqua running on physiologic parameters other than oxygen uptake and heart rate as well as responses in special populations. Questions have also been raised regarding differences between shallow-water and deep-water exercise. The increasing interest in aquatic exercise and research will help us answer these questions and expand the use of aquatic exercise in rehabilitation and fitness.

REFERENCES

1. Edlich RF, Towler MA, Goitz RJ, et al: Bioengineering principles of hydrotherapy. J Burn Care Rehabil 8:580–584, 1987.
2. Brennan DK, Wilder RP: Aqua Running: An Instructor's Manual. Houston, TX: Houston International Running Center, 1999.
3. Wilder RP, Brennan DK: Physiologic responses to deep water running in athletes. Sports Med 16:374–380, 1993.
4. Frangolias DD, Rhodes EC: Metabolic responses to mechanisms during water immersion running and exercise. J Sports Med 22:38, 1996.

5. American College of Sports Medicine: Guidelines for graded exercise testing and prescription, 4th ed. Philadelphia: Lea & Febiger, 1991.
6. Butts NK, Tucker M, Smith R: Maximal responses to treadmill and deep water running in high school female cross country runners. Res Q Exer Sports 62:236–239, 1991.
7. Butts NK, Tucker M, Greening C: Physiologic responses to maximal treadmill and deep water running in men and women. Am J Sports Med 19:612–614, 1991.
8. Svedenhag J, Seger J: Running on land and in water: comparative exercise physiology. Med Sci Sports Exerc 24:1155–1160, 1992.
9. Town GP, Bradley SS: Maximal metabolic responses of deep and shallow water running in trained runners. Med Sci Sports Exerc 23:238–241, 1991.
10. Michaud TJ, Brennan DK, Wilder RP, et al: Aqua running and gains in cardiorespiratory fitness. J Strength Cond Res 9(2):78–84, 1995.
11. Navia AM: Comparison of energy expenditure between treadmill running and water running [thesis]. University of Alabama at Birmingham, 1986.
12. Frangolias DD, Rhodes EC: Maximal and ventilatory threshold responses to treadmill and water immersion running. Med Sci Sports Exerc 27:1007, 1995.
13. Dowzer CN, Reilly T, Cable NT, et al: Maximal physiological responses to deep water and shallow water running. Ergonomics 42:275, 1999.
14. Nakanishi Y: Maximal physiologic responses to deep water running at thermonuclear temperature. Appl Hum Sci 18:31, 1999.
15. Nakanishi Y: Physiologic responses to maximal treadmill and deep water running in young and middle age males. Appl Hum Sci 18:81, 1999.
16. Melton-Rogers S: Cardiorespiratory responses of patients with rheumatoid arthritis during bicycle riding and running in water. Phys Ther 76:1058, 1996.
17. Bishop PA, Frazier S, Smith J, et al: Physiologic responses to treadmill and water running. Physician Sportsmed 17:87–94, 1989.
18. Ritchie SE, Hopkins WG: The intensity of exercise in deep water running. Int J Sports Med 12:27–29, 1991.
19. Yamaji K, Greenly M, Northey DR, et al: Oxygen uptake and heart rate responses to treadmill and deep water running. Can J Sports Sci 15:96–98, 1990.
20. Michaud TJ, Rodriguez-Zayas J, Andres FF, et al: Comparative exercise responses of deep water running and treadmill running. J Strength Cond Res 9:104–109, 1995.
21. DeMaere JM, Ruby BC: Effects of deep water running and treadmill running on oxygen uptake and energy expenditure in seasonally trained cross-country runners. J Sports Med Phys Fitness 37:175, 1997.
22. Gehring MM, Keller BA, Brehm BA: Water running with and without a flotation vest in competitive and recreational runners. Med Sci Sports Exerc 29:1374–1378, 1997.
23. Eyestone ED, Fellingham G, George J, et al: Effect of water running and cycling on maximum oxygen consumption and 2-mile run performance. Am J Sports Med 21:41–44, 1993.
24. Wilber RL, Moffat RJ, Scott BE, et al: Influence of water run training on the maintenance of physiological determinants of aerobic performance. Med Sci Sports Exerc 28:1056–1062, 1996.
25. Bushman BA, Flynn MG, Andres FF, et al: Effect of four weeks of deep water run training on running performance. Med Sci Sports Exerc 29:694–699, 1997.
26. Quinn TJ, Sedory DR, Fisher BS: Physiological effects of deep water running following a land-based training program. Res Q Exerc Sport 65:386–389, 1994.
27. Borg GV: Psychophysical basis of perceived exertion. Med Sci Sports Exerc 14:377–387, 1982.
28. Carlton RL, Rhodes EC: Critical review of the literature on rating scales for perceived exertion. Sports Med 2:198–222, 1985.
29. Brown SP, Chitwood LF, Beason KR, et al: Physiological correlates with perceived exertion during deep water running. Percept Mot Skills 83:155–162, 1996.
30. Wilder RP, Brennan DK, Schotte DE: A standard measure for exercise prescription for aqua running. Am J Sports Med 21:45–48, 1993.
31. American College of Obstetricians and Gynecologists: Exercise during pregnancy and the postpartum period (Technical Bulletin 189). Washington, DC: American College of Gynecology, 1994.

Chapter 8
Aquatic Rehabilitation for the Treatment of Neurologic Disorders

David M. Morris, MS, PT

Injury or disease affecting the central or peripheral nervous system can result in a wide variety of primary movement problems involving motor, sensory, perceptual, cognitive, and behavioral systems. Additionally, primary impairments (e.g., paralysis or spasticity) can lead to secondary movement problems that do not result directly from the nervous system lesion but rather develop over time. For example, paralysis resulting directly from spinal cord injury can lead, over time, to joint tightness and limited range of motion (ROM). Both primary and secondary impairments often significantly contribute to functional problems including walking, reaching, and general execution of activities of daily living (ADLs). Aquatic rehabilitation offers a unique, versatile approach for treating these impairments and the disabilities they create. Such programs range from skilled therapy to wellness services.[1]

The need for neurorehabilitation services has increased. Improved technology and medical management have allowed more individuals to survive head injuries, brain tumors, strokes, birth injuries, and premature birth.[2-4] In addition, longer life expectancies may account for the increased prevalence of neurologic disorders. Currently, our health care system requires increased accountability by the rehabilitation professional, especially with regard to reimbursement for services. Therefore, neurorehabilitation professionals must seek ever more effective treatment strategies. Aquatic rehabilitation has been advocated by many as a useful treatment modality for patients with neurologic disorders.[5-14] The unique properties of water, particularly its buoyancy and turbulence, enable the design of effective and versatile treatment programs.[5-8, 15, 16] Specific benefits of the aquatic environment include weight relief and ease of movement. These characteristics allow safe movement exploration, strengthening, and functional activity training, often before patients can perform the same activities on land. Also, the supportive properties of water allow easy handling of patients by aquatic therapy professionals. In this chapter, the problems encountered by patients with neurologic disorders, the general principles guiding neurotreatment, and aquatic neurorehabilitation approaches are examined. For the purposes of this chapter, neurologic disorders include stroke, head injury, spinal cord injury, cerebral palsy, brain tumors, and Parkinson's disease.

DESCRIPTION OF NEUROLOGIC DISORDERS

Problems encountered during the treatment of patients with neurologic disorders can be classified according to the International Classification of Impairments, Disabilities, and Handicap (ICIDH).[17] According to the ICIDH, an impairment is any loss or abnormality of an organ, structure, or function. Impairments commonly encountered with neurologic disorders are listed in Table 8-1. A disability is any reduction, partial or total, in the capacity to carry out a functional activity within the range considered normal for the average human being. Typical disabilities include walking, performing transfers, and reaching. A handicap is an externally imposed disadvantage that limits or prevents the fulfillment of usual social roles, depending on age, sex, and culture. Typical neurologic handicaps include physical barriers, attitudinal barriers, lowered expectations (the patient's), and fear (the patient's). The application of aquatic rehabilitation approaches can influence neurologic disorders at any or all of these levels.

Rehabilitation of Patients with Neurologic Disorders

The physical rehabilitation approach to examination and management of persons with neurologic disorders has evolved through the years. These changes, occurring in response to societal and technologic advances, have been outlined by Gordon, Horak, and others.[2-4]

Motor Control Models

Assumptions about how humans create and control movement profoundly influence the way patients are examined and managed. Three motor control models—the reflex model, the hierarchical model, and the systems model—have received the most attention from the rehabilitation professional community.[2-4] The reflex model

Table 8-1. Common Impairments Associated with Neurologic Dysfunction

Muscle weakness
  Paresis
  Paralysis
Abnormalities of muscle tone
  Spasticity
  Rigidity
  Hypotonia
Coordination problems
Activation and sequencing problems
Timing problems
Scaling problems
Involuntary movements
  Dystonia
Associated movements
  Tremor
Choreiform and athetoid movements

assumes that human movement occurs in response to sensory input to the central nervous system (CNS). For example, when a person is sitting in a car that quickly accelerates, sensory input into the vestibular system facilitates forward neck and trunk flexion and protective extension of the arms. These movements counterbalance backward displacement and prevent the individual from falling back into the car seat. In studies with animals whose sensory endings were intentionally destroyed, the animals still exhibited coordinated, purposeful movement[18] as well as the ability to move in anticipation of a postural disturbance (feed-forward control).[19] Therefore, a reflex model does not fully explain the production of skilled movement.

The hierarchical model views the CNS as a top-down control pattern in which the higher centers of the cerebral cortex control the lower centers of the brainstem and spinal cord. The lower centers are in charge of more primitive, reflex types of movement; the higher centers control the more complex, voluntary types of movement. Limitations of this model cited have been based on studies in which experimentally induced lesions of the midbrains of cats (i.e., disruption of connections between higher and lower CNS structures) failed to prohibit coordinated, purposeful movement.[20] Reflexive movements may appropriately override voluntary movements for functional purposes in normal humans. For example, when one steps on a nail, the injured foot reflexively withdraws while the supporting limb extends. A purely hierarchical view of motor control appears inaccurate.

Unlike the reflex and hierarchical models, the systems model does not regard the CNS as being solely responsible for motor control. In this model, movement results from interaction among many different kinds of systems, including environmental, musculoskeletal, sensorimotor, and cognitive. No particular system is always in control of others; instead, which is more important depends on the task at hand. In addition, the movement exhibited cannot be explained as a mere additive effect of each individual system. In other words, resulting movements occur secondary to interactions between the systems. There are problems with this view of motor control. The underlying systems whose unique interactions result in movement have yet to be well defined, and the relationship of these systems to neuroanatomic structures is not well understood.[2-4]

Neurorehabilitation Models

The intervention approaches used by rehabilitation professionals are many and varied. Most, however, can be easily aligned with one of three models of neurorehabilitation.[2-4] In the early days of neurorehabilitation, most patients served by therapists had poliomyelitis. The prevalent rehabilitation model was a muscle reeducation model wherein therapists strengthened weak musculature and provided orthopedic support or bracing for body segments to which strength would not return. Patients with neurologic disorders were treated in a similar manner. Many professionals were dissatisfied with the muscle reeducation approach. The plasticity (ability to recover) of the CNS was not considered, and patients with neurologic disorders often had more difficulty with patterns of movement and could not isolate specific muscle actions. This led to a general shift to a neurotherapeutic facilitation approach.

Developed in the 1950s, the neurotherapeutic facilitation model was the basic philosophy followed by many theorists, including the Bobaths, Knott and Voss, Ayres, Rood, and Stockmeyer. Treatment approaches developed from this model dominated the field of neurorehabilitation for the next 30 years and still have a strong influence on neurorehabilitation practices. With this model, therapists facilitate normal (or desirable) movement patterns by providing sensory input. Careful steps are taken to inhibit abnormal muscle tone and to avoid abnormal movement patterns and primitive reflexes.

Dissatisfaction with this model arises from the apparent lack of functional carryover; that is, the avoidance of primitive or abnormal movement patterns does not necessarily produce normal functional movement. Also, the patient's role was largely passive, responding to the therapist's sensory input. Finally, the model explained neurologic movement disorders as the result of an aberrant CNS, but it failed to take into account musculoskeletal and environmental influences on movement.

In recent years, another major shift has occurred. Research of contemporary movement science indicates that functionally oriented neurotreatment, in which patients are more active problem solvers, may be more effective than treatments based on earlier models.[4] This has led many rehabilitation experts to endorse a task-oriented approach to neurorehabilitation. Strategies based on this school of thought incorporate the practice of specific functional tasks. Patients learn to develop effective, efficient compensatory strategies to carry out these skills. They also learn adaptability by performing these tasks under a variety of musculoskeletal and environmental constraints (e.g., on different surfaces, with different obstacles to avoid, or in different lighting). More attention is placed on the patient's ability to perform a task than on which specific movement pattern is used. Like the other neurorehabilitation models, a task-oriented model has dissatisfying aspects. Many patients receiving neurotreatment have a limited ability to participate as active problem solvers due to major physical or mental impairments. Also, it is difficult to retrain a person's ability to anticipate the need for a particular motor strategy.

To review,

1. The muscle reeducation model does not consider incorporating any of the principles of the reflex, hierarchical, or systems models of motor control.
2. The neurotherapeutic facilitation model assumes reflex and hierarchical principles of motor control.
3. The task-oriented approach incorporates principles from all three models of motor control.

As the field of neurorehabilitation has evolved, rehabilitation professionals have expanded their views regarding examination and management of persons with neurologic disorders. All three of the aforementioned neurorehabilitation approaches can be used effectively, depending on a particular patient's problems and goals. A working knowledge of the assumptions underlying these models, however, is crucial for correct execution of these strategies.

AQUATIC NEUROREHABILITATION

Aquatic rehabilitation approaches have been promoted for treating patients with neurologic disorders.[5-14] The guiding principles of each and their relationship to general neurorehabilitation approaches are described later in this section. First, general principles for aquatic neurorehabilitation are discussed.

General Guidelines for Treatment Design

A number of factors must be considered when aquatic rehabilitation programs are designed. In the author's opinion, the factors discussed in the following are most influential in aquatic treatment design for neurologically impaired patients.[12, 14]

Depth of the Water

Because buoyant support increases as more of the body is submerged, patients who have difficulty standing can perform exercises more easily in deeper water. Therefore, exercises should be performed first in deeper water with a progression to more shallow depths. One exception to this guideline is arm exercises. Performing such activities in shallow water may prevent patients from submerging the entire upper extremity to maximize buoyancy assistance to movement or resistance from the water's drag.

Unilateral versus Bilateral Movements

The resistant drag produced with movement in the water increases effort for the patient.[15, 16] When a submerged extremity is moved, the increased effort challenges the stability provided by the moving individual's trunk and proximal segments. This increased effort can be minimized if the patient moves only one extremity, particularly if the other extremity is used to provide additional stability (e.g., holding on to the side of the pool or standing on the pool's floor). As the patient's ability to stabilize improves, bilateral movements should be attempted. Regarding resistive force produced and challenging proximal stability, asymmetric bilateral movements (e.g., moving the right shoulder into flexion while simultaneously moving the left shoulder into extension) are generally easier than symmetric bilateral movements (e.g., both shoulders moving into flexion simultaneously).

Distal Stabilization

When the distal end of a moving body segment is contacting an object with stable properties, the patient performing the activity can incorporate the support into his or her ability to stabilize.[12] Therefore, these distal end–stable activities are generally easier to accomplish than when the distal end of a moving body segment moves free of stabilization (distal end–free). Stability-providing objects may or may not be fixed and stationary. For example, although a free-floating buoyant ring is not fixed to the side of the pool, it still provides stability. Examples of distal end–stable aquatic activities include resting a hand on a kick board and moving across the surface of the water in shoulder-horizontal abduction-adduction or performing most Bad Ragaz Ring Method (BRRM) activities. Distal end–free aquatic activities are performed without the additional distal support from an external source. Examples of these activities include performing a swimming stroke or deep-water running.

Speed and Excursion of Movement

As a person immersed in water slightly increases the speed of his or her movement, the resistance encountered dramatically increases. Similarly, as patients move through greater ROM, the difficulty of the activity also increases. Therefore, patients should begin activities slowly and through small ROM and gradually increase both as skill allows. A general guideline is to instruct patients to move as quickly and as far as they can and still do the activity in a comfortable, correct manner. Improper movement patterns are an indication that the patient is exceeding his or her abilities of speed and excursion.

Patient's Position

As on land, certain body positions assumed in the water are easier to control than others. Unfortunately, many patients automatically assume the least stable positions when allowed to do so. Campion[7, 8] described four positions commonly assumed during therapeutic pool activities: the ball, cube, triangle, and stick positions. These positions are listed from the most to least stable. Although the ball position is the most stable, it is probably the least used during patient care. Instead, the cube is the most practical for use with patients. By submerging the body, assuming a sitting position, and extending the arms, the patient positions the trunk and extremities in a manner that maximizes the buoyant support provided by the water (Fig. 8-1). As the patient gains more skill and independence, he or she can assume the triangle position (Fig. 8-2) and the stick position (Fig. 8-3), in which less of the body is submerged and supported by buoyant forces. Less-skilled patients should

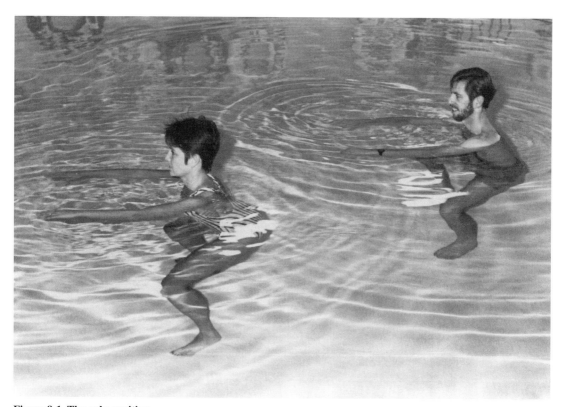

Figure 8-1. The cube position.

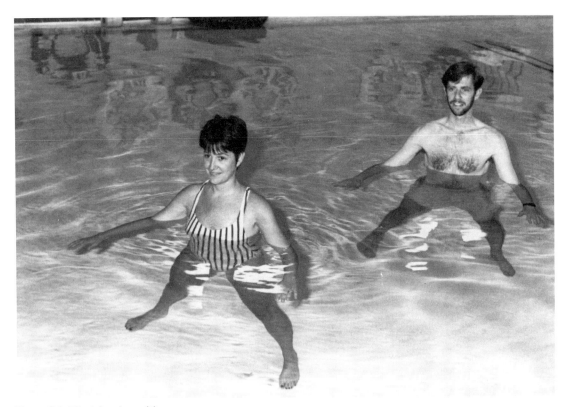

Figure 8-2. The triangle position.

first attempt activities in a more stable position and move toward performing activities in less stable positions as skill progresses.

Water Shiatsu

Water Shiatsu (Watsu) was developed by Harold Dull at Harbin Hot Springs in Middletown, California.[21, 22] Dull describes the technique as Zen Shiatsu principles applied to people floating in the water. Watsu was created as a wellness technique; it was not originally intended for patients with neurologic disorders. Rehabilitation therapists have applied the approach to patients with a variety of physical disorders, however, and reports indicate clinical success.[21, 23] Based on Eastern medicine theory, Watsu stretches the body's meridians (pathways of energy). Through stretching, these pathways are believed to be brought closer to the body's surface, where energy can be released. These effects are enhanced by rotational movements that release blocked energy from joint articulations. Additionally, the slow rhythmical rotational movements used reduce hypertonicity through tone-inhibiting vestibular stimulation. As a completely passive recipient, the patient experiences profound relaxation from the water's support and the continual, rhythmic movement that flows gracefully from one position to the next. The stretches comprise specifically described transitions and sequences of movement including the basic moves, head cradle sequence, near leg over sequence, far leg

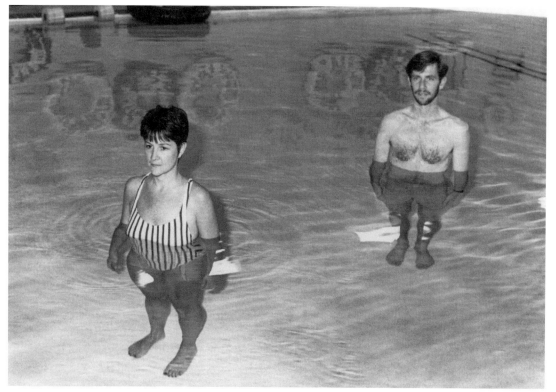

Figure 8-3. The stick position.

over sequence, and saddle sequence.[21, 22] In general, the therapist stabilizes or moves one segment of the body while movement through the water, resulting in a drag effect, stretches another segment. After the transitions and sequences are learned, therapists are encouraged to vary them according to the needs and limitations of the patient.

Water Shiatsu for Patients with Neurologic Disorders

Patients with neurologic disorders often exhibit ROM limitations resulting from soft-tissue restrictions.[4, 24, 25] These limitations can negatively influence functional recovery by preventing patients from moving into positions that are biomechanically efficient. Also, many tone and voluntary movement disorders are magnified when muscle tissue becomes shortened, creating increased resistance to movement.[4, 24, 25] The application of Watsu to these tight body segments can improve flexibility. Also, persons with neurologic dysfunction may have a lowered threshold to muscle contraction due to hyperexcitability at the spinal level.[4, 24, 25] As a result, involuntary movements or sustained voluntary contractions can interfere with the normal, reciprocal active movement needed for functional skill. When applied using slow, rhythmic rotational movements, stimulation to the vestibular system sends inhibitory input down the lateral vestibulospinal tract of the spinal

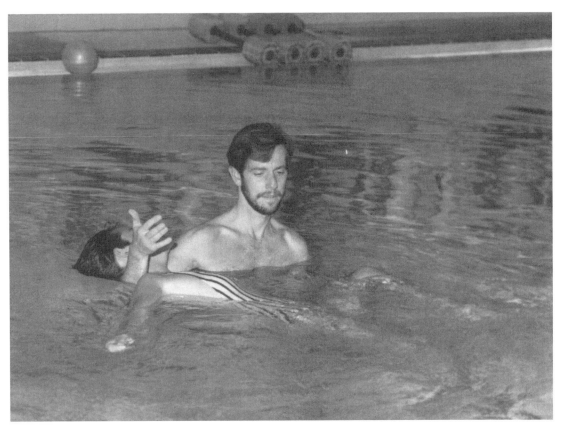

Figure 8-4. Using a Water Shiatsu maneuver, the therapist increases hip rotation flexibility.

cord, resulting in full body relaxation and muscle tone reduction. This technique is particularly helpful when applied at the beginning of a treatment session, preparing the patient to move in a less restricted fashion during more active portions of the treatment session. Maneuvers that may have specific applications to patients with neurologic impairments are the near leg rotation (promoting internal and external hip rotation) (Fig. 8-4), the leg push (promoting hip extension), and the accordion (promoting hip and trunk flexion).[21, 22] Vogtle and associates[23] published a case report concerning the application of Watsu for six adults with cerebral palsy and severe hypertonicity, ROM limitations, joint contractures, and pain. For each of the participants, 45 minutes of Watsu delivered two times per week for 8 weeks led to an increase in joint ROM and a decrease in some painful joints. Additionally, their caregivers reported that their burden of care (e.g., dressing and performing transfers) was reduced and that the participants were sleeping through the night without pain, whereas sleepless nights because of pain had been a problem before the intervention. Watsu can be best described as a muscle reeducation approach because specific impairments (usually tight muscles and joints) are targeted for treatment with little regard to the models of motor control. However, the vestibular stimulation component of Watsu is characteristic of a neurotherapeutic facilitation approach.

Bad Ragaz Ring Method

The BRRM was developed in the 1930s in Bad Ragaz, Switzerland.[6, 26, 27] The technique has been modified through the years and has been dramatically influenced by proprioceptive neuromuscular facilitation (PNF), a therapeutic exercise technique used in many clinical settings. BRRM is similar to PNF in that the therapist guides the patient through specific patterns of movement to increase strength and ROM. Both techniques include passive or active movements for the arms, legs, and trunk and may use unilateral or bilateral patterns. Of the bilateral patterns, some are symmetric (both sides of the body moving in the same direction) and some are asymmetric (each side moving in a different direction).

In both BRRM and PNF, the therapist gives the patient specific movement instructions (e.g., "bring your right knee to your left shoulder") and encourages a movement progression of distal to proximal segments of the body. In BRRM, the patient is floating either prone or supine in the water with flotation support at the neck, hips, and, for some unilateral tasks, the extremities. The therapist places his or her hands on designated spots on specific segments of the patient's body while instructing the patient to move in the desired direction (Fig. 8-5). The therapist thus serves as a point of stability from which the patient moves, generating resistance from the turbulent drag effects of the surrounding water. Generally, resistance to movement is encountered in every direction of movement (i.e., flexion and extension) because the body is completely surrounded by water. Unlike PNF, in which the therapist manually applies graded resistance to the patient's movements, the BRRM allows the patient to determine the amount of resistance encountered based on speed of movement and the resulting turbulent drag of the water. Using this method, therapists can increase the difficulty of the activity by placing their stabilizing hold more distally. Such strategies do not necessarily increase the resistance to movement but do increase the complexity of the activity because the patient must control larger segments of his or her body during the movement. Only in a small portion of the patterns described does the therapist use manual resistance to the patient's movement. Therapists are cautioned to stand in depths of water that allow them to form a stabilizing base for the patient's movements. Water depths above the therapist's eighth thoracic vertebra generally prevent the therapist from maintaining a fixed position, decreasing the effectiveness of the therapeutic application. At times, the therapist may use an overflow principle with the BRRM by stabilizing and resisting one portion of the body to encourage activity in another.

Use of BRRM for Patients with Neurologic Disorders

The BRRM was designed for a variety of movement problems, mainly musculoskeletal. However, the technique can be effectively applied to the treatment of neurologic impairments that include voluntary movement deficit, weakness, and decreased ROM. Many patients with neurologic disorders lack the ability to stabilize multiple segments of their bodies, even when they are horizontally supported in the water. Therefore, these patients often require additional flotation support around the trunk to ensure safety and security. When working with patients exhibiting voluntary movement deficits, emphasis should be placed on smooth movement through the ROM, as opposed to quick, resistance-generating movement typically

Aquatic Rehabilitation for the Treatment of Neurologic Disorders   **161**

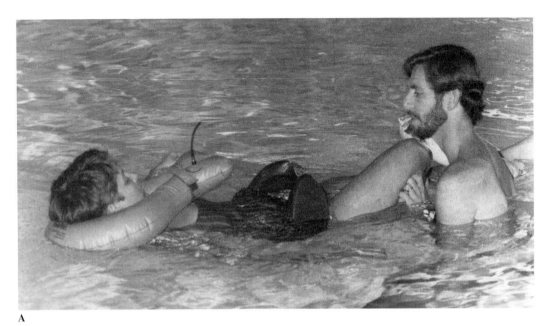

A

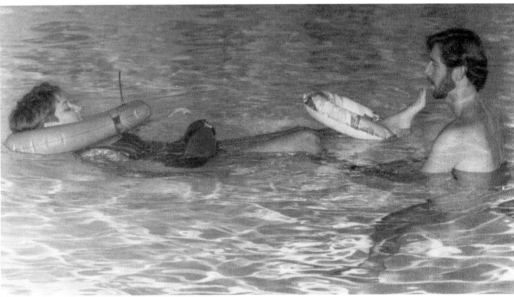

B

Figure 8-5. The therapist uses a Bad Ragaz Ring Method pattern to strengthen or facilitate hip flexion, knee flexion, ankle dorsiflexion, and return. *A*, The patient moves toward the therapist to strengthen/improve hip flexion, knee flexion, and ankle dorsiflexion. *B*, The patient moves away from the therapist to strengthen/improve hip extension, knee extension, and ankle plantar flexion.

used to improve pure strength deficits. Like PNF, facilitation techniques are used to enhance movements (e.g., quick stretch and timing for emphasis) by increasing the efficiency of the CNS with sensory input.

It is common for patients with voluntary movement deficits to have difficulty relaxing muscle groups after a contraction.[4, 24, 25, 28] This prevents subsequent movement from contractions in antagonistic muscle groups. The result is a rigid coactivation of muscles surrounding a joint, preventing movement in any direction. The BRRM can be modified by passively moving the patient in directions where this prolonged contraction occurs, allowing voluntary contraction of the antagonistic muscle. The therapist progressively lessens assistance through the ROM as the patient slowly gains better reciprocal inhibition control (i.e., can voluntarily relax the antagonistic group). Eventually, many patients develop the skill to move smoothly and reciprocally throughout that segment of the body. BRRM resembles a neurotherapeutic facilitation approach in that it encourages improved skill in specific patterns of movement and uses facilitatory techniques to enhance movement.

Halliwick Concept

Developed by James McMillan in the 1930s at the Halliwick School for Girls in England, the Halliwick Concept is based on principles of hydrodynamics and human development.[7, 8, 29–31] The original approach (Ten-Point Program) was intended as a swimming instruction technique, yet many of the Ten-Point Program activities and an elaboration of it (The Logical Approach to Exercise in Water) can be applied to specific therapeutic intervention. In general swimming instruction, each patient is assigned an individual instructor. This patient-instructor pair becomes one of a group of pairs, usually consisting of four to six pairs per group. Games are often used to teach skills and reinforce the principles of the method. For a specific therapeutic intervention, however, activities are often conducted with each patient individually. The Halliwick Concept, best described as a neurotherapeutic facilitation-rehabilitation technique, follows a disengagement principle. Therapists or instructors use activities to facilitate patterns of movement with careful consideration of the activity's level of difficulty and the amount of manual guidance provided. Specifically, the therapist starts with easy activities and guides the patient manually to ensure correct execution of the movement. As the patient becomes more skilled with the movement, the therapist reduces the amount of assistance provided (disengaging) and increases the activity's level of difficulty. Activities are made more difficult by modifications in the patient's position and the therapist's handling techniques. Finally, when the patient masters the activity, the therapist creates turbulence around the patient's body to challenge skill and subsequently reinforce learning. Activities used in the Ten-Point Program are designed with consideration of general principles outlined in Table 8-2. These general principles can be described as part of four phases, as follows:

Phase 1: Adjustment to Water

1. Mental adjustment and disengagement. Developing the patient's comfort while in the water is stressed. This is accomplished through proper handling of patients

Table 8-2. The Ten-Point Program of the Halliwick Concept

Phase 1: Adjustment to water
  1. Mental adjustment and disengagement

Phase 2: Balance control
  2. Sagittal rotation control
  3. Vertical rotation control
  4. Lateral rotation control
  5. Combined rotation control
  6. Use of upthrust
  7. Balance in stillness
  8. Turbulent gliding

Phase 3: Movement in water
  9. Simple progression
  10. Swimming progression

and education about the effects of water on their movements. As a result, patients should never be fearful in the water.

The disengagement principle is used to plan and execute all activities. This progression is believed to best teach and reinforce skill. Activities (e.g., sitting or standing) are easier to accomplish than those in horizontal positions (e.g., prone or supine). Therefore, the approach uses vertical positions earlier in skill development. Because this is the opposite of how skill is developed in a gravity environment (e.g., infants gain skill in the supine position before sitting and standing), the Halliwick Concept is said to use a reversed developmental sequence.

Phase 2: Balance Control

Using the skills of rotation control, patients can change their position in the water. Head movements are emphasized because they greatly influence the position of the body in the water.

2. Sagittal rotation control. Movements in the sagittal plane are encouraged (lateral head/trunk flexion).
3. Vertical rotation control. Movements in a frontal plane are encouraged (e.g., moving from supine to upright to prone). These motions are usually controlled with neck flexion and extension.
4. Lateral rotation control. Movements in a longitudinal plane are encouraged (e.g., rolling from supine to prone). These movements are usually controlled with neck rotation.
5. Combined rotation control. A corkscrew-like motion is encouraged, which combines both vertical and lateral rotation control (e.g., rolling from prone to supine, then coming up into an upright position). When mastered, patients can always achieve a position in the water where they can breathe.
6. Use of upthrust. Patients are taught to control the amount of buoyant support the water provides. Examples include extending the arms and holding one's breath to encourage floating. Conversely, bringing the arms closer to the body and blowing air out promotes sinking.

7. Balance in stillness. Patients are taught to assume and hold a position in the water while turbulence challenges their steadiness.
8. Turbulent gliding. When the patient is able to assume and hold horizontal positions (e.g., supine), the therapist creates turbulence around the patient to move him or her through the water. This assisted movement readies the patient for more independent control of movement through the water.

Phase 3: Movement in Water

9. Simple progression. Before learning specific swimming strokes, patients are encouraged to move themselves through the water in the easiest manner possible. Usually bilateral, symmetric movements are attempted (e.g., elementary backstroke) before bilateral, asymmetric movements (e.g., back crawl stroke).
10. Swimming progression. Specific swimming strokes are approached. At this time, many therapists rely on principles from other schools of thought (e.g., American Red Cross Adapted Swimming Instruction) to promote skill.

Water-specific exercises are developed using principles of the Logical Approach to Exercise in Water and are based on principles of fluid mechanics and neurophysiology. The approach outlines six basic treatment objectives, three rotational planes about which the patient will work, five starting postures, four exercise patterns, seven treatment techniques, and therapeutic swimming instruction.

Use of the Halliwick Concept for Patients with Neurologic Disorders

Use of the Halliwick Concept for swimming instruction is ultimately therapeutic for all people because of the conditioning effects inherent in this form of exercise. It is particularly helpful for individuals with impairments and disabilities caused by neurologic disorders. The approach can also be used to influence movement problems directly; for example, patients believed to be dominated by extensor movement patterns may benefit from gaining skill in vertical rotation control in an anterior direction (Fig. 8-6). Such a movement helps the patient to actively control flexor musculature and inhibit extensor musculature. Skill gained through balance-in-stillness activities may carry over and influence postural stability during functional activities (Fig. 8-7).

Task-Type Training Approach

A task-type training approach (TTTA) for aquatic rehabilitation has been documented for patients who have survived a stroke.[12–14, 32] For this book, the guidelines and principles of the TTTA are extended to the treatment of all patients with neurologic disorders. The TTTA can best be described as a task-oriented approach: Emphasis is placed on influencing the patient's disability by working in functional positions with functional activities. In addition, patients are encouraged to become active problem solvers of their movement difficulties as opposed to passive recipients of manual and verbal input from therapists. Notably, the TTTA is not a treatment technique but a set of principles to guide therapists in designing treatment

Aquatic Rehabilitation for the Treatment of Neurologic Disorders 165

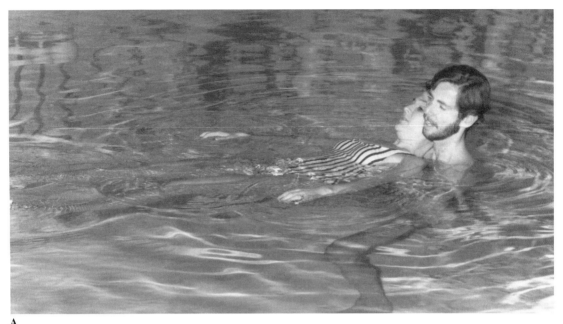

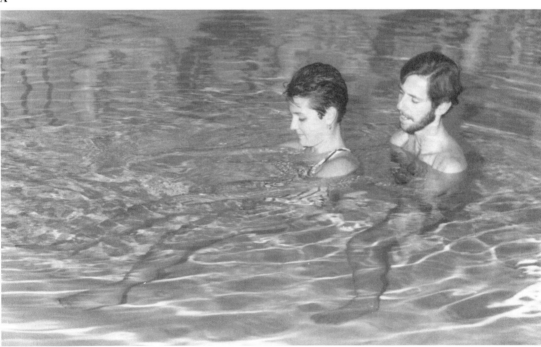

Figure 8-6. Using the Halliwick Concept, the therapist assists the patient to gain vertical rotation control in the water. Using her head to lead, the patient uses vertical rotation to move from a supine to a cube position.

166 COMPREHENSIVE AQUATIC THERAPY

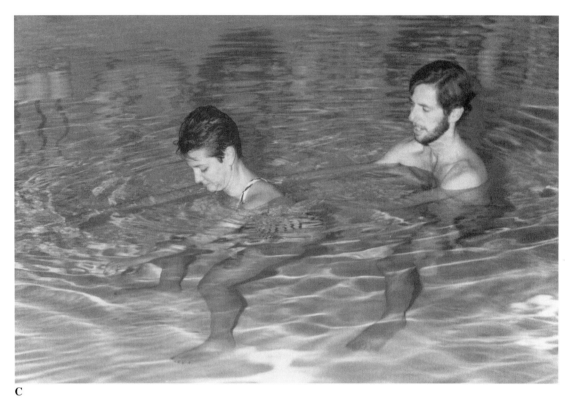

C

Figure 8-6. *Continued.*

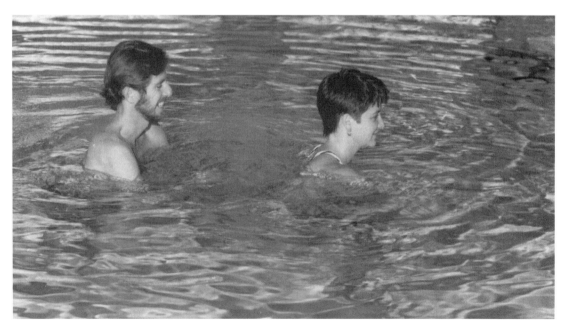

Figure 8-7. Using the Halliwick Concept, the therapist follows a balance-in-stillness principle by creating turbulence behind the patient and challenging the patient's stability.

Table 8-3. General Principles of the Task-Type Training Approach

Work in the most shallow water tolerated.
Practice functional activities as a whole.
Systematically remove external stabilization provided to patients.
Encourage stabilizing muscle contractions in upright positions with movement of selected body segments.
Encourage quick, reciprocal movement.
Encourage active movement problem solving.
Gradually increase the difficulty of the task.

programs for their patients' disabilities (Table 8-3). The general principles are as follows:

1. **Work in the most shallow water tolerated.** The buoyant support of the water allows patients to stand independently and move in a functional manner for the first time. Patients can actively and aggressively work to improve their skill with functional tasks. The ultimate goal is for the functional improvement to carry over to gravity-influenced land activities; therefore, the effect of buoyant support should be systematically removed as patients demonstrate skill with functional activities. Performance indicators, such as the inability to maintain an erect trunk while standing or the inability to maintain knee extension in supporting lower extremities, may show that deeper water is better for functional activity practice.

2. **Practice functional activities as a whole.** Although some treatment programs address strengthening or stretching of specific body segments or facilitating specific movement patterns, the TTTA encourages practice of activities that are identical to or closely approximate the land functional activities to be improved. This principle is based on a specificity-of-training principle that a functional skill must be practiced to be learned.[33, 34] When performed as a whole, the entire functional skill must be mastered, including control of moving body segments and appropriately graded contraction of stabilizing body segments.

3. **Systematically remove external stabilization from patients.** The patient may need to hold on to the pool wall or the therapist's manual assistance may be necessary in the earlier stages of a TTTA. This externally applied stabilization should be quickly removed as he or she gains independent control over the functional activity. Thus, the therapist minimizes the patient's dependence on outside support for functional skills.

4. **Encourage stabilizing contractions in upright positions with movement of selected body segments.** Vertical or upright positions (e.g., sitting and standing) are positions of function and should be used as much as possible.[4] Stereotypical strategies for maintaining postural stability in upright positions have been identified. Patients with neurologic disorders typically have difficulty using these strategies to maintain their balance, so they are encouraged to relearn these maneuvers in a safe but challenging environment, the water. As patients move their extremities in or above the water, their center of balance is challenged. Prevention of falling requires use of effective postural stability strategies (Fig. 8-8). The patient is forced to solve problems actively to redevelop these strategies, with attention given to contracting the appropriate muscles in the proper sequence and with the appropriate force of contraction.

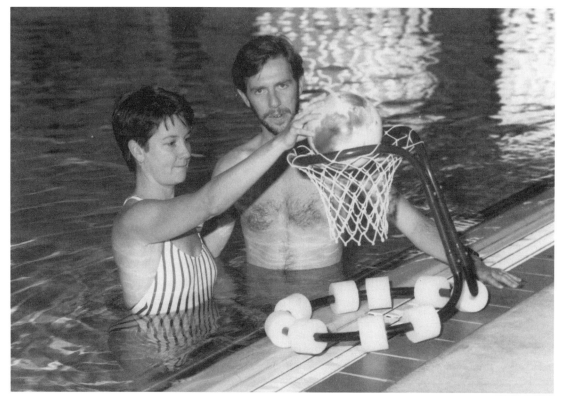

Figure 8-8. The patient practices using postural stability strategies while putting the ball into the basket.

5. **Encourage quick, reciprocal movement.** After many types of neurologic insults, neural shock produces a period of inactivity in which many forms of deconditioning occur. Studies indicate that many patients with neurologic disorders have a predominance of slow-twitch muscle fibers in their skeletal muscles, indicating that a conversion from fast- to slow-twitch fibers has occurred.[35] Some believe that this muscle fiber change contributes to the slow, labored movement typically seen in patients with neurologic disorders.[35] Many functional activities require rhythmic, reciprocal movements along with quick movement changes to maximize the use of inertial forces. Movement in this manner ensures smooth and efficient execution of functional activities. Weakness, ROM limitations, and other voluntary movement deficits prevent patients with neurologic disorders from moving effectively in a gravity environment; the supportive and assistive properties of water dramatically increase the likelihood of their doing so. Therefore, whenever possible, quick, reciprocal movements should be practiced (e.g., marching in place or pedaling the legs while supine). Such practice may produce a conditioning effect that will positively influence the impairments that constrain patients with neurologic disorders to slow, labored movements.

6. **Encourage active movement problem solving.** Motor learning research suggests that healthy humans learn movement skills better when they actively participate in the learning process.[33, 36] For example, when subjects are given less feedback on their performance and are required to practice many and varied activities, they must become more reliant on their own ability to critique and modify their

performance, leading to more active participation. Studies of patients with neurologic disorders have come to similar conclusions. For this reason, patients should be encouraged to critique their performance and propose movement solutions to their problems. Open-ended questions such as "How did you do that time?" and "How can you improve your next attempt?" should be used whenever possible. When working with patients with neurologic disorders in the pool, several factors may make the use of such principles difficult. Many patients with neurologic disorders have difficulty critiquing their performance because of physical (i.e., sensory) and cognitive (i.e., perceptual) impairments. In this case, the therapist must provide minimal guiding feedback regarding the patient's performance.

7. **Gradually increase the difficulty of the task.** Task characteristics can be modified to increase or decrease the challenge of a functional activity. Gentile[37] provided a taxonomy to describe task characteristics that make a task more or less difficult. For example, introducing intertrial variability to a task or changing task requirements from trial to trial increases the skill required to execute the task. A therapist could use this strategy when performing balance training with a patient. While passing a ball with a patient attempting to remain standing, the therapist could throw the ball to the same spot, with the same speed and at the same time (no intertrial variability). Conversely, the task could be made more challenging by varying the speed, timing, and location (intertrial variability). Another variable that could be altered within the taxonomy is the use of body stability activities (e.g., the patient is not required to move from one location) or body transport activities (e.g., the patient is required to move one location to another during the task execution). Using such a progression with balance training, the patient would be asked to pass the ball from one location. Later, the patient would be asked to pass the ball while walking forward.

CONCLUSION

Challenges in the delivery of care to patients with neurologic disorders encourage rehabilitation professionals to explore many approaches to neurorehabilitation. Anecdotally, aquatic rehabilitation has been effectively used to improve many impairment- and disability-related problems for these patients. Aquatic neurorehabilitation approaches must be carefully chosen and based on functional principles. Research is needed to examine the effectiveness of these approaches and study the carryover of aquatic therapeutic activities to land. Such endeavors will improve the delivery of aquatic rehabilitation to patients with neurologic disorders.

CASE STUDY

The patient is a 24-year-old male who sustained a traumatic brain injury in a motor vehicle accident 5 months previously. He is presently an outpatient at the rehabilitation center. He is alert and oriented, is able to follow simple directions, and can talk, although his speech is difficult to understand. He does appear to lack safety awareness. He has heterotopic bone in his right knee and both elbows. He has a thin build and is 6 feet, 4 inches tall.

Subjective Evaluation

The patient states that he has been living in his parents' one-story home since his accident. His family has a house on a nearby lake, and he has always enjoyed swimming; he wants to walk again.

Objective Evaluation

Passive ROM	Right (degrees of)	Left (degrees of)
Shoulder flexion	90	105
Shoulder abduction	90	95
Elbow flexion	90	90
Elbow extension	−90	−35
Wrist flexion	WNL*	WNL
Wrist extension	WNL	0
Hip flexion	70	80
Hip extension	−13	0
Hip abduction	10	15
Knee flexion	WNL	WNL
Knee extension	−30	0
Ankle dorsiflexion	−10	0

*WNL, within normal limits.

Active Movement

The patient exhibits active movement throughout his upper extremities through available ROM. He does move in a moderate flexor synergy pattern, however. He exhibits active movement throughout both lower extremities through available ROM with moderate influence of an extensor synergy pattern. He exhibits clonus in both ankles in standing.

Functional Activities

The patient performs standing pivot transfers with maximum to moderate assistance of one person, requires minimal assistance with sitting balance, ambulates 25 feet with a platform walker, and needs assistance from a maximum of three people to hold him upright and guide walker.

Gait Deviations

The patient can advance both lower extremities but requires assistance in stance on the right lower extremity to extend his knee. He also adducts both legs during swing.

Other

He exhibits poor sitting posture with forward head and flexed trunk. He requires constant verbal cues to sit erect and is unable to hold this position for more than 1 minute.

Impression

The patient is a good candidate for aquatic physical therapy because he is able to follow directions, is motivated, and is comfortable in the water. Treatment will be focused on improving ROM and movement control at an impairment level and improving transfers, sitting, and gait at a disability level.

The patient's major problems are as follows:

1. Dependent for ADLs, including ambulation
2. Limited active and passive ROM
3. Voluntary movement deficits in all extremities
4. Poor sitting posture

Long-Term Goals (4 Weeks)

1. The patient is able to perform standing pivot transfer with minimal assistance of one person. (In water, the patient will be able to perform an independent standing pivot transfer in 4-foot depth.)
2. The patient is able to ambulate 50 feet with a rolling platform walker and moderate assistance of one person. (In water, the patient is able to ambulate in 4-foot–deep water with moderate assistance of one person with the therapist standing at the patient's side, supporting the patient at the waist and holding on to the patient's right hand.)
3. The patient sits independently in 3-foot–deep water and can hold an erect posture with less than three verbal cues for 3 minutes.
4. Patient and family education is completed.

Plan

Patient will be seen three times a week for aquatic physical therapy, including therapeutic exercise, ADL training, and patient and family education. He will also be seen three times a week for physical therapy on land.

Treatment Program

General Considerations

Before treatment with this patient is begun, a thorough orientation to the program should be conducted for the patient and his family. The patient's lack of safety awareness is of great concern, and the therapist should prevent potential problems by setting firm ground rules to be followed while the patient is in the therapeutic pool setting. Because the patient's family does own a house on a lake, and they may be visiting on the weekends, basic water safety concepts should be discussed with the entire family. For example, the patient should be discouraged from participating in any water activity, whether recreational, exercise, or swimming, outside of the therapeutic setting until he has acquired basic swimming skills and has been approved for such activities by an appropriate professional. This discussion is important because families may try to duplicate activities they have observed at the therapeutic pool, unaware of the risks involved.

The patient's stature has both positive and negative implications for program planning. His height and thin build reduce the effects of buoyant support, which will make handling more difficult and provide less buoyancy-assisted movement for the patient. Conversely, the patient's increased body density may allow enough weight bearing to inhibit hypertonicity and provide added sensory input during standing activities.

Treatment of Impairments and Disabilities

Water Shiatsu. The use of Watsu with this patient can prove to be beneficial for several reasons. First, the stretching effects provided by the activities can positively influence the soft-tissue compliance of muscle and joint structures, resulting in increased active ROM and improved quality of voluntary muscle activity. Maneuvers particularly appropriate for this patient include the leg push (promoting hip extension) and the arm-leg rock (promotes hip flexion and stretches the anterior chest wall). Therapists should be aware, however, that these maneuvers may be hindered by and will have little effect on joint contractures resulting from heterotopic bone formation. The Watsu maneuvers used may need to be modified to accommodate these restrictions.

Another benefit provided by Watsu includes the tone reduction and relaxation provided by vestibular stimulation. When Watsu is applied in a slow, rhythmic manner, the steady movement stimulates vestibular receptors, which reduce general body muscle tone through the lateral vestibulospinal tract. Care should be taken to keep Watsu activities with this patient at slow, steady speeds. Quick, jerky movements may actually increase muscle tone.

Watsu is best applied early in the treatment session (i.e., the first 15 minutes). In this way, the increased ROM, relaxation, and reduced hypertonicity will contribute to success with the treatment activities to follow.

Bad Ragaz Ring Method. Activities of the BRRM can be used with this patient to improve voluntary movement control. The therapist should select extremity exercise patterns that encourage movement away from the pathologic synergy patterns exhibited by the patient (i.e., flexor synergy in the upper extremities and extensor synergy in the lower extremities). Additionally, trunk exercise patterns can be used to improve dynamic and static trunk control. Specifically, the upper extremity pattern of shoulder flexion, abduction, and external rotation can be used to improve arm elevation without the influence of the flexor synergy pattern. Similarly, the lower extremity pattern of hip flexion, abduction, internal rotation, knee flexion, and ankle dorsiflexion can be used. This pattern also moves out of the predominant extensor synergy pattern and carries over to an improved swing phase of that leg during gait.

The trunk pattern of lateral trunk flexion with lower trunk and pelvic extension and rotation to one side (with bilateral hip extension) is beneficial for this patient. Improved control with these movements carries over to most antigravity functional skills (e.g., sitting, standing, and ambulating).

Because voluntary movement deficits are present with this patient (i.e., synergistic movement patterns), emphasis should be placed on smooth controlled movement through the ROM. Less concern should be placed on generating resistance by moving quickly. A moderate number of sets with reduced repetitions (e.g., five sets of five repetitions of each exercise) may be best with this patient because fatigue usually reduces quality of movement. Such an exercise schedule allows frequent rest periods.

Halliwick Concept. Principles of the Halliwick Concept can be applied to the direct treatment of this patient's impairments and disabilities. Specifically, the disengagement principle can be applied to improving balance in standing. Early sessions include practice holding the cube position in water with the therapist's assistance through proximal handholds (e.g., support provided at the patient's trunk). Once the patient is able to hold this position without therapist support, he can be challenged by turbulence created around his body. As he becomes independent with this skill, the activity can be made more difficult by moving to a less stable position (e.g., the triangle). The position change may require reapplication of the therapist's support through handling. Ultimately, activities become more challenging until he assumes a stick position independently while turbulence is created around him.

Task-Type Training Approach

Treatment to reduce disability can follow the principles of a TTTA and should be focused on three functional skills: sitting, transfers, and ambulation.

Sitting. Sitting activities can begin in a water depth such that the patient is submerged no higher than midchest level. This is generally the shallowest area of the pool. External stabilization can be provided by the therapist's hand or by a flotation device such as a large inner tube. As the patient gains skill in maintaining independent sitting balance, the external support should be gradually removed. For example, two small flotation rings can be used to progress from the large inner tube. The patient can then be asked to move the small rings in a variety of directions to challenge his ability to maintain sitting balance. These movements should be performed slowly at first and progress to quick reciprocal movements. Once the patient has progressed away from using any buoyant support, he can be challenged by engaging in a "pass-the-ball" game requiring use of the upper extremities. The game can be made progressively more difficult by introducing intertrial variability (e.g., passing the ball at different times, speeds, and locations at random).

Transfers. Two chairs can be placed in shallow water to practice standing pivot transfers. At first, the chairs can be placed beside and facing the pool wall. The patient uses the wall to balance as he executes the transfer. He can also use the therapist's outstretched arm for additional support. As the patient's skill improves, the activity can be practiced in progressively shallower water. External stabilization can be reduced by moving away from the wall. Intermediately, the patient can use a float (e.g., inner tube) for support during activity execution. Ultimately, the patient should perform the activity without any stabilizing support. Intertrial variability can be introduced by varying the height of the chairs or the distance between the two.

Ambulation. An early TTTA activity can include standing at the pool wall in chest-deep water. The patient holds on to the wall with both hands for support.

Single-limb stance activities begin with the patient flexing one hip with the knee bent and returning to the pool floor. The therapist blocks the stance knee and provides support at the patient's stance hip if needed. When one leg up is achieved, the patient is asked to alternate lifts between legs to perform a marching activity. The patient should be encouraged to march as quickly as his skill allows. As soon as he demonstrates moderate skill with the activity, he should be asked to reposition so that his side is next to the pool wall. If he is able, he should be asked to kick the leg farthest from the wall with his knee extended. This activity not only strengthens the kicking leg but also challenges the patient's ability to stabilize throughout the stance leg and trunk.

As the patient progresses to taking steps, stabilization is provided with the therapist's handheld assistance or through some flotation device (e.g., kick boards, stabilizer bar, or inner tube). The handheld assistance provided with the TTTA is different from that provided with more facilitation-oriented approaches, such as the Halliwick Concept. With facilitation-oriented approaches, the therapist guides the patient to improve the quality of his movement. Handheld assistance provided with the TTTA, however, is more fixed, supplying a stability point to be manipulated by the patient. Generally, the therapist's handheld assistance is more stabilizing and should be applied first. The patient is encouraged to increase his walking speed as his skill progresses. As he achieves independent ambulation, activity difficulty is increased by moving to shallower water, adding upper extremity requirements (e.g., passing a ball) and introducing intertrial variability (e.g., changing directions and stopping and starting on command).

REFERENCES

1. Norton CO, Jamison LJ (eds): A Team Approach to the Aquatic Continuum of Care. Boston, MA: Science & Technology Books, 2000.
2. Gordon J: Assumptions underlying physical therapy intervention: theoretical and historical perspectives. In Carr JH, Shepherd RB, Gordon J, et al (eds): Movement Science: Foundations for Physical Therapy in Rehabilitation. Rockville, MD: Aspen, 2000.
3. Horak FB: Assumptions underlying motor control for neurologic rehabilitation. In Lister J (ed): Contemporary Management of Motor Control Problems: Proceedings of the II STEP Conference. Alexandria, VA: Foundation for Physical Therapy, 1990.
4. Shumway-Cook A, Woollacott MH: Motor Control: Theory and Practical Applications. Philadelphia: Lippincott, 2001.
5. Skinner A, Thompson A (eds): Duffield's Exercise in Water, 3rd ed. New York: Churchill Livingstone, 1983.
6. Davis BC, Harrison RA: Hydrotherapy in Practice. New York: Churchill Livingstone, 1988.
7. Campion MR: Hydrotherapy in Pediatrics. Oxford, UK: Heinemann Medical Books, 1985.
8. Campion MR: Adult Hydrotherapy: A Practical Approach. Oxford, UK: Heinemann Medical Books, 1990.
9. Gehlsen GM, Grigsby SA, Winant DM: Effects of an aquatic fitness program on the muscular strength and endurance of patients with multiple sclerosis. Phys Ther 64:653, 1984.
10. Garvey LA: Spinal cord injury and aquatics. Clin Manage 11:21, 1991.
11. Hurley R, Lyons-Olski E, Sweetman NA, et al: Neurology and aquatic therapy. Clin Manage 11:26, 1991.
12. Morris DM: Aquatic rehabilitation of the neurologically impaired client. In Ruoti RG, Morris DM, Cole AJ (eds): Aquatic Rehabilitation. Philadelphia: Lippincott, 1997, pp 105–125.
13. Morris DM: Aquatic neurorehabilitation. Neurol Rep 19(3):22–28, 1995.
14. Morris DM: Aquatic rehabilitation for the treatment of neurologic disorders. J Back Musculoskel Rehabil 4:297, 1994.

15. Becker BE: Biophysiologic aspects of hydrotherapy. In Becker BE, Cole AJ (eds): Comprehensive Aquatic Therapy. Boston, MA: Butterworth-Heinemann, 1997, pp 17–48.
16. Becker BE: Aquatic physics. In Ruoti RG, Morris DM, Cole AJ (eds): Aquatic Rehabilitation. Philadelphia: Lippincott, 1997, pp 15–24.
17. International Classification of Impairments, Disabilities, and Handicaps. Geneva, Switzerland: World Health Organization, 1980.
18. Taub E: Motor behavior following deafferentation in the developing and motorically mature monkey. Adv Behav Biol 18:675, 1976.
19. Evarts EV, Shinoda Y, Wise SP: Neurophysiological Approaches to Higher Brain Function. New York: Wiley, 1984.
20. Shik M, Orlovsky GM: Neurophysiology of locomotor automatism. Physiol Rev 56:465, 1976.
21. Dull H: WATSU: Freeing the Body in Water. Middletown, CA: Harbin Springs Publishing, 1993.
22. Dull H: WATSU. In Ruoti RG, Morris DM, Cole AJ (eds): Aquatic Rehabilitation. Philadelphia: Lippincott, 1997, pp 333–352.
23. Vogtle LK, Morris DM, Denton BG: An aquatic program for adults with cerebral palsy living in group homes. Phys Ther Case Rep 1:250–259, 1998.
24. Craik RL: Abnormalities of motor behavior. In Lister MJ (ed): Contemporary Management of Motor Control Problems: Proceedings of the II STEP Conference. Alexandria, VA: Foundation for Physical Therapy, 1990, p 155.
25. Ballantyne B: Factors contributing to voluntary movement deficits and spasticity following cerebral vascular accidents. Neurol Rep 15:15, 1991.
26. Garrett G: Bad Ragaz Ring Method. In Ruoti RG, Morris DM, Cole AJ (eds): Aquatic Rehabilitation. Philadelphia: Lippincott, 1997, pp 289–292.
27. Boyle AM: The Bad Ragaz Ring Method. Physiotherapy 67:265, 1981.
28. Sahrmann S, Norton BJ: The relationship of voluntary movement to spasticity in the upper motor neuron syndrome. Ann Neurol 2:460, 1977.
29. Martin J: The Halliwick Method. Physiotherapy 67:288, 1981.
30. Campion MR: Water activity based on the Halliwick Method. In Skinner A, Thompson A (eds): Duffield's Exercise in Water, 3rd ed. London: Bailliere Tindall, 1983, p 180.
31. Cunningham J: Halliwick Method. In Ruoti RG, Morris DM, Cole AJ (eds): Aquatic Rehabilitation. Philadelphia: Lippincott, 1997, pp 305–331.
32. Morris D: The use of pool therapy to improve functional activities of adult hemiplegic patients. In Forum Proceedings on Issues Related to Strokes. Alexandria, VA: Neurology Section, American Physical Therapy Association, 1992, pp 45–48.
33. Winstein CJ: Designing practice for motor learning: clinical implications. In Lister MJ (ed): Contemporary Management of Motor Control Problems: Proceedings of the II STEP Conference. Alexandria, VA: Foundation for Physical Therapy, 1991, p 65.
34. Winstein CJ, Gardner ER, McNeal DR, et al: Standing balance training: effect on balance and locomotion in hemiparetic adults. Arch Phys Med Rehabil 70:755, 1989.
35. McComas AJ, Sica RE, Upton AR, et al: Functional changes in motoneurons of hemiparetic patients. J Neurol Neurosurg Psychiatry 36:183, 1973.
36. Schmidt RA: Motor learning principles for physical therapy. In Lister MJ (ed): Contemporary Management of Motor Control Problems: Proceedings of the II STEP Conference. Alexandria, VA: Foundation for Physical Therapy, 1991, p 49.
37. Gentile AM: Skill acquisition: action, movement, and neuromotor processes. In Carr J, Shephard R (eds): Movement Science: Foundations for Physical Therapy Rehabilitation, 2nd ed. Rockville, MD: Aspen, 2000.

Chapter 9
Spine Pain: Aquatic Rehabilitation Strategies

Andrew J. Cole, MD, Michael Fredericson, MD,
Jim Johnson, MD, Marilou Moschetti, BSc, PTA
Richard A. Eagleston, and Steven A. Stratton

Physicians tell many patients with spinal injuries and disorders to swim for rehabilitation, exercise, and pain management, but the role that an aquatic environment plays in spine rehabilitation has not been explored fully. Water's unique properties make it ideal for rehabilitation of patients with spinal pain, and various methods may be used to integrate water-based programs into comprehensive training regimens.

BACKGROUND

In the United States, aquatic activity is the most common participation sport and is an extremely popular exercise for recreation, competition, and rehabilitation.[1] More than 38,000 people are involved with U.S. Masters Swimming, and more than 2,000 centers use aquatic techniques for rehabilitative purposes (U.S. Masters Swimming Web site [http://www.usms.org], 2001). The rising popularity of aquatic activities has resulted in increasing numbers of spinal and associated musculoskeletal injuries.

Land exercises, swimming, and inappropriate aquatic rehabilitation programs can cause new spinal injuries or exacerbate preexisting spinal disorders, but properly designed aquatic programs can help rehabilitate patients with spinal injuries. Aquatic stabilization techniques and swimming programs can be used with aggressive, comprehensive, land-based spine-stabilization programs or as the sole rehabilitative tool.[2] The success or failure of aquatic therapy candidates is not determined by swimming skills alone because swim-stroke proficiency is not a model for successful treatment.

DIAGNOSIS AND TREATMENT

The workup and diagnosis of spinal pain require a thorough understanding of anatomy, physiology, and activity-specific functional biomechanics. After carefully obtaining a history, with close attention to the specific mechanism of injury, a physician performs a thorough yet directed neurologic and musculoskeletal examination of the injured structure and its contiguous supporting elements. A functional evaluation is conducted in which the patient reproduces a painful motion. Finally, ancillary testing is ordered, and the correct final diagnosis is confirmed.

An understanding of anatomy and stroke-specific functional biomechanics allows thorough treatment plans and complete rehabilitation programs to be developed. A rehabilitation program addresses the primary injury, whether spinal or peripheral joint, as well as secondary sites of dysfunction.[3-6]

Recognition of the functional relationship between the spine and peripheral joints is critical to ensure optimal treatment outcomes. Peripheral joint dysfunction can set off a cascading series of motion changes throughout the spinal axis. The cervicothoracic and thoracolumbar transition zones, in particular, are commonly affected because they are the junctions of the more mobile and less mobile sections of the spine.[7] Figure 9-1 presents the motion cascade originally described by Cole

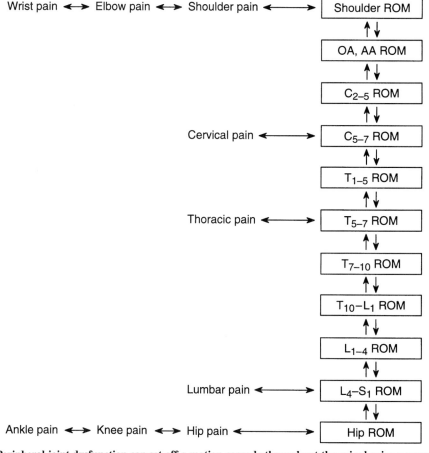

Figure 9-1. Peripheral joint dysfunction can set off a motion cascade throughout the spinal axis; conversely, spine dysfunction can create peripheral joint dysfunction (ROM, range of motion; OA, occipitoatlantal; AA, atlantoaxial; C, cervical; T, thoracic; L, lumbar; S, sacral). (Courtesy of AquaTechnics Consulting Group, Inc., Aptos, CA.)

and Herring.[8] In a swimmer, for example, a shoulder injury such as rotator cuff tendonitis results in guarding and decreased range of shoulder motion.[3, 8–11]

The swimmer's arm cannot abduct and extend as it would[12] during normal recovery, resulting in decreased body roll, increased lumbar segmental motion, and an abnormally low head position from which to breathe.[2] Compensatory adaptive changes then occur. Such changes include crane breathing (increased cervical suboccipital extension and rotation, cervical extension [C2 to C7], and cervical rotation [C2 to C7] (Fig. 9-2), as well as more extension and rotation from C3 to C5.[2] To compensate, the C5 to T1 segment becomes hypomobile, and mid- and low-cervical pain results. Compensatory hypermobility begins from T2 to T5 and hypomobility from T5 to T7 and T10 to L1. Primary cervical, thoracic, and lumbar injuries and pain influence the spinal axis in a similar fashion. Hip,[13] pelvis, and lumbar spine pain result in hypomobility at L4 to S1 and ultimately at the T10 to L1 transition zone. Adaptive changes proceed up the axis and may set the stage for compensatory changes in shoulder mechanics that eventually cause a shoulder injury. Identifying the initial injury is important so that treatment can eliminate that problem as well as secondary compensatory sites of dysfunction.[3, 8, 14]

When prescribing rehabilitation plans, it is important to recognize that physiologic and psychological needs vary among patient populations. Highly competitive athletes, for example, require alternative training regimens during their rehabilitation programs to maintain peak flexibility, strength, and aerobic conditioning. The requirements for recreational athletes may be more flexible. Competitive athletes require specific training schedules and goals to compete effectively during particular athletic seasons, but the needs of weekend athletes are usually not as rigorous. Specific patient goals are met by tailoring workups and rehabilitation programs to

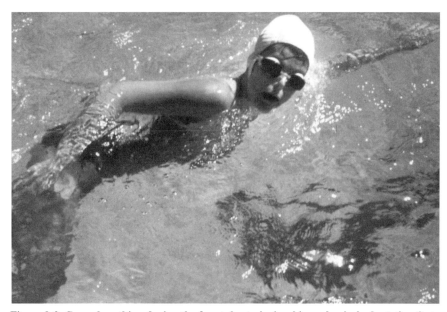

Figure 9-2. Crane breathing during the freestyle stroke is a biomechanical adaptation that improves access to air by increasing capital and cervical spine extension and rotation. Such breathing can occur for a variety of reasons, the most common being poor body roll. (Courtesy of AquaTechnics Consulting Group, Inc., Apots, CA.)

REHABILITATION PROGRAMS

The aquatic rehabilitation programs reviewed here are based on dynamic lumbar, thoracic, and cervical stabilization techniques that have been described for land programs.[16, 17] Dynamic land-based stabilization training is a specific type of therapeutic exercise that can help patients gain dynamic control of segmental spine forces; eliminate repetitive injury to motion segments, that is, discs, zygapophyseal joints, and related structures; encourage healing of injured motion segments; and possibly alter the degenerative process. The underlying premise is that motion segments and supporting soft tissues react to minimize applied stresses and reduce risk of injury.[16, 17] The goals of aquatic stabilization exercise and swimming programs incorporate these elements but take into account the unique properties of water so that the risk of spinal injury is reduced. Aquatic stabilization programs help to develop patients' flexibility, strength, and body mechanics so that a smooth transition to aquatic stabilization swimming programs or other spine-stabilized aquatic activities may occur. Such programs can help first-time swimmers and patients who previously swam (Table 9-1).[2, 8, 11, 18, 19]

REHABILITATION ENVIRONMENT: LAND VERSUS WATER

Accurate diagnosis of patients' spinal injuries and observation of their initial responses to land-based or aquatic stabilization programs help to determine further treatment with therapeutic exercises. A transition from dry to wet exercise conditions eliminates dry-land risks, establishes a supportive training environment, provides a new therapeutic activity, decreases the risk of peripheral joint injury, and allows a return to prior activity. Moving from dry to wet environments also should be considered if patients cannot tolerate axial or gravitational loads, if they require increased support in the presence of strength or proprioceptive deficit[20] or if they are at risk of a compression fracture due to decreased bone density.[21] Remaining in a water-supported environment is appropriate if a dry environment exacerbates symptoms or if patients prefer water. Transition from a wet to a dry environment should occur if rehabilitation is going well in the water but patients must return to land to meet functional training needs efficiently and attain their ultimate competitive goals.[18, 22] Table 9-2 lists specific contraindications for aquatic rehabilitation.[11, 23, 24]

Spinal rehabilitation programs offer advantages that are directly related to the intrinsic properties of water—namely, buoyancy, resistance, viscosity, hydrostatic pressure, temperature, turbulence, and refraction. We have described these properties elsewhere.[2, 11, 18, 25, 26] Graded elimination of gravitational forces through buoyancy

Table 9-1. Benefits of Aquatic Stabilization Programs

Minimization of segmental trunk motion and shear forces
Reinforcement of lumbar control
Encouragement of hip, knee, and ankle propulsion
Development of head and neck stability
Establishment of arm control and strength

Table 9-2. Contraindications for Aquatic Rehabilitation

Fever
Cardiac failure
Urinary infections
Bowel or bladder incontinence
Open wounds
Infectious diseases
Contagious skin conditions
Excessive fear of water
Uncontrolled seizures
Colostomy bag or catheter used by patient
Cognitive or functional impairment that creates a hazard to the patient or others in pool
Severely weakened or deconditioned state that poses a safety hazard
Extremely poor endurance
Severely decreased range of motion that limits function and poses a safety hazard

Source: AquaTechnics Consulting Group, Inc., Aptos, CA.

allows patients to train with decreased, yet variable, axial loads and shear forces. In essence, water increases the safety margin of patient postural error by decreasing the compressive and shear forces on the spine. Motion velocity can be controlled by water resistance, viscosity, buoyancy, and training devices. Buoyancy increases the range of training positions. The psychological outlook of swimmers may be enhanced because rehabilitation occurs in their competitive environment. Many believe that water reduces pain because of the sensory overload generated by hydrostatic pressure, temperature, and turbulence.[19, 27–40]

AQUATIC SPINE-STABILIZATION TECHNIQUES

The spine-stabilization principles discussed for land programs also apply to aquatic programs. Certain exercises that can be performed on land cannot be reproduced in water and vice versa. Aquatic programs can be designed for patients who cannot train on land and for those whose land training has reached a plateau. Eagleston first described aquatic stabilization in 1989.[41]

We have developed eight core aquatic stabilization exercises with four levels of difficulty that provide graded training of stabilization skills.[2, 11, 18, 25, 26] Programs must be customized to meet the needs of each patient's unique spinal pathologic condition, related musculoskeletal dysfunctions, and comfort with the aquatic environment. Also, patients who have had joint replacements require particular care during positioning in the water, because the replacements can change the center of buoyancy and may cause patients to sink due to high specific gravity.[42] When one program is mastered, a more advanced program is provided. Eventually, if a patient wants to begin a swimming program, a series of transitional aquatic stabilization exercises are initiated. These help to establish a spine-stabilized swimming style that minimizes the risk of further spinal injury and helps to maximize swimming performance.[18, 25]

Wall Sit

The wall sit exercise develops isometric strength primarily in the quadriceps and hamstring group. It also trains abdominal muscles to hold the appropriate neutral spine posture.[11, 18, 25]

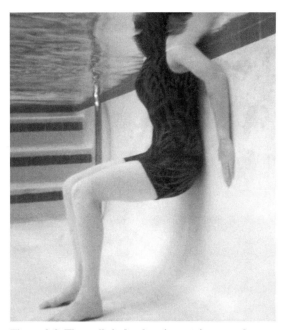

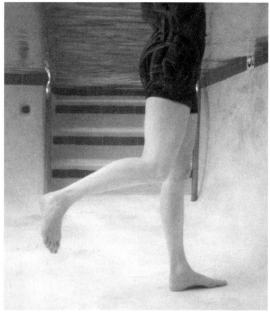

Figure 9-3. The wall sit develops isometric strength, primarily in the quadriceps and hamstring groups. Abdominal muscles are trained to hold the appropriate neutral spine posture. (Courtesy of AquaTechnics Consulting Group, Inc., Aptos, CA.)

Figure 9-4. Modified Superman level I. (Courtesy of AquaTechnics Consulting Group, Inc., Aptos, CA.)

- Level I: Supported by the pool wall, the patient maintains the vertical position with hips and knees in 90-degree flexion. This position is held for 1 minute (Fig. 9-3). Patients with knee problems may need to modify this exercise to provide less flexion at the knee joint.
- Level II: The patient holds the level I position for 2 minutes.
- Level III: The patient holds the position for 3 minutes.
- Level IV: The patient holds the position for 5 minutes.

Modified Superman

The modified Superman exercise trains the ipsilateral hip flexors, extensors, and contralateral gluteus medius and increases isometric strength in abdominal and paraspinal stabilizers.[11, 18, 25]

- Level I: Facing the pool wall, the patient stands and holds on to the edge of the pool with both hands. Movement is unilateral, one leg at a time, with the knee flexed at 45 degrees. The hip is actively extended to 20 degrees and then returned to the neutral position. The movement pattern continues for 60 seconds at 50% of maximum velocity (Fig. 9-4).
- Level II: Level II is performed exactly like level I, but the knee is maintained in full extension and the movement pattern continues for 2 minutes at 70% of maximum velocity (Fig. 9-5).

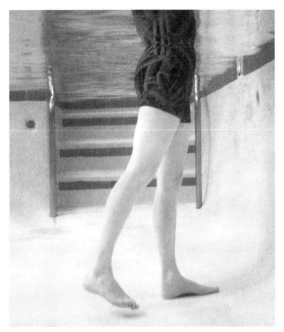
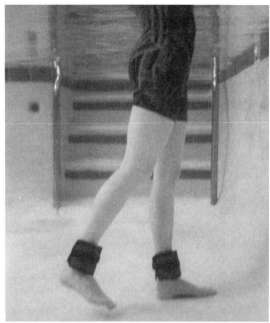

Figure 9-5. Modified Superman level II. (Courtesy of AquaTechnics Consulting Group, Inc., Aptos, CA.)

Figure 9-6. Modified Superman levels III and IV. (Courtesy of AquaTechnics Consulting Group, Inc., Aptos, CA.)

- Level III: Level III is performed exactly like level II, but a 3-pound cuff is applied to each ankle. This movement pattern continues for 2 minutes at 50% of maximum velocity (Fig. 9-6).
- Level IV: Level IV is performed exactly like level III, but the pattern continues for 3 to 5 minutes at 85% of maximum velocity.

Water Walking Forward

The water walking forward exercise isometrically strengthens the abdominal muscles and muscle groups that maintain proper posture. Isotonic strengthening occurs in muscles that are dynamically involved in gait.[11, 18, 25]

- Level I: The patient begins in the standing position, unsupported, with the water depth at the xyphoid level. Elbows are extended with the palms at the sides and forward. The patient water walks for 3 minutes at 50% of maximum velocity (Fig. 9-7).
- Level II: Level II provides an incrementally greater challenge for all muscle groups described in level I. The arms are abducted to 45 degrees and hand mitts are used. The patient walks for 5 minutes at 70% of maximum velocity (Fig. 9-8).
- Level III: Level III further enhances resistive training. Hand paddles are used, and the patient walks for 10 minutes at 85% of maximum velocity (Fig. 9-9).
- Level IV: The patient walks forward and backward with water shoes, 3-pound ankle weights, or both. A piece of Plexiglas (36 × 24 inches) or a kick board held vertically beneath the water surface increases the resistance. The exercise is performed for 10 minutes at a velocity of 90% to 100% of maximum velocity (Fig. 9-10).

184 COMPREHENSIVE AQUATIC THERAPY

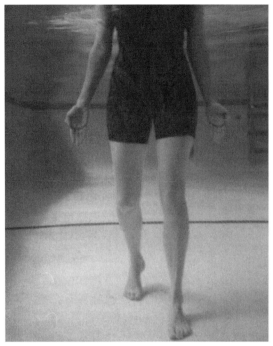

Figure 9-7. Water walking forward level I. (Courtesy of AquaTechnics Consulting Group, Inc., Aptos, CA.)

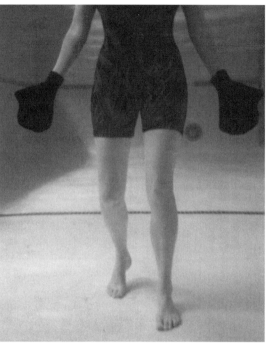

Figure 9-8. Water walking forward level II. (Courtesy of AquaTechnics Consulting Group, Inc., Aptos, CA.)

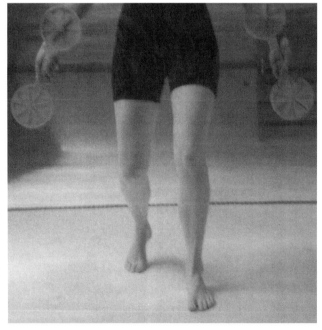

Figure 9-9. Water walking forward level III. (Courtesy of AquaTechnics Consulting Group, Inc., Aptos, CA.)

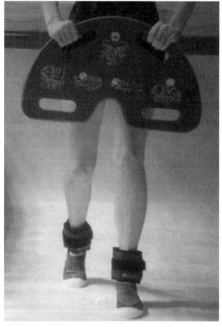

Figure 9-10. Water walking forward level IV. (Courtesy of AquaTechnics Consulting Group, Inc., Aptos, CA.)

Water Walking Backward

Water walking backward, like the previous exercise, provides similar strengthening, but with greater emphasis on isometric paraspinal muscle conditioning.[11, 18, 25]

- Level I: The patient begins in the standing position, unsupported, with the water depth at the xyphoid level. Elbows are kept extended with the palms at the sides and forward. The patient water walks backward for 3 minutes at 50% of maximum velocity (Fig. 9-11).
- Level II: Level II provides an incrementally greater challenge for all muscle groups described in level I. The arms are abducted to 45 degrees, and hand mitts are used. The patient walks backward for 5 minutes at 75% of maximum velocity (Fig. 9-12).
- Level III: Level III further enhances resistive training. Hand paddles are used, and the patient walks backward for 10 minutes at 85% of maximum velocity (Fig. 9-13).
- Level IV: The patient walks forward and backward with water shoes, 3-pound ankle weights, or both. A piece of Plexiglas (36 × 24 inches) or a kick board held vertically beneath the water surface increases the resistance. The exercise is performed for 10 minutes at a velocity of 90% to 100% of maximum velocity (Fig. 9-14).

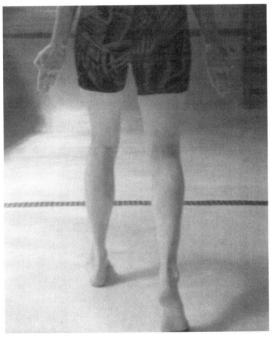

Figure 9-11. Water walking backward level I. (Courtesy of AquaTechnics Consulting Group, Inc., Aptos, CA.)

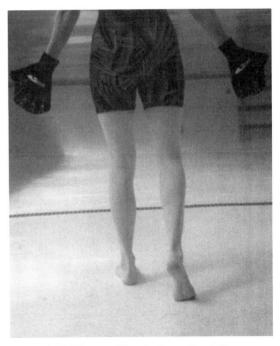

Figure 9-12. Water walking backward level II. (Courtesy of AquaTechnics Consulting Group, Inc., Aptos, CA.)

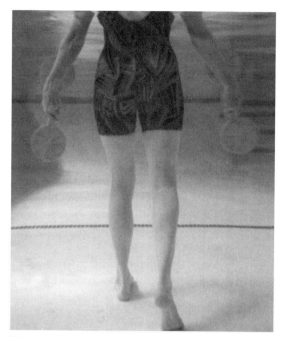

Figure 9-13. Water walking backward level III. (Courtesy of AquaTechnics Consulting Group, Inc., Aptos, CA.)

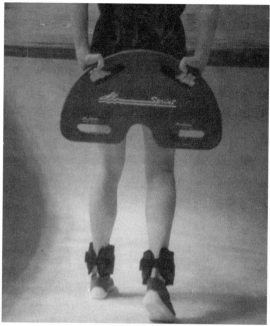

Figure 9-14. Water walking backward level IV. (Courtesy of AquaTechnics Consulting Group, Inc., Aptos, CA.)

Supine Sculling

Supine sculling simultaneously initiates strengthening in the upper and lower extremity muscle groups. Posterior and anterior muscle groups of the lower extremities, gluteals, shoulder complex, and paraspinals are incrementally challenged.[11, 18, 25]

- Level I: The patient wears a flotation jacket to support the torso and a flotation collar for the neck while being maintained in a supine, supported position by the therapist. The upper extremities simultaneously perform a sculling figure-eight movement at the hip, while the lower extremities initiate a flutter kick. This exercise is performed for 1 minute at 50% of maximum velocity (Fig. 9-15).

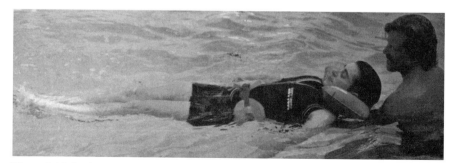

Figure 9-15. Supine sculling level I. (Courtesy of AquaTechnics Consulting Group, Inc., Aptos, CA.)

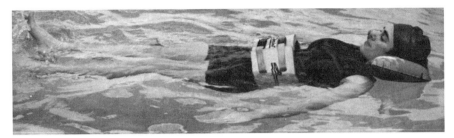

Figure 9-16. Supine sculling level II. (Courtesy of AquaTechnics Consulting Group, Inc., Aptos, CA.)

- Level II: A flotation belt is substituted for the flotation jacket, and the cervical flotation support is maintained. The therapist supervises but does not support the patient. Arms are abducted to 40 degrees, and the flutter is increased in intensity. This exercise is performed for 3 minutes at 70% of maximum velocity (Fig. 9-16).
- Level III: Hand mitts and short blade fins are added. The flotation belt continues to be used, but the cervical support device is eliminated. This exercise pattern is performed for 5 minutes at 85% of maximum velocity (Fig. 9-17).
- Level IV: The flotation device is eliminated. Short-blade fins and hand mitts are used. Sculling and kicking are performed for 30 seconds followed by 15 seconds of rest. The exercise is performed at 90% to 100% of maximum velocity; 12 sets are performed (Fig. 9-18).

Wall Crunch

Wall crunch exercises train muscles activated in the wall sit and additionally challenge the contralateral gluteal, ipsilateral hip flexor, and paraspinal muscles.[11, 18, 25] To co-activate the deeper paraspinal, oblique, and transversus abdominis muscles, the abdominal "hollowing" technique is recommended. The patient is instructed to contemplate his or her navel and gently pull it up and against the spine. During the performance of this technique, the rib cage should be slightly elevated without restriction of natural, relaxed breathing. A depression of the rib cage or a protrusion of the abdominal wall usually indicates that the technique has been performed

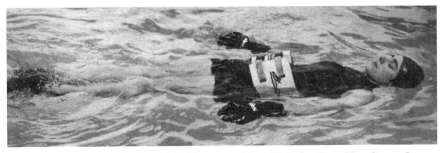

Figure 9-17. Supine sculling level III. (Courtesy of AquaTechnics Consulting Group, Inc., Aptos, CA.)

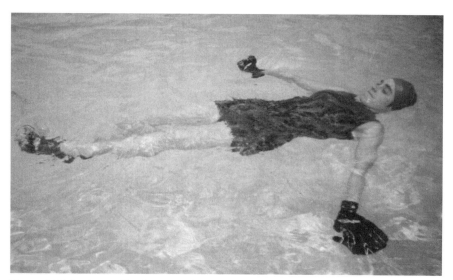

Figure 9-18. Supine sculling level IV. (Courtesy of AquaTechnics Consulting Group, Inc., Aptos, CA.)

incorrectly and the rectus abdominis rather than the deeper abdominal muscles are predominating in the co-contraction pattern.[43]

- Level I: The patient stands with the spine against the pool wall flexes one hip to 90 degrees with the knee at 90-degree flexion. One hand provides isometric resistance, and the isometric contraction is held for 5 seconds. Ten repetitions at 50% of maximum velocity are performed (Fig. 9-19).
- Level II: The patient stands with the spine against the pool wall and the arms hooked over the pool ledge and simultaneously flexes both hips to 90 degrees with knees at 90-degree flexion. The position is held for 10 seconds; 10 repetitions at 70% of maximum velocity are performed (Fig. 9-20).
- Level III: The patient stands in the same position as level II and flexes both hips simultaneously to 90 degrees with the knees at full extension. Three-pound weights are attached to the ankles. The position is held for 10 seconds. Twenty repetitions at 50% of maximum velocity are performed (Fig. 9-21).
- Level IV: This level is performed the same way as level III; however, there is no isometric hold. The motion is continuous for 3 minutes at 50% of maximum velocity.

Quadruped

The quadruped exercise is performed in the prone position, with the patient using a snorkel and mask to avoid the struggle for air while training arm and leg mechanics. A patient who is unfamiliar with the proper use of a snorkel and mask may be taught by a therapist in shallow water. The patient must perform all skills comfortably before proceeding, including correct recovery from a prone position to a standing position. The therapist should not leave the patient unattended while using this equipment in the therapy pool.[11, 18, 25]

Spine Pain: Aquatic Rehabilitation Strategies **189**

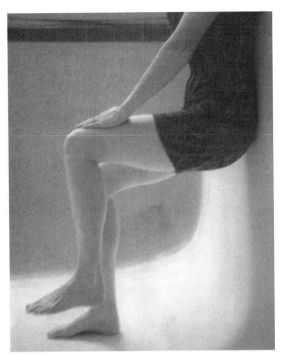

Figure 9-19. Wall crunch level I. (Courtesy of AquaTechnics Consulting Group, Inc., Aptos, CA.)

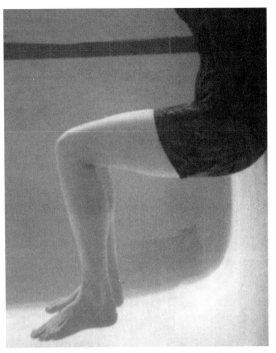

Figure 9-20. Wall crunch level II. (Courtesy of AquaTechnics Consulting Group, Inc., Aptos, CA.)

Quadruped level I activities for legs only challenge lumbar spine stabilizer groups isometrically and lower extremity hip flexors and extensors isotonically and for arms only, level I activities challenge lumbar spine stabilizer groups isometrically and upper extremely shoulder groups that reproduce flexion and extension isotonically.

- Level I: The patient begins in a semisupported prone position with a flotation belt at hip level. The therapist supports the legs and hips. The patient moves the

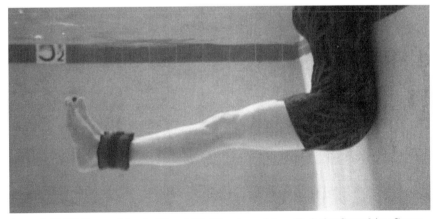

Figure 9-21. Wall crunch levels III and IV. (Courtesy of AquaTechnics Consulting Group, Inc., Aptos, CA.)

arms simultaneously, with the elbows extended, from 0- to 180-degree forward flexion. This motion is performed for 1 minute at 50% of maximum velocity (Fig. 9-22A). Next, the therapist supports the arms and instructs the patient simultaneously to move the legs from 0-degree hip position to 90-degree hip- and knee-fixed position (Fig. 9-22B). This motion is performed for 1 minute at 50% of maximum velocity.

- Level II: The flotation device is removed, and the therapist supports the patient's hips. Alternating arm movements are performed in a pattern similar to level I for 3 minutes at 50% of maximum velocity (Fig. 9-23A). The legs are then trained in an alternating pattern through the same range of motion as in level I (Fig. 9-23B). This occurs for 3 minutes at 50% of maximum velocity.
- Level III: Level III increases the training intensity by requiring greater independence during activity. Therapist support is removed, but a flotation device is used (Fig. 9-24). The patient performs simultaneous, alternating upper and lower extremity patterns, as in level II, for 3 minutes at 70% of maximum velocity.
- Level IV: Weights are added to ankles and wrists for an additional challenge, and a flotation device is placed at the waist to prevent sinking (Fig. 9-25). The movement pattern is the same as that of level III, but it continues for 5 minutes at 70% of maximum velocity.

When the patient can perform the quadruped, the log-roll swims (a transition exercise to spine-stabilized swimming) is introduced.

Log-Roll Swim

The log-roll swim exercise teaches spine-stabilized movement, thus eliminating segmental rotation through the spinal axis. The patient, supported at the hip with a small flotation belt, uses a snorkel and mask to ease breathing. The therapist may fix strapping tape to the lumber spine to give proprioceptive cues and to help to avoid segmental spine movement.[11, 18, 25]

- Level I: The therapist instructs the patient to float in a prone position, with the knees flexed to 25 degrees and the arms at 0-degree flexion (Fig. 9-26). The cervical spine is maintained at approximately 20 degrees of flexion. Proper breathing and relaxation are emphasized. Upper extremity movement of the entire shoulder complex begins with small, rotatory movements of the lower arms under the chest, as if the patient is rototilling water. The hips are maintained at 25 degrees of flexion. Small flexion-extension knee movements are initiated simultaneously with small, rotatory arm movements. Both movements cause propulsion. A lateral rocking movement is taught so that the patient "log-rolls" in the water. This motion minimizes the amount of segmental stress placed across each motion segment in the lumbar spine. The patient performs the exercise pattern for 5 minutes at 50% of maximum velocity. Lateral flexion and rotation must be avoided.
- Level II: Level II begins with the upper extremities performing scouping movements under the body (Fig. 9-27). Each arm is lifted in an arc for recovery above the head just like the freestyle stroke, and the hand enters the water to repeat the cycle. The log-roll pattern must be maintained. When upper body motion is correctly performed, level I kicking is added. This exercise continues for 5 minutes at 50% of maximum velocity.

Spine Pain: Aquatic Rehabilitation Strategies 191

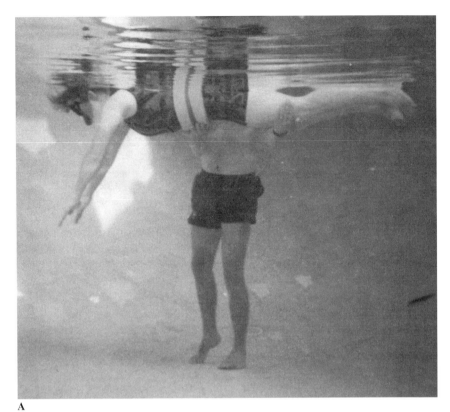

A

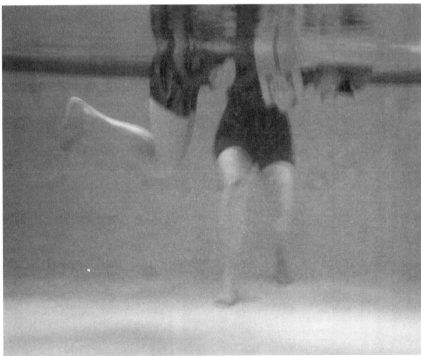

B
Figure 9-22. Quadruped level I. (Courtesy of AquaTechnics Consulting Group, Inc., Aptos, CA.)

192 COMPREHENSIVE AQUATIC THERAPY

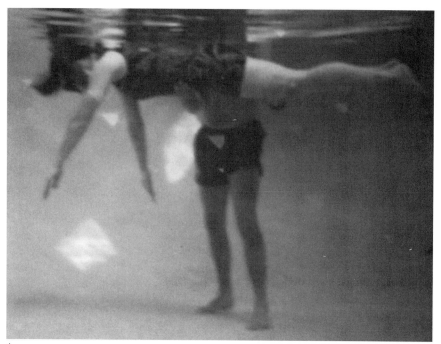

A

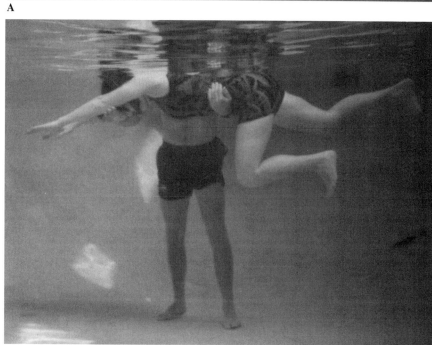

B

Figure 9-23. Quadruped level II. (Courtesy of AquaTechnics Consulting Group, Inc., Aptos, CA.)

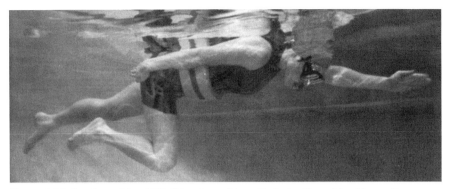

Figure 9-24. Quadruped level III. (Courtesy of AquaTechnics Consulting Group, Inc., Aptos, CA.)

- Level III: The level II exercise continues, but the arm motion advances to normal freestyle, and kicking begins from the hip rather than the knee (Fig. 9-28). The pattern continues for 5 minutes at 50% of maximum potential velocity.
- Level IV: Level IV is similar to level III, but the flotation belt is eliminated and short-blade fins are added (Fig. 9-29). This pattern continues for 10 minutes at 80% of maximum potential velocity.

At this point, the patient can eliminate the mask, snorkel, and fins and can begin a spine-stabilized swimming program.

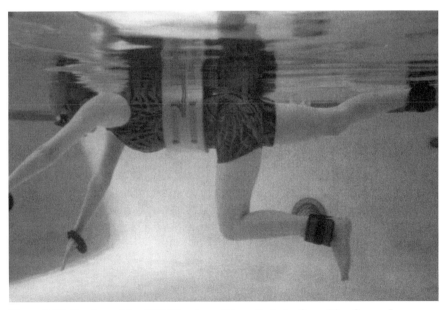

Figure 9-25. Quadruped level IV. (Courtesy of AquaTechnics Consulting Group, Inc., Aptos, CA.)

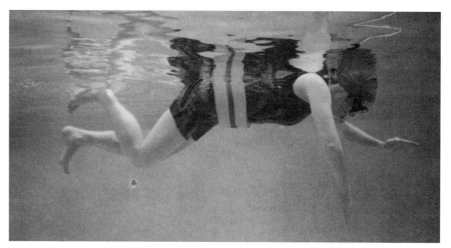

Figure 9-26. Log-roll swim level I. (Courtesy of AquaTechnics Consulting Group, Inc., Aptos, CA.)

SPINE-STABILIZED SWIMMING PROGRAMS

Once a patient's stabilization skills have progressed to the point at which swimming is possible, a thorough analysis of stroke technique and its effect on spine motion is critical.[44] The following overview focuses on lumbar spine injury and indicates the role that the cervical spine plays in the mechanics of lumbar aquatic motion.

Analysis of stroke mechanics, like gait analysis, should be done in an ordered, sequential manner so that all deficits and their relationships are carefully and fully scrutinized. Typically, we begin the analysis at the head and work distally.

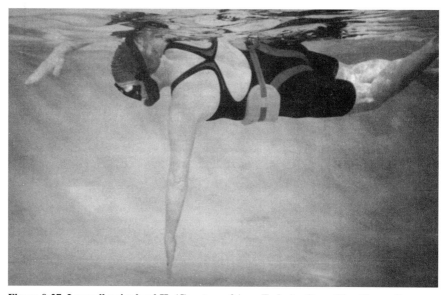

Figure 9-27. Log-roll swim level II. (Courtesy of AquaTechnics Consulting Group, Inc., Aptos, CA.)

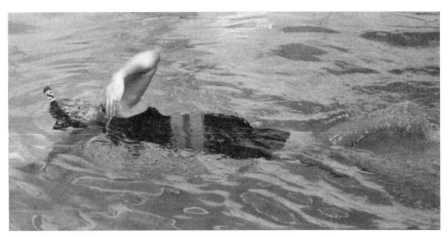

Figure 9-28. Log-roll swim level III. (Courtesy of Aqua Technics Consulting Groups Inc., Aptos, CA.)

Prone Swimming

In prone swimming, the patient's head should be midline and the cervical spine should be kept in the neutral position along the sagittal plane because excessive extension causes the legs and torso to drop in the water, and excessive flexion can cause a struggle for air.[2, 3, 11, 18, 44] The eyes should be looking down as opposed to forward to help maintain the head in neutral position. There should be no craning (suboccipital cervical extension and rotation) or cervical extension and rotation (C2 to C7) (see Fig. 9-2). Breathing should occur by turning the head, that is, by rotating the head along the axial plane. The body should rotate at least 45 degrees from its long axis equally with each stroke, which contributes to proper breathing mechanics and is essential to minimize dysfunctional cervical positioning and subsequent pain.

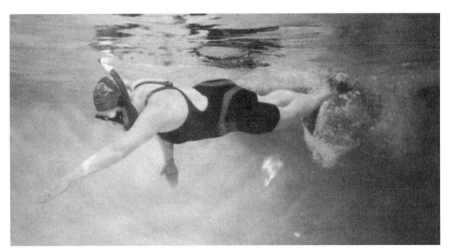

Figure 9-29. Log-roll swim level IV. (Courtesy of AquaTechnics Consulting Group, Inc., Aptos, CA.)

Table 9-3. Swimming Stroke Phases (Freestyle)

I. Catch phase
   A. Hand entry
   B. Hand submersion (ride)
II. Pull phase
   A. Insweep
   B. Outsweep
   C. Finish
III. Recovery phase
   A. Exit
   B. Arm swing

Source: AquaTechnics Consulting Group, Inc., Aptos, CA.

The upper-body arm position is evaluated by stroke phase (Table 9-3). Freestyle is made up of three phases—catch, pull, and recovery. The catch phase includes finger (not thumb) first hand entry with immediate "grabbing" of the water. The pull phase incorporates early, mid, and late components in a straightline path in relation to space. The previously taught S-shaped pull phase was based on a two-dimensional model and is not necessary if there is adequate body rotation. The recovery phase includes the hand exit just above the waist with the palm facing the swimmer. This maintains the shoulder in external rotation and less prone to impingement.[41]

Body balance is difficult to learn and to explain but is the most important skill in maintaining a neutral spine position. The body's center of mass is around the pubis but the center of buoyancy is at the sternum. The lungs filled with air float the body, but the mass and density of the legs tend to bring the body down feet first. The swimmer must learn to use the counterbalance of the weight of the head and press the center of buoyancy into the water to float the legs. Mostly, the swimmer must play with the balance in the water and try to find the best dynamic position to maintain the whole "vessel" at or near the surface on the same horizontal plane. Floating drills with the hands at the side are the best way to learn this technique.[45]

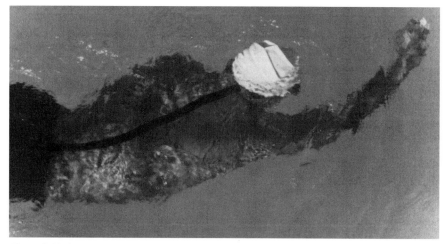

Figure 9-30. This swimmer's arm abducts beyond 180 degrees during the entry phase of freestyle. This stroke defect creates lateral lumbar flexion (*line*) and lumbar segmental rotation. (Courtesy of AquaTechnics Consulting Group, Inc., Aptos, CA.)

Several stroke defects can cause poor lumbar mechanics. If the arm abducts beyond 180 degrees, lateral lumbar flexion and rotation occur (Fig. 9-30). During the pull phase, decreased body rotation can cause lateral lumbar flexion and rotation that stress the lumbar motion segments, particularly the annular fibers surrounding the nucleus pulposus. Inadequate strength in the triceps during the finish phase results in low arm recovery, which in turn generates secondary lateral flexion and rotation through the lumbar spine. During recovery, inadequate body roll causes the neck to crane, which results in a struggle for air and accompanying lateral flexion and rotation through the lumbar spine.[2, 3, 8, 11, 18, 44]

Trunk motion is monitored closely for any primary or secondary lumbar flexion, both sagittal and coronal, or for axial rotation. If flexion and rotation are not corrected by simple changes in stroke mechanics, additional proprioceptive cues can be provided by taping the lumbar spine region. The tape pulls on the skin each time the lumbar spine moves in a segmental manner, that is, when the patient generates excessive lumbar rotation or lateral lumbar flexion[19] (Fig. 9-31). Table 9-4 delineates how these and other primary peripheral joint freestyle stroke defects and secondary effects can create abnormal spine mechanics during swimming and can cause or exacerbate a painful spine dysfunction.

Flip turns are discouraged. Instead, the patient uses a stabilized turn in which a vertical position is reached before turning. This vertical position allows the patient to stabilize the spine when preparing to change direction. Eventually, a horizontal spin is incorporated into the turn, and the vertical position is eliminated. Flip turns may then be resumed.[2, 11, 18, 25]

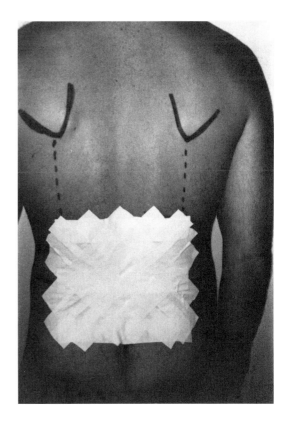

Figure 9-31. Waterproof strapping tape applied to the lumbar spine reinforces lumbar proprioceptive awareness and helps to minimize lumbar rotation and lateral flexion. (Courtesy of AquaTechnics Consulting Group, Inc., Aptos, CA.)

Table 9-4. Freestyle Stroke Defects

Primary Peripheral Joint Stroke Defect	Secondary Effect	Spine Reaction
Head high	Lower body sinks	Increased cervical extension
		Increased lumbar extension
Head low	Upper body sinks	Increased lumbar flexion
Crane breathing	Lower body sinks	Increased cervical and suboccipital extension
	Contralateral shoulder sinks	Increased cervical rotation
		Increased lumbar lateral flexion and rotation
Crossover hand entry	Lateral body movement	Increased lumbar lateral flexion and rotation
Wide hand entry	Contralateral shoulder roll	Increased cervical rotation
		Increased lumbar lateral flexion and rotation
Inefficient pull power	Upper body sinks	Increased cervical rotation
	Difficulty breathing	Increased cervical extension
		Increased lumbar extension
		Increased lumbar lateral flexion and rotation
Increased hip flexion	Decreased kick propulsion	Increased cervical extension
	Lower body sinks	Increased lumbar extension
		Increased lumbar lateral flexion and rotation
Crossover kick	Decreased kick propulsion	Increased cervical extension
	Increased hip roll	Increased lumbar extension
	Lower body sinks	Increased compensatory lumbar lateral flexion and rotation
Increased knee flexion	Decreased kick propulsion	Increased cervical extension
	Lower body sinks	Increased lumbar extension
Increased ankle dorsiflexion	Decreased kick propulsion	Increased cervical extension
	Increased hip roll	Increased lumbar extension
	Lower body sinks	Increased compensatory lumbar lateral flexion and rotation

Source: AquaTechnics Consulting Group, Inc., Aptos, CA.

Supine Swimming

It is best to start with a simple kicking program, with the patient in the supine position and arms at the side, because adequate stabilization can be maintained easily. The use of fins is often suggested to improve propulsion. In the supine position, extension of the cervical spine induces lumbar extension. In contrast, cervical flexion causes the patient to "sit" in the water, with lowered leg position and decreased propulsion. Extreme cervical extension or flexion is avoided in favor of a more neutral, stabilized cervical posture.[2, 3, 11, 18, 44]

Problems with stroke technique usually can be solved with simple changes in stroke mechanics or by adding adaptive equipment. For example, struggling for air can be resolved by the addition of a mask and snorkel. Trunk position can be improved by using the taping technique already described. Poor propulsion can be remedied by use of appropriate fins. Hand paddles can provide better kinesthetic awareness of hand and arm position.[2, 11, 18]

Spinal Pain in Swimmers

Repetitive microtrauma from swimming is a primary cause of spinal injury. If the average competitive swimmer swims 5,000 yards freestyle per day, 5 days each week, using 15 strokes per pool length, and breathes every other stroke, he or she performs approximately 600,000 arm movements, 300,000 cervical spine rotations, and 600,000 lumbar rotatory movements per year. Supplementary land-based flexibility and strength programs without attention to proper spinal mechanics can cause or contribute to spine injury and pain.[5] Mutoh and associates[46] retrospectively studied 66 elite Japanese aquatic athletes, including competitive swimmers, divers, water polo players, and synchronized swimmers. The lower back was the most common site of injury for all four groups; 37.1% of the 19 competitive swimmers had chronic low-back pain. This finding is similar to Mutoh's 1983 study,[47] in which 33% of the 51 Japanese swimmers he studied had low-back pain. Mutoh's findings are in contradistinction to a 1980 study in which shoulder pain was the most common orthopedic problem in competitive swimming.[48] A more recent retrospective study by Cole and colleagues[49] of 325 competitive swimmers from the 1996 to 1997 season found that for the 214 swimmers who were injured, shoulder injuries were most common (38%) with back problems a close second (23%). There was a linear increase of back pain with advancing age. Although all spinal structures are presumably at risk during swimming activities, the biomechanics of certain strokes predispose particular structures to increased risk.

Biomechanics of Spinal Injury in Swimmers

Of the four competitive strokes, freestyle and backstroke most increase lumbar segmental axial rotation and torque force, thereby placing the annulus fibrosus in particular jeopardy.[50–53] In elite swimmers, this risk factor would seem to decrease in importance because of improved stroke technique. Although they are trained to roll their bodies as a unit (nonsegmentally),[2, 8, 11, 54, 55] thus minimizing torque force across individual lumbar motion segments and also decreasing head drag forces, elite swimmers probably subject these segments to greater force per stroke. Paradoxically, they increase the chance of injury due to repetitive microtrauma.[44, 50, 57–60] (S. Kenney, personal communication, 1991). Risk of lumbar facet pain increases with strokes such as the butterfly and breaststroke, which include an accentuated lumbar extension (Fig. 9-32).[55] When performing these strokes, elite athletes, in particular, are at risk because of an exaggerated undulation that increases sagittal motion (i.e., extension and flexion). This undulation compounds the risk of facet injury due to repetitive microtrauma. Even with the breaststroke, traditionally a controlled swimming style, recent advances in stroke technique have resulted in a significant increase in sagittal plane motion by emphasizing undulatory rather than linear, plane horizontal motion (S. Kenney, personal communication, 1991). Although injury to the pars interarticularis may be seen more frequently in

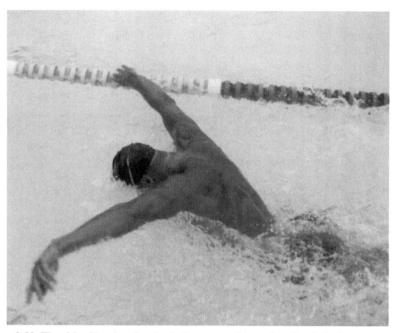

Figure 9-32. The risk of lumbar facet pain increases with strokes that include an accentuated lumbar extension, such as the butterfly. (Courtesy of AquaTechnics Consulting Group, Inc., Aptos, CA.)

competitive divers,[57] many swimmers with a quiescent spondylolysis may develop symptoms due to the repetitive extensions that occur with breaststroke, butterfly, starts, and turns. Furthermore, the risk of development of spondylolysis is particularly high in adolescents in whom the spine is developing, which supports recommendations against excessive training in this age group.

Although injuries to the thoracic spine seem to occur less frequently and appear to be more easily rehabilitated, these structures are nonetheless at risk. Most commonly seen is thoracic facet pain, especially with strokes that generate a great degree of increased segmental rotatory motion at particular thoracic motion segments, such as freestyle and backstroke. The extension required in butterfly and breaststroke may cause facet joint dysfunction and pain. The pain, which may be caused by inflammation, results from repetitive facet compression, distraction, and shear forces.[3, 8, 11] We believe that during the pull phase, compressive forces are generated by the ipsilateral latissimus dorsi, scapular retractors, and long thoracic spinal extensor muscle groups. Ipsilateral thoracic spinal muscle groups produce an extension to counter the flexion of the latissimus dorsi. The contralateral thoracic spinal muscle groups stabilize the thoracic spine, preventing untoward lateral flexion toward the pull-phase side. Passive distractive forces affect the ipsilateral facet during the recovery phase due to activation of the ipsilateral scapular protractors, relaxation of the scapular retractors, inactivation of the latissimus dorsi, and relative relaxation of the thoracic spinal extensor muscle groups.[9, 18, 54, 58, 59]

Thoracic costovertebral joints may be injured as a result of significantly increased vital capacity and enhanced motion of the chest wall and ribs. These joints may be compromised further by arm elevation and the consequent increase in tension on the rib system. Additionally, faulty stroke mechanics resulting in increased rotation through the thoracic spine may contribute to costovertebral joint pain.[18, 54]

The cervical spine is subjected continuously to repetitive microtrauma from the mechanics of breathing. Annular as well as facet injuries are most commonly seen with the freestyle stroke because of the significant rotation required for side-breathing.[3, 18, 54] Occasionally, a side-breathing technique is used during the butterfly, also placing the cervical segments at increased risk. Extension, which is seen with breaststroke and butterfly (Fig. 9-33), increases the chance of cervical posterior element injury, resulting in cervical facet pain. Cervical extension can also increase intradiscal pressure, compromising the intervertebral disc.[60] Although the backstroke requires little rotation for breathing, exceptional stabilization of the cervical segments in a relatively neutral position is needed to reduce drag forces. As a result, fewer intrinsic cervical segmental injuries tend to occur from this stroke, but muscular strain to the cervical dynamic stabilizing soft tissues, such as the paraspinal muscle groups, is common. There is significant risk of catastrophic cervical spine injury caused by impact loading.[61–64] The greatest potential for this type of injury is found in faulty start mechanics and, less commonly, with impact loading of the cervical spine during a missed turn, particularly during the backstroke, in which the swimmer cannot see the oncoming wall or may fail to observe overhead warning flags.[18, 54]

Patients with Scheuermann's kyphosis were found to develop increased pain during swimming, particularly when they used the butterfly stroke, in a study by Wilson and Lindseth.[65] Of the four competitive strokes, the butterfly includes the greatest end-range extension of the diseased, less mobile thoracic motion segments. Increased pectoral and associated chest and abdominal muscle contractions during the pull phase of a butterfly stroke may cause compressive forces that further damage anterior column structures.[66] Because these muscles are also significantly active during the pull phase of the freestyle and breaststroke,[27, 28, 55, 56, 67] repetitive end-range extension microtrauma may be the primary biomechanical source of pain in

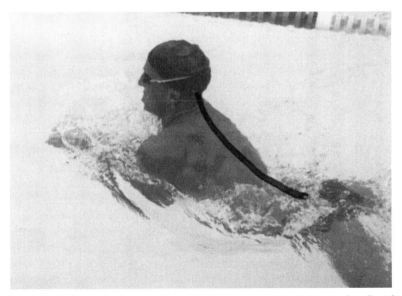

Figure 9-33. Breaststrokes requires repetitive end-range cervical extension *(line)* for breathing. This increases the risk of cervical posterior element injury that can produce facet pain. (Courtesy of AquaTechnics Consulting Group, Inc., Aptos, CA.)

the butterfly. Although kyphotic patients can be managed conservatively with daily use of braces, additional time out of their braces was suggested to allow continued swimming. When the butterfly was avoided, no deleterious change was noted.[65] Additionally, because of the swimmer's horizontal position in the water and the buoyant effect of the water, the axial compressive forces on the spine[27] are reduced significantly. This positioning and buoyancy may significantly mitigate mechanical risk factors that may cause this condition to progress.

The prevalence of idiopathic scoliosis in adolescents is approximately 2% to 3%.[68] In the athletic population, the average frequency of idiopathic scoliosis has been reported to be 2% and of functional scoliosis to be 33.5%.[69] The higher incidence of functional scoliosis in the athletic population may be due to larger unilateral torque forces developed in particular activities, such as serving and throwing.[29] More recent work by Becker[70] (personal communication, 1991), who screened 336 swimmers at the Junior Olympic Swimming Championships, East, in 1983, showed a 6.9% incidence of idiopathic scoliosis and 16% incidence of functional scoliosis. The 6.9% figure is roughly three times the reported incidence of structural idiopathic scoliosis, but the 16% figure is less than the incidence reported by Krahl and Steinbruck.[69] One hundred percent of the functional curves, however, were toward the dominant-hand side, which, according to Yeater and associates,[68] consistently produces greater pull-phase peak forces than those for the nondominant side. Further studies summarized by Becker[70] revealed histologic and morphologic changes in the paraspinal and gluteus muscles, secondary adaptation of supporting vertebral soft tissues, and adaptive changes in muscles to meet specific repetitive functional demands. However, if curve progression is truly facilitated by the asymmetric functional demands that swimming places on the spine, then a therapeutic exercise program could theoretically be designed to counter them. Moreover, exercise alone is not sufficient to inhibit the progression of scoliotic curve,[70] and it remains to be shown whether exercise can accelerate curve progression. Additionally, the most recent advances in swimming techniques, especially in the freestyle, emphasize symmetric motion (e.g., alternate-side breathing) and minimize repetitive unilateral torsion and lateral flexion. Proper coaching should help to further deemphasize the potential effect of a stronger, dominant side on the spine. We believe that swimming is not contraindicated for adolescents with functional or idiopathic scoliosis. We recommend appropriate training by the patients' therapists and coaches, who should know swimming technique and mechanics. In fact, with proper technique, aquatic activity may help patients with scoliosis.

CONCLUSION

Repetitive microtrauma from aquatic rehabilitation and from land-based flexibility and strength programs that are performed without attention to proper spinal mechanics can cause or contribute to spinal injury and pain. Because the spinal axis is essentially a force transmitter for peripheral joint motion, both direct spinal injury and altered biomechanics at sites distant from the spine can change spinal mechanics and cause dysfunction and pain. A series of aquatic stabilization exercises that incorporate the intrinsic properties of water and enhance rehabilitative efforts have been designed. When these exercises are mastered, injured patients can soon advance to spine-safe swimming or other high-level aquatic training activites.[71] Swimming programs, in particular, require that close attention be paid to proper swim-stroke biomechanics and to the effect that abnormal mechanics may have on the spine. This attention ensures the most rapid rehabilitation of painful spinal disorders.

Acknowledgment

The authors thank Carolinda E. Hill (Scientific Publications office, Baylor Research Institute, Dallas, Tex) for reading and editing the manuscript.

REFERENCES

1. Canadian Olympic Association: Canadian Olympic Association Report. Canada, Autumn, 1982.
2. Cole AJ, Moschetti ML, Eagleston RA: Getting backs in the swim. Rehabil Manage 5:62, 1992.
3. Cole AJ, Farrell JP, Stratton SA: Cervical spine athletic injuries: a pain in the neck. In Press J (ed): Physical Medicine and Rehabilitation Clinics of North America. Philadelphia: WB Saunders, 1994, p 37.
4. Press JM, Herring SA, Kibler WB (eds): Rehabilitation of Musculoskeletal Disorders: The Textbook of Military Medicine. Borden Institute, Office of the Surgeon General (in press).
5. Kibler WB, Chandler TJ, Pace BK: Principles of rehabilitation after chronic tendon injuries. In Renstrom AFH, Leadbetter WB (eds): Clinics in Sports Medicine. Philadelphia: WB Saunders, 1992, p 661.
6. Herring SA: Rehabilitation of muscle injuries. Med Sci Sports Exerc 22:453, 1990.
7. Paris S: The spine and swimming. In Hockschuler S (ed): Spine: State of the Art Reviews. Philadelphia: Hanley & Belfus, 1990, p 351.
8. Cole AJ, Herring SA: The role of the physiatrist in the management of lumbar spine pain. In Tollison DC (ed): The Handbook of Pain Management, 2nd ed. Baltimore, Md: Williams & Wilkins, 1994, p 85.
9. Scovazzo M, Browne A, Pink M, et al: The painful shoulder during freestyle swimming: an electromyographic cinematographic analysis of twelve muscles. Am J Sports Med 19:577, 1991.
10. Cole AJ, Reid M: Clinical assessment of the shoulder. J Back Musculoskel Rehabil 2:7, 1992.
11. Cole AJ, Moschetti ML, Eagleston R: Lumbar spine aquatic rehabilitation: a sports medicine approach. In Tollison DC (ed): The Handbook of Pain Management, 2nd ed. Baltimore, Md: Williams & Wilkins, 1994, p 386.
12. Kadaba MP, Cole AJ: Intramuscular wire electromyography of the subscapularis. J Orthop Res 10:394, 1992.
13. Wilder RP, Sobel J, Cole AJ, et al: Overuse injuries of the hip and pelvis in sports. J Back Musculoskel Rehabil 4:236, 1994.
14. Kibler WB: Clinical aspects of muscle injury. Med Sci Sports Exerc 22:450, 1990.
15. Saal J: Rehabilitation of the injured athlete. In DeLisa J (ed): Rehabilitation Medicine: Principles and Practice. Philadelphia: JB Lippincott, 1988, p 840.
16. Saal JA, Saal JS: Later stage management of lumbar spine problems. In Herring S (ed): Physical Medicine and Rehabilitation Clinics of North America. Philadelphia: WB Saunders, 1991, p 205.
17. Saal JA: Dynamic muscular stabilization in the nonoperative treatment of lumbar pain syndromes. Orthop Rev 19:691, 1990.
18. Cole AJ, Campbell DR, Berson D, et al: Swimming. In Watkins RG (ed): The Spine in Sports. St Louis: Mosby, 1996, p 362.
19. Cole A, Eagleston R, Moschetti ML, et al: Lumbar torque: a new proprioceptive approach. Poster presented at the Annual Meeting of the North American Spine Society, Keystone, Colo, August 1–3, 1991.

20. Minor MA, Hewett JE, Webel RR, et al: Efficacy of physical conditioning exercise in patients with rheumatoid arthritis and osteoarthritis. Arthritis Rheum 32:1396, 1989.
21. Goldstein E, Simkin A, Epstein L, Peritz E: The influence of weight-bearing water exercises on bone density of post-menopausal women (in press).
22. LeFort SM, Hannah TE: Return to work following an aquafitness and muscle strengthening program for the low back injured. Arch Phys Med Rehabil 75:1247, 1994.
23. Cole AJ: When to call for help. J Phys Ed Recreation Dance Jan:55, 1993.
24. Reister VC, Cole AJ: Start active, stay active in the water. J Phys Ed Recreation Dance Jan:52, 1993.
25. Cole AJ, Moschetti ML, Eagleston RA: Swimming. In White AH (ed): Spine Care. St Louis: Mosby, 1995, p 727.
26. Cole AJ, Moschetti ML, Eagleston RA: The water scale: a classification system for aquatic exercise. Manuscript in preparation, 1997.
27. Miller F: Fluids. In College Physics, 4th ed. New York: Harcourt, Brace, Jovanovich, 1977, p 271.
28. Piette G, Clarys JP: Telemetric EMG of the front crawl movement. In Terauds J, Bedingfield W (eds): Swimming III. Baltimore, Md: University Park Press, 1979, p 153.
29. Kuprian W: Physical therapy for sports. Philadelphia: Saunders, 1982, p 377.
30. Councilman J: The Science of Swimming. Englewood Cliffs, NJ: Prentice Hall, 1968.
31. Martin R: Swimming: force on aquatic animals and humans. In Vaughan CL (ed): Biomechanics of Sport. Boca Raton, Fla: CRC Press, 1989, p 35.
32. Costill D, Cahill P, Eddy D: Metabolic responses to submaximal exercise in three water temperatures. J Appl Physiol 22:628, 1967.
33. Kirby RL, Sacamano JT, Balch DE, Kriellaars OJ: Oxygen consumption during exercise in a heated pool. Arch Phys Med Rehabil 65:21, 1984.
34. Kolb M: Principles of underwater exercise. Phys The Rev 37:361, 1957.
35. Kreighbaum E, Barthels K: Biomechanics: A Qualitative Approach for Studying Human Movement, 2nd ed. Minneapolis, Minn: Burgess, 1985, p 421.
36. Martin WH III, Montgomery J, Snell PG, et al: Cardiovascular adaptations to intense swim training in sedentary middle-aged men and women. Circulation 75:323, 1987.
37. McArdle W, Katch F, Katch V: Energy expenditure during walking, jogging, running and swimming. In McArdle W, Katch F, Katch V (eds): Exercise physiology: energy, nutrition, and human performance. Philadelphia: Lea & Febiger, 1986, p 158.
38. Panjabi M, Abumi K, Duranceau J, Oxland T: Spinal stability and intersegmental muscle forces: A biomechanical model. Spine 14:194, 1989.
39. Shirazi-Adl A, Ahmed A, Shrivastava S: Mechanical response of lumbar motion segment in axial torque alone and combined with compression. Spine 11:914, 1989.
40. Constant F, Collin JF, Guillemin F, Boulangé M: Effectiveness of spa therapy in chronic low back pain: a randomized clinical trial. J Rheumatol 22:1315, 1995.
41. Eagleston R: Aquatic stabilization programs. Presented at the Conference on Aggressive Nonsurgical Rehabilitation and Lumbar Spine and Sports Injuries, Mar 23, 1989, San Francisco Spine Institute, San Francisco.
42. Brewster NT, Howie CR: That sinking feeling. BMJ 305:1579, 1992.
43. Richardson CA, Jull GA: Concepts of assessment and rehabilitation for active lumbar stability. In Boyling JD, Palastonga N, Grieve GP (eds): Modern Manual Therapy: The Vertebral Column. New York: Churchill Livingstone, 1984, pp 705–719.
44. Maglisco E: Swimming Even Faster. Sunnyvale, Calif: Mayfield, 1993.
45. Johnson JN, Gauvin J, Fredericson M: Swimming biomechanics and injury prevention. Physician Sports Med (in press).
46. Mutoh Y, Miwako T, Mitsumasa M: Chronic injuries of elite competitive swimmers, divers, water polo players, and synchronized swimmers. In Ungerecht VB, Wilke K (eds): Swimming Science. Champaign, Ill: Human Kinetics Books, 1988, p 333.
47. Mutoh Y: Mechanism and prevention of swimming injury. Jpn J Sports Sci 2:527, 1983.
48. Richardson A, Jobe F, Collins H: The shoulder in competitive swimming. Am J Sports Med 8:159, 1980.
49. Cole AJ, Johnson JN, Fredericson M: Injuries in competitive swimmers: a retrospective study of injury site and incidence. Manuscript in preparation.

50. Bogduk N, Twomey LT: Clinical Anatomy of the Lumbar Spine, 2nd ed. New York: Churchill Livingstone, 1991.
51. Farfan H: Effects of torsion on the intervertebral joints. Can J Surg 12:336, 1969.
52. Farfan HF, Cossette JW, Robertson GH, et al: The effects of torsion on the lumbar intervertebral joints: the role of torsion in the production of disc degeneration. J Bone Joint Surg [Am] 52:468, 1970.
53. Goldstein JD, Berger PE, Windler GE, Jackson DW: Spine injuries in gymnasts and swimmers: an epidemiologic investigation. Am J Sports Med 19:463, 1991.
54. Cole AJ, Moschetti ML, Eagleston RE: Spine pain: aquatic rehabilitation strategies. J Back Musculoskel Rehabil 4:273, 1994.
55. Ruoti RG, Morris DM, Cole AJ: Aquatic Rehabilitation. Philadelphia: Lippincott, 1997.
56. Cole AJ, Weinstein S: Lumbar spine pain: a clinical approach. Andover Medical Publishers, 1995.
57. Rossi R: Spondylolysis, spondylolisthesis and sports. J Sports Med Phys Fitness 18:317, 1978.
58. Nuber GW, Jobe FW, Perry J, et al: Fine wire electromyography analysis of muscles of the shoulder during swimming. Am J Sports Med 14:7, 1986.
59. Pink M, Perry J, Browne A, et al: The normal shoulder during freestyle swimming: an electromyographic and cinematographic analysis of twelve muscles. Am J Sports Med 19:569, 1991.
60. White A: Clinical anatomy and biomechanics. Presented at the meeting of the Cervical Spine and Upper Extremity in Sports and Industry, Apr 1, 1990, San Francisco Spine Institute, San Francisco.
61. Bailes JE, Herman JM, Quigley MR, et al: Diving injuries of the cervical spine. Surg Neurol 34:155, 1990.
62. Good R, Nickel V: Cervical spine injuries resulting from water sports. Spine 5:502, 1980.
63. Kewalramani L, Taylor R: Injuries to the cervical spine from diving accidents. J Trauma 15:130, 1975.
64. Kiwerski J: Cervical spine injuries caused by diving into water. Paraplegia 18:101, 1980.
65. Wilson F, Lindseth R: The adolescent swimmer's back. Am J Sports Med 10:174, 1982.
66. Benson D, Wolf A, Shoji H: Can the Milwaukee brace patient participate in competitive athletics? Am J Sports Med 5:7, 1977.
67. Clarys JP, Piette G: A review of EMG in swimming: explanation of facts and/or feedback information. In Hollander AP, Huijing PA, deGroot G (eds): Biomechanics and Medicine in Swimming. Champaign, Ill: Human Kinetics Books, 1983, p 153.
68. Yeater RA, Martin RB, White MK, Gilson KH: Tethered swimming forces in the crawl, breast, and back strokes and their relationship to competitive performance. J Biomech 14:527, 1981.
69. Krahl H, Steinbruck K: Sportsachaden and Sportverletzungen and der Wirbelsaule. Arztebl: Deutsch, Berlin, Germany, 1:9, 1978.
70. Becker TJ: Scoliosis in swimmers. In Ciullo JV (ed): Clinics in Sports Medicine. Philadelphia: WB Saunders, 1986, p 149.
71. Wilder RP, Brennan D, Schotte DE: A standard measure for exercise prescription for aqua running. Am J Sports Med 21:45, 1993.

Chapter 10
Hydrotherapeutic Applications in Arthritis Rehabilitation

Bruce E. Becker, MD, and Gwendolyn Garrett, MS, OTR

The healing benefits of warm water immersion probably have been known since prehistorical times. The early medical writings of the Greeks and Romans reveal the widespread usage of water immersion for medicinal purposes for a variety of ills, including arthritis. Observations have been made through history that immersion in thermal mineral waters resulted in shrinking of peripheral edema, reduction of joint pain, and improvement in joint mobility. Hydrotherapy combined with heat is among the oldest rehabilitative treatments for arthritis.[1] Today, passive and active treatments in a warm-water environment play a significant and distinct role in the rehabilitation of patients with arthritis.

The rheumatic diseases affect the joints, muscles, and connective tissues of the body and appear to be a result of a complex of interacting mechanical, biologic, biochemical, and enzymatic feedback loops.[2] The word *arthritis* literally means joint inflammation. The precise mechanisms causing these structures to be attacked are incompletely understood and, in some instances, seem to be triggered by a preceding infectious process, in others by a sudden autoimmune response, and in some cases perhaps as a response to joint stress. There is considerable individual variation in symptom magnitude, joint involvement, and disease duration. A symptom complex of joint swelling, pain, stiffness, inflammation, and limitation of range of motion (ROM) is typically produced, irrespective of cause. The most prevalent forms of the disease are osteoarthritis, a degenerative joint disease in which one or many joints undergo degenerative changes, including loss of articular cartilage and the formation of osteophytes, and rheumatoid arthritis, an autoimmune disease that produces both acute inflammatory and progressive joint damage.[3] With osteoarthritis, age is the most significant risk factor, but as with many other forms of arthritis, the condition may result from anatomic or metabolic predisposition. More commonly, the pathogenesis is simply unknown. There are thought to be more than 100 types of arthritis, including ankylosing spondylitis, fibromyalgia, lupus erythematosus, and juvenile rheumatoid arthritis.[3] Most of these are chronic conditions for which there is no definitive cure but a series of medical management options. Left untreated, many are progressive and can cause significant impairment, disability, and handicap over time. For the great majority of arthritides, medical management can be very helpful in controlling symptom magnitude, limiting progression of the disease, and reducing disability. The typical approach is (1) to control the underlying disease and reduce symptoms, (2) to preserve and maintain function through activity modulation and adaptation, and (3) to prevent disability through activity regulation, joint protection, and lifestyle adjustment.

DEMOGRAPHICS OF ARTHRITIS

Arthritis and other rheumatic conditions are the number one cause of disability and the most common clinical complaint in the United States.[4] In 2001 the Centers for Disease Control and Prevention (CDC) estimated the current prevalence at 17.5%.[5] The same studies show that nearly 3% of the population is functionally limited by their arthritis. In 1994, Guccione[6] stated that 60 million adults in the United States were thought to have some form of osteoarthritis, an estimate much higher than the one previously suggested by the Arthritis Foundation. As the general population ages, the number of persons with arthritis will continue to rise. Overall, women are more commonly affected than men; of the 40 million persons who have arthritis today, 23 million are female, and health care consumption and disability are quite proportional to the sex disparity.[7] Arthritis strikes children and those in their twenties and thirties, and pathologic joint changes are essentially universal by age 70.

The direct and indirect costs of arthritis and chronic joint symptoms are great. Billions are spent annually on physician costs, radiology and laboratory fees, hospitalization, surgery, therapy, medication, and medical equipment. The CDC has estimated that one in every three adults in the United States has arthritis or chronic joint symptoms, comprising a total of 70 million people, and thus arthritis is the number one cause of disability in Americans.[4] Despite advanced technology and current research efforts, arthritis still accounts for 427 million days of lost work annually and is the leading cause of industrial absenteeism in the United States.[8]

DISEASE EFFECTS

The rheumatic diseases share common signs and symptoms: pain, general stiffness, joint inflammation, swelling, and diminished ROM.[9] The primary impairments associated with arthritis are the alterations of normal structures and functions of bones, muscles, and joints of the musculoskeletal system. Deformities and loss of function in arthritis are caused by changes in articular and periarticular tissues directly or indirectly related to the disease process. Early tissue changes cause pain and stiffness that interfere with movement before there is actual loss of function.[10] Muscles and joints tend to become stiff, tense, and weak. Tense muscles press on nerve endings, also making movements painful and difficult. Persistent pain causes restricted joint motion and inhibition of muscle contraction, which results in further loss of joint mobility and disuse atrophy of adjacent muscle groups. This leads to a weakening of the muscles essential to joint protection and a vicious cycle of lack of activity and loss of function. Inactivity causes substantial weakness and loss of tissue from all elements of the musculoskeletal system. Deficits such as poor endurance and fatigue associated with aerobic deconditioning are viewed as reversible functional losses for the patient with arthritis.

The weakness associated with arthritis may have multiple origins. Joint effusion has been shown to decrease active strength across the joint.[11] Strength may be

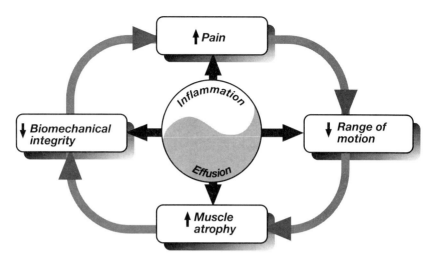

Figure 10-1. Cycle of arthritic dysfunction. (Adapted from Hicks JE: Exercise for patients with inflammatory arthritis. J Musculoskel Med 10:40, 1989.)

reduced because of decreased biomechanical integrity, with consequent reflex inhibition of the joint effector muscles.[12] Pain-induced inactivity leads to deconditioning and atrophy.[12] The medical management of arthritis may involve medications that create muscle atrophy, such as corticosteroids, even with low-dose regimens.[13-15] The arthritic process may involve muscle directly, producing an inflammatory myopathy and consequent diminished strength.[16] Other causes have also been found to cause muscle weakness, including nerve involvement, muscle fiber type alteration, and cellular metabolic process changes. Figure 10-1 demonstrates the vicious cycle that an active arthritic process can develop. These changes include loss of bone, muscle, and connective tissue; a reduction in joint ROM, muscle strength, and endurance; and a marked decline in fitness.[17] Prolonged inactivity results in loss of flexibility and physical capacity, deconditioning, and deterioration of functional abilities, such as reaching overhead, dressing, getting up from the toilet, and walking.

As limiting as the loss of physical functioning may be, arthritis also affects other, nonphysical aspects of a person's life: the way he or she feels about himself or herself and others and how he or she works, sleeps, eats, and relaxes.[18] These changes in lifestyle can lead to depression, social isolation, and an inability to fulfill social, family, and societal roles. Through proper treatment, however, symptoms and disease progression can often be managed or diminished.

EXERCISE IN ARTHRITIS

Many believe that exercise and rest are the cornerstones of the overall medical management of arthritic diseases. The incorporation of exercise as an essential part of the management of patients with arthritis dates at least to Roman times. Although exercise may or may not change the progression of the underlying rheumatic process in a given individual, it can play an invaluable role in keeping muscle strength and joint ROM as normal as possible without further damaging diseased intra- and extraarticular tissues, aiding contracture prevention, slowing down other deformities, and by preventing much of the loss of function.[19] Specific goals of exercise for these populations include maintaining strength and endurance, preserving joint motion, retaining the ability to perform activities of daily living, preserving bone density, and reducing pain.[20]

Beals[21] said, "Rheumatoid patients as a group have lower than expected aerobic capacity and physical performance, and their overall muscle strength is 60% below that of age-matched control subjects," concluding that "such patients tolerate well-tailored strengthening and endurance programs, with gains in physical performance levels in as brief a time as six weeks." Long-term exercise regimens over many years in patients with rheumatoid arthritis have proved to be well tolerated with resultant improvement in functional and other outcome measures.[22, 23]

Because patients with arthritis have decreased endurance, these individuals should participate in some form of aerobic exercise to enhance their overall fitness. Studies have demonstrated the benefits of aerobic exercise for many conditions, including fibromyalgia pain,[24] rheumatoid arthritis,[25–27] lupus erythematosus,[28] and osteoarthritis.[29] Hampson and colleagues[30] found that patients with arthritis who participate in exercise programs are more likely to effectively manage their osteoarthritic symptoms through low-impact exercise than with medications.

The properties of the aquatic environment make aquatic exercise and swimming (forms of low-impact exercise) good ways to manage arthritic symptoms. This contention has been substantiated in two studies of patient groups with nonacute rheumatoid arthritis and osteoarthritis participating in water exercise. In a Danish study, Danneskiold-Samsøe and coworkers[31] found markedly increased isometric and isokinetic muscle strength of the quadriceps in subjects with rheumatoid arthritis after only moderate training in the pool.[31] Other gains included an increase in aerobic capacity and freedom of movement and a higher degree of self-help in activities of daily living. Bunning and Materson[29] found pool therapy to be effective for patients with osteoarthritis, concluding that aquatic exercise should be the cornerstone of treatment for severe arthritis. Patients who participated in the study exhibited significant improvements in aerobic capacity, ambulation distances, and physical activity levels. The use of group exercise also allowed increased socialization, counteracting the isolation that many patients with arthritis feel. The overall benefits of aquatic exercise programs can include reduction of joint swelling, a decrease in joint stiffness and muscle soreness, which enhances the opportunities for active motion, improvement or maintenance of joint flexibility, increased muscle strength, improved coordination, increased endurance, and improved ability to perform daily tasks.

Aquatic therapy programs in a heated pool are effective for patients with arthritic conditions for many reasons. Water's remarkable properties of heat transmission, buoyancy, resistance, and hydrostatic pressure provide a medium in which passive and voluntary exercise can be carried out with minimal stress and freedom, producing multiple therapeutic benefits. These biologic effects have been well described in earlier chapters.

Immersion and exercise in water of therapeutic temperatures (92 to 96°F) facilitate relaxation and the stretching and strengthening of muscles, ligaments, and tendons. Water has a very high capacity for specific heat, which means it absorbs or transfers heat very efficiently. Application of heat produces the following benefits in arthritic conditions:

- Decreased joint stiffness[32]
- Increased collagen extensibility in tendons[33]

- Pain relief[34]
- Pain threshold elevation[35]
- Muscle spasm relief[36]
- Increased circulation[37]
- Increased diuresis and cell metabolism[38]

Although warm water has been the traditional means of treating patients with arthritic conditions, and research has validated its utility, more recent surprising research has shown clinical results from cool-water immersion. Nobunaga and coworkers[39] at Kyushu University in Japan studied the effects of cold-water bathing (13°C) on activity indices of morning stiffness and joint pain, grip strength, ease with activities of daily living, plasma norepinephrine levels, serum adrenocorticotropic hormone and cortisone levels, and a number of measures of immunosuppression. Significant gains in the activity indices were noted, along with significant elevations of norepinephrine. A mild immunosuppressive effect was noted in the population bathing in cold water, with lowered immune complexes and lymphocyte subgroups. The control group, which had bathed in warm water (40°C) for comparable times, showed similar index reduction curves but lower performance levels throughout the treatment sessions. Only slight elevation of norepinephrine levels was noted in the warm-water control group, and no immunosuppressive effect was found.

Water's buoyancy offsets body weight and supports painful and weakened structures. The density of water supports the immersed human body. When submerged to neck level, a person's apparent body weight is about one tenth of his or her weight on land, which enables the individual with weakness to move more comfortably. People with atrophied muscles are allowed complete freedom of movement due to their virtual weightlessness. When gradation of weight-bearing activities is desired, exercise can begin in deep water, where the lower extremities carry no weight and buoyancy unloads the compressive forces on the spine. For a gradual increase in weight bearing, activities can be moved to progressively more shallow water. Patients recovering from lower extremity joint replacement surgery, such as total hip replacement and total knee replacement, benefit tremendously from this approach. Passive ROM movements to prevent joint deformities and contractures are much easier to conduct in the aquatic environment. The use of buoyancy can be structured to assist, support, or resist motions of the extremities or trunk while ambient body weight is reduced. Water's viscosity acts as resistance to movement. As turbulence and speed of movement increase, so does resistance. The patient can use lightly resistive aquatic equipment to develop muscle strength and endurance.

Hydrostatic pressure assists in reduction of edema. Edema, a major symptom of rheumatic conditions, can stretch intraarticular joint structures and produce pressure in the joint capsule. The pressure of periarticular edema is one of the factors that triggers pain with joint movement, which is a key factor in the initial loss of ROM and the development of joint stiffness.

The benefits available with whirlpool therapy are increased through the use of the larger therapeutic pool, which permits the following:

- Simultaneous treatment of multiple joint problems
- Deeper immersion in the vertical position
- Heat transference though total body immersion
- A much broader range of therapeutic exercise
- Swimming for conditioning

- Ambulation training
- Popular medical spa techniques, such as the Bad Ragaz Ring Method (BRRM)
- Cost-effective group treatments versus more costly one-on-one therapy treatments

Given the current trends in population aging and the high age-related incidence of arthritis in our society, the construction of more therapeutic pools might be one of America's most worthwhile undertakings.

PROGRAMS

The aquatic environment presents a cost-effective and versatile option for occupational and physical therapists to expedite the goals of rehabilitation for a disease as pervasive as arthritis. Medically supervised water therapy interventions are available to the individual with arthritis. The primary goals of treatment are the same for most of the rheumatic diseases:

- Mobilization of joints
- Strengthening of muscles
- Conditioning
- Reeducation of function
- Patient education about activity pacing, joint protection, and disease management
- Instruction in self-directed exercise regimens

Aquatic therapy techniques are not simply adaptations of conventional land-based therapeutic exercise programs. The aquatic environment allows a different approach to achievement of therapeutic goals for a variety of arthritic conditions, using water's properties of buoyancy, heat absorption, pain reduction, and resistance to assist rehabilitative goals at each stage of the arthritic process. The approach is determined by whether the condition is acute, subacute, or chronic; inflammatory or noninflammatory; and unifocal or multifocal. Other considerations specific to the individual diagnosis also affect the management approach.

Acute Arthritis Management

Traditional medical management for acute episodes or flares consists of rest, immobilization, and medication for pain. Some evidence has surfaced in patients with acute rheumatoid arthritis participating in partial weight-bearing water exercise that regular exercise can decrease joint pain and inflammatory activity.[40] This effect may be due to endorphin release and in part to edema reduction. In the acute stages, therefore, gentle ROM exercise, strengthening, and endurance goals can be pursued in the therapeutic pool along with the passive benefits of pain relief, muscle relaxation, and decreased joint stresses. Uninvolved joints can also be exercised, and joints in a less acute phase of disease may show therapeutic benefit.

For acute flares, some modifications of the aquatic therapy technique are recommended. These include keeping the number of repetitions low (three to five repetitions), with therapist supervision or positioning to keep buoyancy or active patient motions from forcing the joints into extreme ROM. In the acute phase of treatment, it is important to educate the patient on joint protection principles in the use of equipment, handrails, and grab bars. Because movement is easier in water due to the lack of weight on joints and reduced pain, there can be a tendency to overdo; therefore, it is important to pace the activity and keep sessions short to avoid overfatiguing the patient. The patient should be counseled that if pain occurs after treatment and persists for a period of hours or into the next day, exercise ranges and repetitions should be decreased. For patients with severe cervical joint involvement, a Plastizote collar or a mask and snorkel can be used in prone horizontal activities and swimming to prevent pain, cervical joint hypermobility, or even subluxation. When patients are febrile with a temperature elevation of more than 1°C, admission into the therapeutic pool is generally not advisable.

Subacute and Chronic Arthritis Management

Treatment programs for patients with subacute and chronic arthritis can include one-on-one techniques with the therapist as well as more general exercises and activities designed to improve functional capacity. These include: passive mobilization and relaxation; buoyancy-assisted, -supported, or -resisted exercise; and strength training, conditioning, and functional training for posture, balance, and mobility. Patients may be positioned in the seated, standing, horizontal supine, or prone flotation setup positions or suspended in deep water. Treatment may be carried out on an individual basis or in groups.

Mobilization of Joints

The goal of mobilization of joints and stretching muscles, ligaments, and tendons is common to many treatment protocols recommended for patients with arthritis.[39] ROM exercises can help maintain joint movement, relieve stiffness, promote synovial fluid production and quality, and restore flexibility. The buoyancy and warmth of the water promote both general and specific relaxation of the muscle groups around painful joints.[31, 41, 42] Once the patient achieves this optimal state, exercise can progress from passive ROM movements performed by the therapist, to active assisted ROM exercise, to active patient exercise, and then to resistive exercise.

Passive Technique

Mobilization of joints with contractures involves stretching fibrous tissue, but care must be taken not to overstretch periarticular structures, which may cause local recurrence of pain and inflammation.[17] It is essential that the therapist control joint mobilization techniques as well as limit range and activity in a specific joint. Receiving feedback from the patient about the effects of the last treatment is essential. After a session of joint mobilization, one can expect the joint to be a little sore for a few hours, but this should subside within 24 hours. Harrison[1] said, "In a joint that is both stiff and painful, the only way the therapist can be assured of achieving the desired effect is by isolating the movement with adequate fixation." This may mean positioning the patient on a pool chair, bench, or water plinth, or working with a patient in a flotation setup with the therapist providing stabilization, as in the BRRM. Joint mobilization and joint oscillations can then be performed with accuracy.

Halliwick Method techniques (e.g., rocking, swaying, and snaking) may also be incorporated into passive treatment sessions to promote patient relaxation and elongation and traction to the spine, and to decrease muscle guarding and splinting before exercise.

Active Assisted Exercise

In active assisted exercise, the individual moves the limb actively but may need some assistance in moving it through its full excursion. Treatment programs should begin with one-on-one techniques with the therapist, who can position the patient for the best use of buoyancy and assist the limb through controlled available joint ROM. BRRM exercise using proximally controlled handholds is excellent for this purpose.

Active Exercise

In active exercise, the patient can move the body or body part through the water with control throughout the available joint ROM. General exercises and activities based on improving functional patterns of motion can be performed independently in specific positioning setups or in groups in the shallow water. Improving coordination of precise functional motions, with supervision and cueing as to proper use of body mechanics and joint protection principles, is perhaps best done in the water. The therapist can readily observe spinal alignment and movement patterns in functional tasks, while the density and viscosity of the water slows down movements for observation and analysis. Many types of arthritis cause deformities that alter normal biomechanical alignment, and therefore postural deviations are quite common. The therapist is present to provide skilled corrections and modifications of active exercise. From poolside, careful attention to true body position is essential because the refractive properties of the water may create distortion that masks actual body posture. This is an argument for the therapist to stay in the pool until the patient is able to self-correct. Calisthenic exercises, water walking, deep-water exercises, and swimming instruction are modes of active exercise.

Resistive Exercise

Because water has buoyancy, movement is easier due to weight off-loading, but it becomes more difficult against the resistance presented by the viscosity of the water. This resistance varies, depending on factors such as the speed of movement, the surface area of the moving body part, the use of equipment, and the ambient turbulence of the water. The resistance noted with increasing speed of movement is not linear but rather is complex and logarithmic. Viscous damping properties of water make the resistance drop almost instantaneously on cessation of effort. Water offers the patient with arthritis the opportunity for protected, subtle, and gradable increases in resistive exercise to increase muscle strength and muscular endurance. When the body is submerged to the neck, the effect of gravity on joints with impaired integrity is negligible. Muscles can be strengthened through isometric exercises by holding a stable position against the resistance of the water, against

Table 10-1. Sample Progress Report: Upper-Body Aquatic Endurance Exercises

Date	Buoyancy Object	Number of Repetitions	Elapsed Time (min)	Movement Arc (degrees)
10/01/96	Small paddles	20 extensions	80	90–150
10/08/96	Large paddles	10 extensions	75	90–140
10/15/96	Quart jug	15 extensions	55	90–170

therapist-created turbulence, or against a float, or by maintaining a static position while being pushed through the water, as in certain patterns of the BRRM. By moving the body or limb through water, the patient can perform isokinetic resistive exercise to strengthen muscles. Because water is a three-dimensional medium, active exercise in any direction is resistive. A wide variety of aquatic exercise equipment is available to grade and progress the activity. Light weight training of 3 to 10 repetitions in specific muscle groups is indicated to minimize the debilitating effects of many arthritic conditions and to develop and maintain lean muscle mass. Graded isokinetic water activities provide a protective medium to accomplish this aim. It is important to slow the speed of movement through the ROM whenever equipment is added to prevent injury.

BRRM and conventional water exercises performed under a therapist's supervision are also effective in the treatment of patient weakness.[31, 42, 43] Conventional water exercise uses flotation rings, which act as added resistance when the patient performs a motion against the force of buoyancy. This method may generate considerable resistance to the muscles, depending on the buoyant object. The exercise effort may be graded by using progressively more buoyant objects, increasing the number of repetitions, speeding up the movement, and going through larger arcs of movement. Table 10-1 is an example of a grid that might be used to quantify progress.

It is important to quantify exercise movement in arthritis because patients need protection against overload, which requires knowledge of past loads successfully managed. In this way strength is developed while joint tolerances are monitored. The faster the motion away from buoyancy or the more air in the flotation rings, the greater the resistance to movement (Fig. 10-2). In BRRM exercises, the therapist

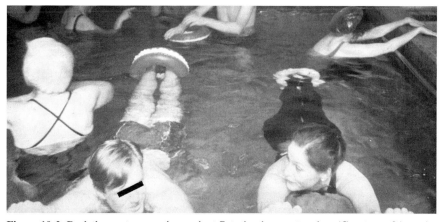

Figure 10-2. Resistive water exercise against flotation in a water ring. (Courtesy of Aquatic Rehabilitation Consultants, Smithfield, VA.)

216 COMPREHENSIVE AQUATIC THERAPY

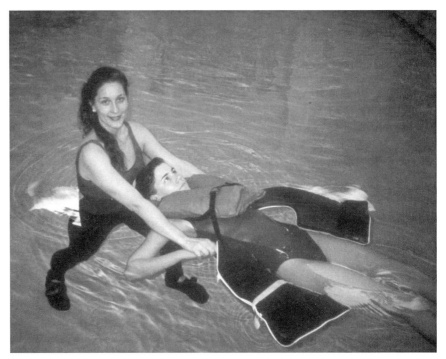

Figure 10-3. Bad Ragaz Ring Method. Arm pattern for bilateral upper extremity. (Courtesy of Aquatic Rehabilitation Consultants, Smithfield, VA.)

acts as a fixator around which the patient works isometrically, supported by floats in supine, prone, or side-lying positions, while moving in straight or diagonal closed chains of movement (Figs. 10-3 and 10-4). Thus, the arms, trunk, and legs can be strengthened using a system of resistance progression readily graded by the aquatic

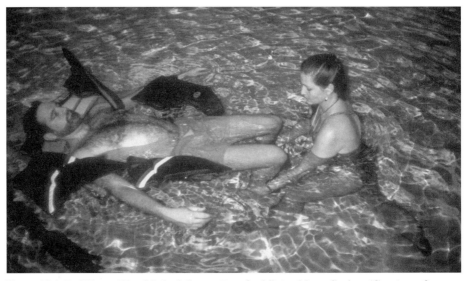

Figure 10-4. Bad Ragaz Ring Method. Leg pattern for bilateral knee flexion. (Courtesy of Aquatic Rehabilitation Consultants, Smithfield, VA.)

therapist trained in this method. A word of precaution is needed: When working with patients who have abnormal joint physiology, the therapist must keep the momentum of initiated movements from proceeding too far by stepping forward into the direction of the joint movement when the movement approaches end ranges (Fig. 10-5).

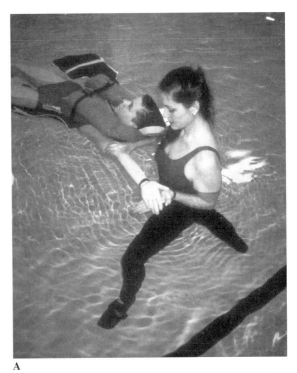

A

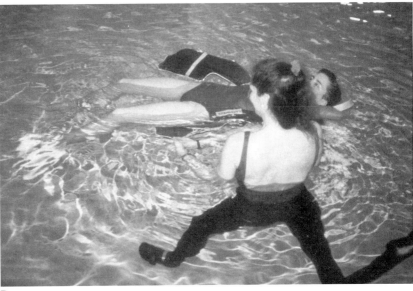

B

Figure 10-5. Therapist breaking resistance in the Bad Ragaz arm pattern by stepping in the direction of the patient's motion. *A*, Starting motion. *B*, Ending motion. (Courtesy of Aquatic Rehabilitation Consultants, Smithfield, VA.)

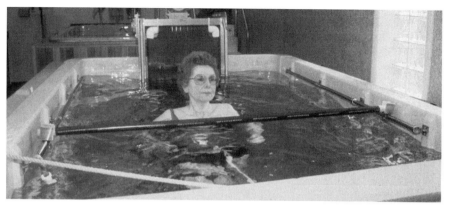

Figure 10-6. Patient with rheumatoid arthritis exercising in a water tank. (Courtesy of Therapeutic Systems, Inc., Doylestown, PA.)

Aerobic Conditioning

Paramount to the prevention and slowing of the progression of many arthritic diseases is the control of joint loading.[2] Water provides a safe, versatile, and protective medium for the deconditioned individual to initiate or enhance his or her cardiovascular capacity. A wide variety of aerobic exercise modes can be conducted in water of varying depths. Deep-water exercise, in which the patient can be suspended with a flotation belt, saddle, or vest in the vertical position at the water's surface, permits a wide range of non–weight-bearing underwater exercises that can be aerobically formatted (Fig. 10-6). Some examples are water running, scissor kicks, cross-country skiing movements, abduction-adduction kicks with and without lower extremity water resistance equipment, such as fins and boots, with simultaneous upper extremity motions of figure-eights, finning, and sculling. Aerobic conditioning of very high intensity can be accomplished even while injured joints are protected.

Shallow water also offers a range of aerobic workout opportunities, such as water walking (Fig. 10-7), water aerobics in which calisthenics are performed in simple straight planes of motion incorporating good body mechanics, and exercising with lightly resistive aquatic equipment. Swimming with adaptations made for adherence to proper postural alignment and joint protection techniques is yet another aquatic aerobic option for the patient with a rheumatic disease. For specific problems, the therapist can design aquatic aerobic circuits using functional tolerances and motions, such as squatting to standing, sitting to standing, trunk flexion to extension, and ambulation (Fig. 10-8).

Reeducation of Function

Improvement and maintenance of joint flexibility, muscle strength, and cardiovascular conditioning improve physical capacity, which translates into improved function. Measurable functional outcome activities, such as supine rolling, coming from supine to sitting, sitting balance, upper extremity movement in sitting, moving from sitting to standing, standing balance, ambulation for flat and uneven terrain, and stair climbing, can be done effectively with skilled therapeutic aquatic therapy intervention. First, the patient performs the activity in the water, and then he or she

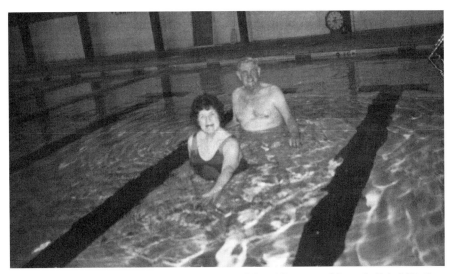

Figure 10-7. Patients with osteoarthritis water walking. (Courtesy of Aquatic Rehabilitation Consultants, Smithfield, VA.)

progresses to land under gravity load. Restoration of the muscles' normal pattern of movement with freedom from pain is the functional outcome measure from which to judge the effectiveness of treatment interventions.

PATIENT EDUCATION

Joint Protection, Pacing, and Management

Exercise groups and aquatic circuits lend themselves well to educationally formatted group treatments, which are cost effective, offer psychological and peer support, and emphasize important patient educational goals. Pacing, joint protection skills,

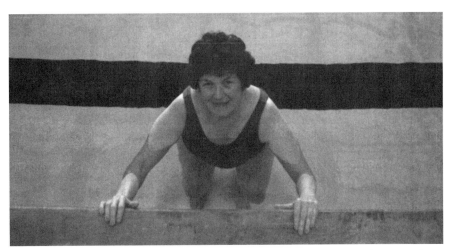

Figure 10-8. Total knee replacement patient performing squats in the pool. (Courtesy of Aquatic Rehabilitation Consultants, Smithfield, VA.)

proper body mechanics, pain management, and self-empowering knowledge of exercise theory can be taught effectively in groups with the goal of long-term maintenance and independent exercise program adherence.[44] Such groups may facilitate exercise adherence while decreasing health care system use and its associated costs.

Community Transitioning

Once discharged from skilled water therapy and rehabilitation programs, patients with arthritis should follow some type of functional maintenance program. Recognizing the importance of water exercise for those who suffer from arthritis, the Arthritis Foundation in cooperation with the YMCA has developed a nationwide Arthritis Aquatics Program. The Arthritis Foundation YMCA Aquatics Program (AFYAP) was developed in 1982 and revised in 1990, 1996, and 2002. The 2002 program has marked differences from the prior programs. Earlier versions emphasized simple ROM exercises in the standing position and water-walking variations. The original program uses 68 ROM and strengthening exercises and an optional endurance-building component; several of these exercises are shown in Appendix A. Swimming skills are unnecessary. The Arthritis Foundation developed other programs, including PACE (People with Arthritis Can Exercise), a community-based group program, and Joint Efforts, a gentle exercise program for sedentary older adults. The PACE program consists of calisthenic exercises in straight planes of motion that promote total body flexibility and gentle aerobic exercises that increase cardiovascular capacity. Water walking, deep-water exercise, and swimming are aerobic modes from which individuals can select (Figs. 10-9 and 10-10). The Plus Program was added to allow for deep-water or feet-off-the-floor exercise. The 2002 version has more emphasis on combination movements as well as interval performance exercise. Balance and cardiovascular improvement join the previous therapeutic goals for the program.

In 2002, two new classes were added to the AFYAP: the Deep Water Program and the Juvenile Arthritis Program. The Deep Water Program is targeted for adults

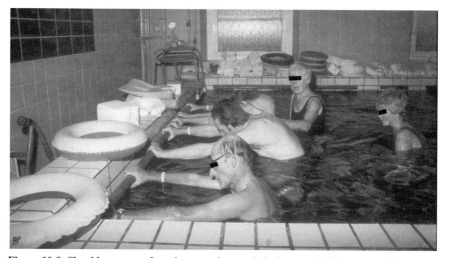

Figure 10-9. Shoulder range-of-motion exercises: ankylosing spondylitis group. (Courtesy of Aquatic Rehabilitation Consultants, Smithfield, VA.)

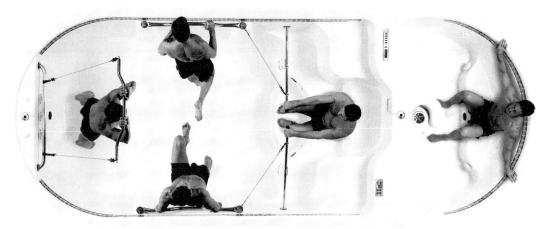

Figure 10-10. Swimming against a gradable resistant current. (Courtesy of Swimex, Inc., Warrington, RI.)

who are familiar with the AFYAP guidelines for exercise and are able to tolerate wearing a flotation device without pain or discomfort, who can exercise without fear or apprehension in water depths where they cannot touch bottom, and who can maintain alignment in vertical and other positions with recovery to vertical while wearing a flotation device. The deep-water class component adds variety and exercise intensity variations and provides a reduced impact and near-weightless environment for participant exercise. Open kinetic chain exercise is appropriate for those who are non–weight-bearing and cannot tolerate joint loading. The program potentially reduces stress on joints, soft tissues, and bones. Sample exercises are illustrated in Appendix B.

The Juvenile Arthritis Program is the first recreational exercise program with therapeutic benefits designed to address the needs of the estimated 285,000 children in the United States who have some form of juvenile arthritis. The program is offered for children younger than 16 years of age and uses the American College of Rheumatology diagnostic criteria and terminology for the individual diseases included under the umbrella of juvenile arthritis. The program accommodates the approach desirable for instructing children. An assessment of the child's mobility, independence, and skill level in and out of the water is made to allow for accommodation of each child's needs and interests. Time is allotted for warmups and play as well as breaks and age-appropriate teaching strategies. Types of exercises are broken down into ROM and flexibility exercises, strengthening exercises, and aerobic endurance exercises. Furthermore, classes are organized into age groupings for young children and teenagers.

These carefully structured recreational programs have incorporated the basic precautions needed to provide safe, effective, low-cost, and medically sound water exercise programs to those who have arthritis. Certification in the content base is available for interested therapists, and training materials are available through the Arthritis Foundation (1330 West Peachtree Street, Atlanta, GA 30309). Information regarding the nearest Arthritis Aquatics Program may be located by calling the arthritis information line at 800-283-7800. The certification process is sufficient so that a medical practitioner may generally feel comfortable referring a patient to the program, and the author's experience has been that patient adherence has been high, therapeutic value significant, and cost to the patient low.

CONCLUSION

The physical properties of water create an ideal environment for the rehabilitation of the patient with arthritis, as has been known and practiced since the beginnings of recorded medical therapeutics. Watching the relief on a patient's face as he or she slips into warm water allows no other conclusion. The physical properties of water address nearly all the causes of arthritic symptoms and allow the patient an opportunity to reduce pain, decrease joint swelling, increase joint movement and strength, and preserve and build functional capacity while in a comfortable relaxing medium. The therapeutic options range from simple warm water immersion, to passive and active underwater exercise techniques, to skilled hydrotherapeutic interventions by an aquatic therapist in individual and group treatments. These therapies can progress into recreational usage of water for exercise maintenance. The therapeutic margin of safety is exceedingly high, permitting self-directed exercise programs and low-cost disease management. The aquatic options beneficial to management of the individual with arthritis are nearly endless, depending only on the imagination and creativity of the individual with arthritis, and his or her therapist or physician.

Appendix A
Arthritis Foundation YMCA Aquatics Program Class Planner Worksheet 1

Sample Program

Exercise Category	Exercise No.	Suggested Name	Comments
Walking (A) 5 min warm-up	1	Forward walking	
	2	Backward walking	
	5	Sidestepping	
Neck exercise (C)	10	Neck rotation	
	11	Neck tilts	
Shoulder exercise (E)	17	Shoulder circles	
	16	Shoulder shrugs	
	18	Flexion/extension	
	22	Abduction/adduction	
	27	Internal/external rotation	
	35	Rope pull	
Trunk stretching exercise (D)	12	Side bends	
Elbow exercise (F)	37	Flexion/extension	
Hip and knee exercise (H)	51	Quadriceps stretch	
	53	Hip and knee	
	55	Flex/extension squats	
	62	Calf stretch	
	59	Leg circles	

Source: Adapted with permission from YMCA Aquatics Instructors Manual. Alpharetta, GA: AFYAP Program Institute, Arthritis Foundation.

Hydrotherapeutic Applications in Arthritis Rehabilitation **223**

Exercise 69—Knee Chest
- Bring both knees toward chest then lower
- May be performed one leg at a time
- Alternate with toes toward knee and away from knee

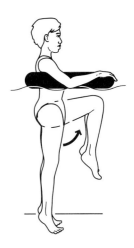

Exercise 70—Bicycle
- Simulate a bicycle movement
- Bicycle forward and backward
- Bicycle with one leg only
- Alternate with point and flex foot position

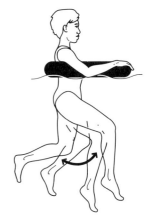

Exercise 71—Forward Scissors
- Legs straight, knees firm but not locked
- Simulate a forward scissors motion (similar to cross country ski movement)
- Alternate with point and flex foot position

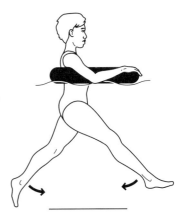

Exercise 72—Side Jacks
- Legs straight, knees firm but not locked
- Open legs to the side, return to center (similar to jumping jack movement)

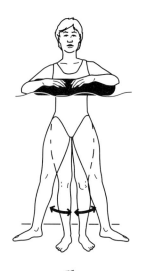

Exercise 73—Scissors
- Legs straight, knees firm but not locked
- Scissor left to right, crossing legs
- Alternate left leg on top, right leg on top
- Alternate with point and flex foot position

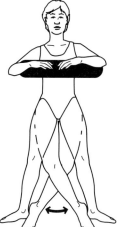

Appendix B
Arthritis Foundation YMCA Aquatic Program for Juvenile Arthritis (AFYAP JA)

Sample Class

1. **Demonstrate use of noodle, hula hoop, and kickboard for games**
2. **Warm up**
   a. Walk forward and backward. Walk in a circle. If class is large enough, walk group in a circle.
   b. Sing "Head, Shoulders, Knees, and Toes." Touch upper body parts, bend knees, and wiggle toes.
   c. Walk side to side with scissor arms.

3. **Games: Select one for each age group**

    Ages 6–11 years   "Musical chairs" with a kickboard or cookie. Choose this game only if you will have access to music.

    Follow the leader or Simon says.

    Scavenger Hunt. Tie a noodle in a knot for a floating basket to gather objects or use a kickboard to balance objects collected.

    Ages 11–14 years Individual kickboard relay race.

    Air ball also known as Sky ball. Use a beach ball.

    Ages 14–18 years Kickboard relay race in teams.

    Water basketball. If no basket hoop is available, use hula hoops for floating "baskets." Use colored visors (two colors) for teams.

4. **Strength and endurance**
    a. Arm scissors and figure eights (3–5 repetitions and build to 8–10).
    b. Kickboard (kicking) for legs or jogging. (Use pool width rather than length of pool for kicking or jogging so that children are moving toward or in shallow water.)

5. **Cool down**
    a. Active stretches if water temperature permits.
    b. Wooden soldier walk.
    c. "Loose walk" to relax limbs.
    d. Hugs and pats (see AFYAP instructor's guide).
    e. Deep breathing and relaxation ("sigh" on exhale).

Source: Drawings reprinted with permission from YMCA Aquatics Instructors Manual. Alpharetta, GA: AFYAP Program Institute, Arthritis Foundation.

REFERENCES

1. Harrison R: Hydrotherapy in rheumatic conditions. In Hyde S (ed): Physiotherapy in Rheumatology. Oxford, UK: Blackwell, 1980.
2. Reed K: Quick Reference to Occupational Therapy. Rockville, Md: Aspen, 1991.
3. Robinson D: Osteoarthritis. In Rubenstein FD (ed): Scientific American Medicine. New York: Scientific American, 1994.
4. Prevalence of self-reported arthritis or chronic joint symptoms among adults in the United States, 2001. MMWR Morb Mortal Wkly Rep 51:948–950, 2002.
5. Prevalence of disabilities and associated health conditions among adults—United States 1999. MMWR Morb Mortal Wkly Rep 50:120–125, 2001.
6. Guccione AA: Arthritis and the process of disablement. Phys Ther 74:408–414, 1994.
7. Verbrugge LM: Women, men, and osteoarthritis. Arthritis Care Res 8:212–220, 1995.
8. Marmer L: Preparing for the arthritis epidemic. Occup Ther Adv 11:54, 1995.
9. Caspers J, Ostle E: Osteoarthritis and rheumatoid arthritis. In Helm, M (ed): Occupational Therapy with the Elderly. New York: Churchill Livingstone, 1987, p 31.
10. Instill J: Reconstructive surgery and rehabilitation of the knee. In Kelly WM, Ruddy S, Sledge CB (eds): Arthritis and Related Disorders. Philadelphia: WB Saunders, 1981.
11. deAndre JR, GC, Dixon AS: Joint distension and reflex muscle inhibition in the knee. J Bone Joint Surg [Am] 47:313, 1965.
12. Herbison GJ, Ditunno JF, Jaweed MM: Muscle atrophy in rheumatoid arthritis. J Rheumatol 14(suppl 15):78–81, 1987.
13. Danneskiold-Samsøe B, Grimby G: The relationship between the leg muscle strength and physical capacity in patients with rheumatoid arthritis, with reference to the influence of corticosteroids. Clin Rheumatol 5:468–474, 1986.
14. Danneskiold-Samsøe B, Grimby G: Isokinetic and isometric muscle strength in patients with rheumatoid arthritis: the relationship to clinical parameters and the influence of corticosteroid. Clin Rheumatol 5:459–467, 1986.
15. Danneskiold-Samsøe B, Grimby G: The influence of prednisone on the muscle morphology and muscle enzymes in patients with rheumatoid arthritis. Clin Sci (Lond) 71:693–701, 1986.
16. Hicks JE: Exercise in patients with inflammatory arthritis and connective tissue disease. Rheum Dis Clin North Am 16:845–870, 1990.

17. Swezey R: Rehabilitation aspects in arthritis. In McCarty DJ (ed): Arthritis and Related Disorders. Philadelphia: Lea & Febiger, 1979, 349.
18. Melvin J: Rheumatic Disease in the Adult and Child: Occupational Therapy and Rehabilitation, 3rd ed. Philadelphia: Davis, 1989.
19. Gerber L: Principles and their application in rehabilitation of patients with rheumatic diseases. In Kelly WM, Ruddy S, Sledge CB (eds): Arthritis and Related Disorders. Philadelphia: WB Saunders, 1981.
20. Namey TC: Exercise and arthritis: adaptive bicycling. Rheum Dis Clin North Am 16:871–886, 1990.
21. Beals C: A case for aerobic conditioning exercise in rheumatoid arthritis. Clin Res 29:780A, 1981.
22. Nordemar R, et al: Physical training in rheumatoid arthritis: a controlled long-term study. I. Scand J Rheumatol 10:17–23, 1981.
23. Nordemar R: Physical training in rheumatoid arthritis: a controlled long-term study. II. Functional capacity and general attitudes. Scand J Rheumatol 10:25–30, 1981.
24. McCain GA: Nonmedicinal treatments in primary fibromyalgia. Rheum Dis Clin North Am 15:73–90, 1989.
25. Ekdahl C: Muscle function in rheumatoid arthritis: assessment and training. Scand J Rheumatol Suppl 86:9–61, 1990.
26. Ekdahl C, et al: Dynamic versus static training in patients with rheumatoid arthritis. Scand J Rheumatol 19:17–26, 1990.
27. Perlman SG, Connell K, Alberti J, et al: Synergistic effects of exercise and problem solving education for rheumatoid arthritis patients. Arthritis Rheum 30(suppl):13, 1987.
28. Robb-Nicholson LC, et al: Effects of aerobic conditioning in lupus fatigue: a pilot study. Br J Rheumatol 28:500–505, 1989.
29. Bunning RD, Materson RS: A rational program of exercise for patients with osteoarthritis. Semin Arthritis Rheum 21(3 suppl 2):33–43, 1991.
30. Hampson SE, et al: Self-management of osteoarthritis. Arthritis Care Res 6:17–22, 1993.
31. Danneskiold-Samsøe B, et al: The effect of water exercise therapy given to patients with rheumatoid arthritis. Scand J Rehabil Med 19:31–35, 1987.
32. Bucklund L, Tiselius P: Objective measurement of joint stiffness in rheumatoid arthritis. Acta Rheumatol Scand 13:275, 1967.
33. Gersten J: Effects of ultrasound on tendon extensibility. Am J Phys Med Rehabil 34:362, 1995.
34. Harris ED Jr, McCroskery PA: The influence of temperature and fibril stability on degradation of cartilage collagen by rheumatoid synovial collagenase. N Engl J Med 290:1–6, 1974.
35. Benson TB, Copp EP: The effects of therapeutic forms of heat and ice on the pain threshold of the normal shoulder. Rheumatol Rehabil 13:101–104, 1974.
36. Figny D, Sheldon K: Simultaneous use of heat and cold in the treatment of muscle spasm. Arch Phys Med Rehabil 43:235, 1962.
37. Harris P: Iontophoresis: clinical research in musculoskeletal inflammatory conditions. J Orthop Sports Phys Ther 4:109, 1982.
38. Epstein M: Renal effects of head-out water immersion in humans: a 15-year update. Physiol Rev 72:63–621, 1992.
39. Nobunaga M, Tatsukawa K, Ishii H, Yoshida F: Balneotherapy for patients with rheumatoid arthritis, especially the effect of cold spring water bathing. In Aigshi OY (ed): New Frontiers in Health Resort Medicine. Noboribetsu, Japan: Hokkaido University School of Medicine Press, 1996, p 109.
40. Scott DL, Wolman RL: Rest or exercise in inflammatory arthritis? Br J Hosp Med 48:445, 447, 1992.
41. Hall J, et al: A randomized and controlled trial of hydrotherapy in rheumatoid arthritis. Arthritis Care Res 9:206–215, 1996.
42. Stenstrom CH, et al: Intensive dynamic training in water for rheumatoid arthritis functional class II—a long-term study of effects. Scand J Rheumatol 20:358–365, 1991.
43. Wyatt FB, et al: The effects of aquatic and traditional exercise programs on persons with knee osteoarthritis. J Strength Cond Res 15:337–340, 2001.
44. Becker B: Motivating adherence in the rehabilitation setting. J Back Musculoskel Med 1:48, 1991.

Chapter 11
Aquatic Strategies in Musculoskeletal Pain

Joseph T. Alleva, MD, Thomas H. Hudgins, MD,
and Marti Biondi, PT

GENERAL PRINCIPLES

Hydrostatic pressure refers to the pressure a fluid creates on an immersed object. It varies with the density of the fluid as well as with the depth of the immersed object. It is a valuable property to exploit for an injured joint. It allows control of joint effusion and provides a source of constant proprioceptive feedback for a particular joint.[1] Consequently, range of motion may improve. From a cardiovascular standpoint, hydrostatic pressure increases preload to the heart and therefore increases cardiac output and the work of breathing.[2,3]

Buoyancy is an upward thrust equal to the weight of fluid displaced by any object. Athletes who have a weight-bearing restriction as a result of injury or surgery will find this invaluable. Immersion to the symphysis pubis will off-load approximately 40% of a patient's body weight, to the umbilicus approximately 50%, and to the zyphoid approximately 60%.[4]

Viscosity is the resistance of fluid flow, and more specifically, the friction between molecules of the liquid that forces them to adhere to each other as well as to the surface of the body moving through it. Turbulent flow refers to the rotary motion of fluid that takes place behind the body as it moves through liquid. The turbulent flow tends to drag the body backward as it attempts to move forward. Turbulent flow depends on multiple factors including size, shape, and speed of the object moving. These properties each provide varying degrees of resistance essential to conditioning and strengthening. This effect can be further amplified by using aquatic devices such as fins and floats.

Hot and cold temperature can cause various physiologic changes. Examples include vasodilatation or vasoconstriction in warm water and cool water, respectively. Warmer temperatures are also thought to prepare muscles for stretching by causing a decrease in gamma fiber activity.[5]

Cardiovascular Benefits of Aquatics for the Athlete

Cardiopulmonary fitness will decline significantly after 2 weeks of detraining. It can decrease to pretraining levels as soon as 10 weeks.[6] There is no reliable research comparing aquatic conditioning programs with their dry land counterparts. One problem with such studies is the obvious difference in environments. Physical properties of water alter temperature regulation, muscles used, and cardiovascular response. However, for an injured athlete it is clear that cardiopulmonary goals can be attained.

It is known that immersion alone will increase central blood volume, cardiac volume, mean stroke volume, and cardiac output.[2] Treadmill running has been shown to positively influence cardiopulmonary fitness as measured through $\dot{V}O_{2max}$, blood lactate levels, respiratory exchange ratio, and perceived exertion. Research has demonstrated an even greater increase in cardiac output in conditioned athletes compared with that in untrained control subjects. These gains are sustained for a longer period of time than in the untrained control group.[7]

AQUATIC REHABILITATION OF THE ANKLE

Functional Anatomy

The talus articulates with the tibia and fibula. It rests upon the calcaneus, which serves posteriorly as the insertion point of the plantar flexors and the major weight-bearing structures. The fibula extends more distally than the tibia and adds to the vulnerability of the lateral aspect of the ankle.[8]

There are three principal lateral ankle ligaments: the anterior talofibular ligament, the calcaneofibular ligament, and the posterior talofibular ligament. They collectively function to provide proprioceptive feedback and lateral ankle stability. It is generally agreed that the anterior talofibular ligament is the weakest of the lateral ligaments and therefore is the most prone to injury.[6] Furthermore, the deltoid complex is stronger in general than the lateral ligamentous complex.[9,10] Essentially, the muscular portion of the leg is broken down into the posterior musculature or the plantar flexors, such as the gastrocsoleus complex, tibialis posterior, and the long toe flexors, and the anterior muscles or the dorsiflexors, such as the tibialis anterior, the long extensors of the toes, and the peroneus tertius. Finally, the lateral musculature or the everters, peroneus brevis and longus, play a critical role during the rehabilitation of the ankle.[10]

Differential Diagnosis of Ankle Pain

Causes of ankle pain in the athlete include ankle sprain, Achilles tendinosis, Achilles tendon rupture, retrocalcaneal bursitis, os trigone pain, plantar fasciitis, and stress fractures.

History and Physical Examination

Ankle sprain is the most common injury in sports and constitutes 7% to 10% of all injuries seen in emergency departments. It occurs most commonly in basketball and soccer.[11] At the time of injury, the most common position of the ankle is inverted, plantar-flexed, and adducted. The ligaments are most vulnerable in this position. Questions about previous ankle injuries, a "pop" or a "snap" at the time of injury, and the ability to bear weight are particularly important to ask during the history taking. The diagnosis can be made by history alone, however a physical examination will determine the severity of the injury. There will be obvious swelling, tenderness, and ecchymosis laterally. Stability should be assessed in the anterior plane (anterior drawer) and in inversion (the talar tilt test). The severity of a tear is graded: macroscopic (I), partial (II), or complete (III). Radiographs should be obtained for patients suspected of having a grade II or III tear. Because fractures occur in 6% to 8% of ankle sprains, anteroposterior, lateral, and mortise views should be obtained.[11]

Rehabilitation of the Ankle

Standard rehabilitation is typically divided into three phases: phase I, the acute phase; phase II, the recovery phase; and phase III, the functional phase. The acute phase focuses on PRICE (protection, rest, ice, compression, and elevation) to limit injury progression. Protection includes use of an air or gel cast as well as taping techniques. Rest typically will include weight bearing as tolerated. During this phase, range of motion (ROM) exercises within a pain-free range are initiated. Ice, compression, and elevation are used to control inflammation and swelling.[12, 13] The aquatics model allows early intervention, particularly for those who had weight-bearing problems due to pain. Aquatic rehabilitation also helps to control effusion due to the hydrostatic property exerted by the water.

The recovery phase focuses on physical rehabilitation of the ankle. Aquatic rehabilitation, like its dry land counterpart, is focused on strengthening the peroneus muscle group and improving plantar flexor flexibility. Proprioceptive retraining is also an integral component of rehabilitation. Use of aquatics offers several advantages. Early entry into phase II because of buoyancy is particularly useful in athletes having difficulty with full weight bearing due to pain or clinical restrictions. Weight bearing can be increased in a graded fashion by performance of exercises in incrementally decreased depths until a transition to a dry land program is achieved. Hydrostatic pressure also helps to control/decrease edema and increase range of motion. Although there are no studies specific to the ankle there are data that demonstrate such a relationship in rehabilitation of the knee. Hydrostatic pressure also complements proprioceptive retraining.[14]

Strengthening of the peroneus longus, brevis, and tertius can be achieved by using viscosity and turbulence (Fig. 11-1). Fins or flotation devices may enhance these effects. Flexibility goals can be achieved by taking advantage of the temperature effects on gamma fiber activity in the gastrocsoleus muscle complex.

AQUATIC REHABILITATION OF THE KNEE

Functional Anatomy

The knee, classified as the largest joint in the body, is situated between its two longest lever arms, making it particularly vulnerable to injury.[15, 16] In addition, the incongruity of the approximating joint surfaces places it at increased risk.[16] The knee complex comprises two functional joints within a single joint capsule: the tibiofemoral and the patellofemoral joints.[16, 17] Considered a modified hinge joint,

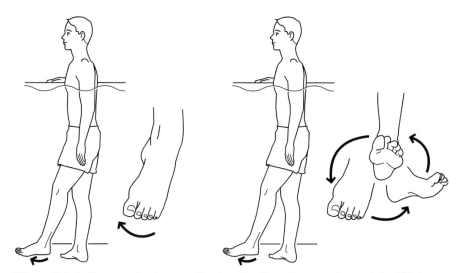

Figure 11-1. Ankle strengthening exercises in water. Inversion, eversion, and dorsiflexion.

the tibiofemoral articulation includes the distal femur, interposed menisci, and the proximal tibia. The primary motions at this joint include flexion/extension, rotation, and minimal abduction/adduction.[18] Because the knee depends on musculotendinous and ligamentous intervention for anterior/posterior stability, there is an increased risk of injury in the sagittal plane.[16] In both repetitive use and traumatic injuries, the ligamentous system, while efficient, is particularly vulnerable.

The patellofemoral joint consists of the articulation of the patellar facets with the corresponding surface of the femur. There is primarily a sliding motion at this joint, occurring simultaneously in the frontal and transverse planes.[16, 17] The patellofemoral joint relationship consists of the intercondylar groove of the anterior femur articulating with the central, vertical ridge of the posterior aspect of the patella.[19] The patella, suspended in the joint capsule and attached to the quadriceps via the quadriceps tendon, lies anteriorly to the tibiofemoral joint. During flexion, the patella slides distally along the femoral groove approximately 7 to 8 cm,[16] until it comes to rest in the intercondylar notch of the femur.

The articular surfaces that make up the tibiofemoral portion of the knee complex include the two convex femoral condyles and the corresponding concave tibial condyles. The menisci, crescent-shaped discs of fibrocartilage, are located on the tibial plateaus. These structures improve the integrity of the relationship between the femoral and tibial condyles and assist with stability at the tibiofemoral joint by interposing tightly between the joint surfaces during maximum extension.[17] Additionally, they distribute the load at the knee during weight bearing, carrying between 40% and 60% of the total load acting on the knee.[17]

Knowledge regarding the relationship between structure and function of the knee complex is essential for proper rehabilitation. Motion at the knee joint produces a functional shortening or lengthening of the lower extremity in open kinetic positions and is responsible for supporting or transferring the body's weight during closed chain activities.[16, 17] The femoral condyles simultaneously roll posteriorly and slide anteriorly to maintain contact with tibial and femoral condyles during flexion.[17] The menisci facilitate joint congruity and function to limit extreme flexion or extension.[16, 17, 18] When the knee is fully extended, the tibial tubercles are lodged in the intercondylar notch of the femur, the menisci are tightly positioned between tibial and femoral condyles, and the ligaments are taut, providing an extremely stable joint.[16, 17] A locking mechanism is initiated when the femoral condyles begin to roll/spin, and this enhances stability.[17]

Structurally, the knee complex involves various dynamic and passive stabilizers designed to enhance its strength in closed chain, flexed positions. Although the knee has many passive stabilizers, the four primary contributors include the anterior cruciate ligament (ACL), the posterior cruciate ligament, the medial collateral ligament, and the lateral collateral ligament, plus the joint capsule. The specific involvement of each of these depends on the joint angle and the plane in which the knee is loaded.[19] In most situations, there are several ligaments working synergistically to provide stability, although one usually has primary responsibility for the load.[16, 19] Dynamically, the muscles that stabilize the knee include the quadriceps, the hamstrings, the pes anserinus, the extensor retinaculum, the popliteus, and the iliotibial band.[17] Muscle activity around joint segments plus compressive forces in weight-bearing positions likewise assist with lower extremity stability in closed chain positions. Although the neuromuscular control process is an integral part of stability,[19] it will be discussed with treatment.

Differential Diagnosis of Knee Pain

The most common cause of knee pain in the athlete is patellofemoral syndrome. Other causes of knee pain include ligament sprain/tear, cartilage/meniscus tear, popliteus tendinitis, plica syndrome, and referred pain from the hip or back.

History and Physical Examination

The patient with patellofemoral/maltracking syndrome will present with vague anterior knee pain with or without an effusion. The discomfort may be recognized acutely but typically has an insidious onset. The pain is exacerbated by descending stairs or squatting, positions that increase the patellofemoral joint reaction force. The athlete may also describe increased discomfort after prolonged sitting with the knees flexed, a positive "theater sign." The ligamentous and meniscal examination is unremarkable, but the examiner may recognize musculoskeletal imbalances such as pes planus, increased pronation, internal rotation of the tibia, increased Q-angle, and weak gluteus medius.

Rehabilitation of the Knee

Immersion can initiate a decrease in compressive joint force,[20, 21] which allows a patient with significant instability in weight bearing to function in a vertical position. As the depth of immersion increases, less body weight is borne through the lower extremities.[20] Patients with weight-bearing restrictions may start ambulating earlier in the pool than on land. However, with fast walking, weight bearing at a specified depth increases by as much as 76%.[22] Physical therapists must, therefore, carefully monitor walking speed so that forces across the knee do not become excessive.

Range of motion can also be improved during aquatic rehabilitation.[21, 23] In a study conducted on patients after ACL repairs, the aquatic group reached normal ROM for both flexion and extension faster than the traditionally treated group.[24] Skeletal unloading, combined with relaxation and decreased pain perception,[21] provides an excellent therapeutic environment for early improvement in motion.

Resistance training can be optimized early in water-based rehabilitation. Although training principles and progressions imitate land-based treatment, water therapy can be used in situations in which closed chain exercises are contraindicated.[23] Deep-water training that can completely unload weight on the knee joint can be used for patients who have weight-bearing restrictions due to surgical intervention or fractures. As a patient is able to progressively increase the amount of weight bearing, workouts can progress to shallow water. This progression provides significant benefit for gait sequencing, weight bearing through the affected limb, promotion of healing, sensory feedback, and articular cartilage nutrition.[23] Work intensity can be modified by using the properties of buoyancy and turbulence, changing speed and/or depth, adding resistance equipment, or changing the position of the affected limb.[21, 23]

Postoperative rehabilitation of the knee usually emphasizes restoring joint ROM. During the acute stage, the therapist must be aware of the possibilities for overexertion, with resultant increased pain.[23] Patients should be instructed to refrain from end-range, painful positions. Flotation equipment that may move a joint past comfortable ROM should be avoided. At this stage, buoyancy can facilitate progressive improvement in ROM. When there are weight-bearing restrictions, deep water is preferable because the athlete can be belted and suspended to perform active knee ROM exercises. For patients with ligamentous laxity, shallow water may prove more comfortable, because partial weight bearing permits better control of the affected joint. An example of this would be an individual with a lax ACL who has been instructed to improve knee ROM. When suspended, there is no ground reactive force and the extension is unimpeded except for the viscosity of the water; thus, hyperextension may occur. Additionally, an individual with a lax ACL should refrain from walking backward because hyperextension is facilitated. Backwards water-walking may be successfully used to help restore full extension.

Progression from the acute stage should use shallow water, dynamic movements, and flotation devices such as a cuff. In addition, therapists should consider hip and ankle positions that facilitate improved knee ROM. Table 11-1 provides a progression of knee ROM activities for both shallow and deep water. Therapists must recognize patients who have a fear of water and adjust the progression accordingly.

Strength training for postoperative rehabilitation may be initiated in the aquatic environment. Buoyancy exercises, initially used to facilitate motion, can be adjusted to resist movements. When weight-bearing status is an issue, deep water can be used. As weight bearing improves, water exercise becomes an integral component of the strength training process. Utilizing progressively shallow water, graduating from bilateral to unilateral stance activities, and progressing to quick transfers and ballistics all have a place in the exercise protocol. Early weight shifts can progress from single leg stance to full unilateral challenges.[23] Use of the contralateral extremity to increase the intensity of the proprioceptive challenge is appropriate, as is use of assistive or resistive equipment to further increase the intensity. Lastly, impact-loading or plyometric training might be required to expedite a return to

Table 11-1. Knee Range of Motion Exercise Progression

I. Acute Stage: Deep-Water Progressions—Client is belted and feet are off the bottom.
   a. Vertical position: bicycling (gentle)
   b. March
   c. Straight leg raise—partial
   d. Transition to shallow water (if appropriate for weight-bearing restrictions)
II. Acute Stage: Shallow-Water Progression—Client begins aquatic therapy in shallow water.
   a. Bilateral quarter squats
   b. Gentle weight shift from involved lower extremity (LE)
   c. Gentle march
   d. Walk forward→*sideways—backward (restricted to forward if this is a patient with an ACL deficit)
   e. Walk with exaggerated heel strike to facilitate extension→exaggerated heel strike and increase step-lengths
   f. Supported unilateral stationary motions with affected LE:
      i. Knee flexion with hip flexed to 90 degrees
      ii. Knee flexion/extension with hip neutral
      iii. Gentle knee flexion with hip neutral to knee extension to hip flexed to 90 degrees—punt
      iv. Gentle proprioceptive neuromuscular facilitation (PNF) Partial patterns to tolerance
III. Minimal Range of Motion Deficits Persist (may be continued with strengthening exercises): Accentuate range of motion for the following actions, holding positions at end range for 5 to 10 seconds and utilizing a cuff or other flotation apparatus
   a. Knee flexion with hip flexed to 90 degrees
   b. Knee flexion/extension with hip neutral: intense for end-range flexion when cuff is applied
   c. Punting action through full range of motion without cuff→cuff through full range
   d. PNF patterns to end range with cuff
   e. Bilateral and unilateral full squats if possible relative to shallowness of pool

*Indicates progress to similar activity.

previous activities. Shoulder-deep water is appropriate for the initiation of these exercises because the task-off phase is assisted but impact at landing is decreased (Fig. 11-2). The patient soon enters the land-based exercise phase, which helps facilitate both the remodeling process and proprioceptive retraining.[19] Table 11-2 provides a progression for strength training and proprioceptive exercises.

AQUATIC REHABILITATION OF THE SHOULDER

Functional Anatomy

The shoulder is a complex ball and socket joint with multiple muscles, tendons, ligaments, and articulations working in concert to keep the humeral head (the "ball") aligned with the glenoid (the "socket") through multiple planes of motion. The vast ROM of the shoulder joint is balanced with stability. The bones, ligaments, and muscles all contribute to stability. The glenoid fossa is a small concave structure in relation to the large convex humeral head. The glenoid is enlarged 75% by the labrum. The relationship of these structures allows more controlled motion.

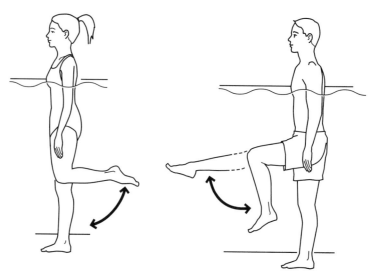

Figure 11-2. Quadriceps and hamstring strengthening in water. One-legged exercises also improve balance and proprioception.

The glenohumeral ligaments help with static stability. The biceps muscle tendon and rotator cuff tendons (supraspinatus, infraspinatus, teres minor, and subscapularis) also help to stiffen the joint capsule, contributing to static stability.

The muscular biomechanics of the shoulder joint can be divided into three basic groups: the scapulohumeral, the scapuloaxial, and the humeroaxial muscles. The scapulohumeral muscles include the deltoid, coracobrachialis, teres major, supraspinatus, infraspinatus, teres minor, and subscapularis. The scapuloaxial muscles include the trapezius, rhomboids, levator scapulae, and serratus anterior. The humeroaxial muscles include the latissimus dorsi and pectoralis. These muscles cross multiple joints including the glenohumeral, acromioclavicular, sternoclavicular, and scapulothoracic joints, which all influence shoulder motion and stability.[25]

The muscles work in force/couples to maintain the center of rotation of the humerus at the glenoid.[26] For instance, the deltoid creates upward force on the humeral head during shoulder abduction, opposing the downward force of the subscapularis and infraspinatus. A scapulothoracic force/couple exists between the levator scapulae and serratus anterior, opposing the middle and lower trapezius with shoulder elevation to control scapular elevation. Internal rotation created by the pectoralis and latissimus dorsi is balanced by external rotation created by the posterior deltoid, infraspinatus, and teres minor to control upper arm rotation.[26, 27]

Differential Diagnosis of Shoulder Pain

Shoulder pain in the athlete may be due to a single traumatic event (macrotrauma) or, more commonly, overuse injury due to soft tissue failure from repetitive microtrauma.[28, 29] Therefore, the differential diagnosis of shoulder pain includes overload injuries such as rotator cuff impingement due to tendinosis/tendonitis, instability, bicipital tendinosis, subacromial bursitis, or adhesive capsulitis. Acute

Table 11-2. Lower Extremity Strength and Proprioceptive Exercise Progression

I. Deep Water: Patients who do NOT have full weight-bearing status.
   a. Bicycling with resistive equipment
   b. March with resistive equipment
   c. Vertical flutter kick
   d. Cross-country skiing action vertically

II. Shallow Water, Phase I (shoulder to waist deep): Patient has full weight-bearing status.
   a. Bilateral quarter squats stationary→*forward→backward→sideways
   b. Stationary unilateral exercises with resistive equipment
      i. Knee flexion/extension with hip at a 90 degrees flexed position
      ii. Knee flexion/extension with hip neutral
      iii. Proprioceptive neuromuscular facilitation patterns
   c. Unilateral stance on affected lower extremity (LE) and using movement in straight plane patterns from nonaffected LE to challenge balance of affected side. Balance exercises performed on kick boards or other flotation devices.
   d. Noodle standing with reversed squats. Balance on noodle either bilaterally or unilaterally.
   e. Step up/down with knee flexion no greater than 90 degrees→side step up/down
   f. Lunges→grapevine
   g. Fast walking→forward with elongated steps→sideways→backward

III. Shallow Water, Phase II: Patient is able to perform unilateral stance position with minimal challenges from unaffected LE and can perform a minisquat on affected LE. NOTE: The following exercises incorporate some power moves. This may not be appropriate for all patients.
   a. Skipping→increase height of excursion, length of excursion or decrease depth
   b. Two-legged hop→increase height of excursion
   c. Single leg hopping for time, depth, or excursion
   d. Water running forward→sideways
   e. Water running intervals: forward, backward, sideways for time or timed/distance
   f. Tethered running: patient is tethered to edge of the pool or to a buddy. Run against each other for time or for speed.

IV. Deep Water, Phase II: These exercises can be interspersed with shallow water activities.
   a. Depth jumping: Patient sinks to the bottom and explodes to the surface in a vertical position. Performed for time or for speed.
   b. Bobs: Patient rebounds repetitively off bottom. Performed for time or for speed.

*Indicates progress to similar activity.

macrotraumatic events include glenohumeral dislocation, acromioclavicular joint sprain, and labral tear.[30]

History and Physical Examination

The history should focus on the onset and duration of pain, exacerbating and relieving factors, and location of pain and any referred discomfort. After a detailed neurologic examination of the upper extremities, the musculoskeletal examination progresses from inspection for any atrophy or bony defects to active and passive ROM, noting any limitations or painful arcs. Finally, provocative maneuvers such as impingement tests, including Hawkins and Neers tests, are performed. The scapulothoracic rhythm is evaluated with the lateral scapular slide test. Kibler[31] showed that asymmetries in performing this maneuver suggest dyskinesis of the scapulothoracic motion, contributing to shoulder pathologic conditions, particularly in athletes performing overhead maneuvers. The musculoskeletal examination also includes an assessment of biomechanical imbalances in the upper extremity kinetic chain.

Rehabilitation of Shoulder Pain

Conservative management of shoulder pain can be divided into three phases: acute, recovery, and functional.[27] Controlling pain and inflammation is the goal during the acute phase, whereas restoring function and normal biomechanics is emphasized during the recovery phase. Lastly, the functional phase will focus on sports-specific training.

Aquatic therapy is indicated at any time along the continuum of rehabilitation when the athlete cannot tolerate the land-based exercises or fails to progress. It may be particularly useful during the acute phase to help reduce muscle spasm, inflammation, and pain.[32] The warmth of the water contributes to increased collagen distensibility, and the buoyancy reduces the stress on painful weight-bearing joints.

With reduction in pain, the athlete is ready to progress to the recovery phase to focus on motion and strength of the shoulder. For example, during rotator cuff rehabilitation, restoring normal ROM occurs before the athlete moves ahead to strengthening exercises during the recovery phase.[33] The goals are to restore normal arthrokinetics, scapular positioning, scapulohumeral rhythm, and scapulothoracic and scapulohumeral strength.[32] For example, a tight posterior capsule may lead to an imbalance of internal/external rotation. Thus, flexibility training may begin with stretching of the posterior capsule with crossed shoulder adduction flexibility. This can be performed on land and in water (Fig. 11-3).

Once ROM is restored, strengthening exercises begin with the spine and scapular stabilizers to provide a base for humeral rotation. Weak abdominal muscles will lead to increased utilization of the latissimus dorsi, resulting in increased humeral internal rotation and decreased external rotation, and, thus, increased propensity for rotator cuff impingement. Weak middle and lower trapezius muscles with tight levator scapulae and rhomboids will lead to excessive downward rotation of the scapula with glenohumeral abduction and increase the chance of impingement.[32] A weak trapezius and serratus anterior will fail to sufficiently raise the acromion during shoulder elevation and retraction. The rotator cuff muscles will be required

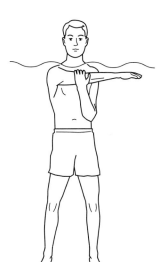

Figure 11-3. Flexibility training for posterior capsule of shoulder in water.

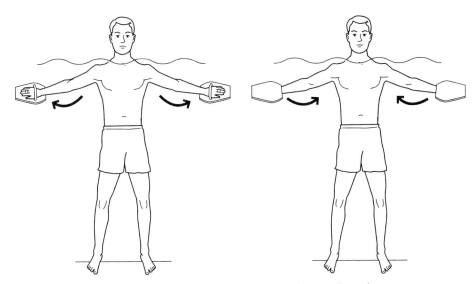

Figure 11-4. Resistance training for shoulder in external and internal rotation.

to work harder to depress the humeral head and avoid compression at the coracoacromial arch; this contributes to an overuse tendinopathy.[25]

One of the advantages of aquatic therapy is that exercises require three-dimensional coordination in the water. Exercises in the pool for the shoulder joint are typically conducted with the water level at the base of the neck. All motion occurs below the surface of the water, which reduces the amount of stress on the shoulder joint due to the antigravity effects of buoyancy. All of these exercises in the pool may be conducted in conjunction with the traditional land exercises in shoulder rehabilitation. Examples include: deep-water walking with arms externally rotated while performing the breaststroke to help restore strength and ROM to the glenohumeral joint; strengthening the scapular stabilizers with use of a mask and snorkel in a prone position; anterior and posterior capsule stretches in the vertical or supine positions using the flotation device with belt (Fig. 11-4); and proprioceptive neuromuscular facilitation exercises using a ball.

REFERENCES

1. Norton C, Shha S: Aquatics versus traditional therapy: contrasting effectiveness for acquisition rates. Phys Ther 73(6 suppl):S10, 1993.
2. Arborelius M Jr, Balldin UI, Lila B, Lundgren CE: Hemodynamic changes in man during immersion with head above water. Aerosp Med 43:592-598, 1972.
3. Hong SK, Cerretelli P, Cruz JC, Rahn H: Mechanics of respiration during submersion in water. J Appl Physiol 27:535-538, 1969.
4. Harrison R, Hillman M: Loading of the lower limb when walking partially immersed. Physiotherapy 78:165, 1992.
5. McGrath A, Johnson A: The effects of hamstring stretching on land versus water physical therapy. J Orthop Sports Phys Ther 73(6 suppl):S30, 1993.
6. Croce P, Gregg J: Keeping fit when injured. Clin Sports Med 10:181-195, 1991.
7. Claybaugh JR, Pendergast DR, Davis JE, et al: Fluid conservation in athletic responses to water intake, supine posture and immersion. J Appl Physiol 61:7-15, 1986.

8. Jenkins D (ed): The leg. In Hollingshead's Functional Anatomy of the Limbs and Back, 6th ed. Philadelphia: WB Saunders, 1991.
9. Lassiter TE Jr, Malone TR, Garrett WE Jr: Injury to the lateral ligaments of the ankle. Orthop Clin North Am 20:629–640, 1989.
10. Safran MR, Benedetti RS, Bartolozzi AR III, Mandelbaum R: Lateral ankle sprains: a comprehensive review: part 1: etiology, pathoanatomy, histopathogenesis, and diagnosis. Med Sci Sports Exerc 31(suppl):S429–S437, 1999.
11. DeLee J, Drez D (eds): Sports injuries of the lower extremity. In Orthopedic Sports Medicine Principles and Practice. Philadelphia: WB Saunders, 1994.
12. Safran MR, Zachazewski JE, Benedetti RR, et al: Lateral ankle sprains: a comprehensive review: part II: treatment and rehabilitation with an emphasis on the athlete. Med Sci Sports Exerc 31(suppl):S439–S450, 1999.
13. Prentice W (ed): Rehabilitation of ankle injuries. In Rehabilitation Techniques in Sports Medicine, 2nd ed. St Louis: Mosby, 1994.
14. Geigle P, Daddona K: The effect of supplemental aquatic physical therapy program on balance and girth for NCAA division III athletes with a grade I or grade II lateral ankle sprain. J Aquat Phys Ther 9:13, 2001.
15. Reider B: The Orthopedic Physical Examination. Philadelphia: WB Saunders, 1999, pp 202–225.
16. Kapandji IA: The Physiology of the Joint, Vol 2, Lower Limb, 5th ed. New York: Churchill Livingston, 1987, pp 64–146.
17. Norkin C, Levangie P (eds): Joint Structure and Function: A Comprehensive Analysis. Philadelphia: FA Davis, 1983, pp 291–323.
18. Gray JC: Neural and vascular anatomy of the menisci of the human knee. J Orthop Sports Phys Ther 29:23-30, 1999.
19. Williams G, Chmielewski T, Rudolph K, et al: Dynamic knee stability: current theory and implications for clinicians and scientists. J Orthop Sports Phys Ther 31:546–566, 2001.
20. Harrison RA, Bulsrode S: Percentage weight bearing during partial immersion in the hydrotherapy pool. Physiother Pract 3:60–63, 1987.
21. Becker BE, Cole AJ (eds): Comprehensive Aquatic Therapy. Boston: Butterworth-Heinemann, 1997, pp 17–45.
22. Harrison RA, Hillman M, Bulsrode S: Loading of the lower limb when walking partially immersed: implications for clinical practice. Physiotherapy 78:164–166, 1992.
23. Ruoti RG, Morris DM, Cole AJ (eds): Aquatic Rehabilitation. Philadelphia: Lippincott, 1997, pp 59–82.
24. Tovin B: Comparison of the effects of exercise in water and on land on the rehabilitation of patients with interarticular anterior cruciate ligament reconstructions. Phys Ther 24:710–719, 1994.
25. Shrode LW: Treating shoulder impingement using the supraspinatus synchronization exercise. J Manipulative Physiol Ther 17:48–53, 1994.
26. Mantone JK, Burkhead WZ, Noonan J: Non-operative treatment of rotator cuff tears. Orthop Clin North Am 31:295–311, 2000.
27. Kibler WB: Functional Rehabilitation of Sports and Musculoskeletal Injuries. Rockville, Md: Aspen, 1998, pp 149–170.
28. Dixit R: Non-operative management of shoulder injuries in sports. Phys Med Rehabil Clin North Am 5:69–79, 1994.
29. Hulstyn MJ, Fadale TD: Shoulder injuries in the athlete. Clin Sports Med 16:663-678, 1997.
30. Murnaghan JP: Adhesive capsulitis of the shoulder: current concepts and treatment. Orthopedics 11:153–158, 1988.
31. Kibler WB: Role of the scapula in the overhead throwing motion. Contemp Orthop 22:525–532, 1991.
32. Woolfenden JT: Aquatic Physical Therapy. Philadelphia: WB Saunders, 1994, pp 209–230.
33. Speer KP, Cavanaugh JT, Warren RF, et al: A role for hydrotherapy in shoulder rehabilitation. Am J Sports Med 21:850–853, 1993.

Chapter 12
Pediatric Aquatic Therapy

Teresa M. Petersen, PT, MS, PCS

DESCRIPTION OF PEDIATRIC AQUATIC THERAPY

Pediatric aquatic therapy (PAT) programs were first described in the 1950s, yet there has been little progress toward objective identification of therapy goals, interventions, and outcomes. The therapeutic picture is further blurred by the multitude of PAT providers representing a variety of disciplines. It is unlikely that a single, all-inclusive description of PAT will develop in the near future. Each provider must work from within his or her professional framework to develop appropriate PAT techniques.

In the last decade, there has been an increase in the number of aquatic research studies, in large part generated by the need to substantiate current aquatic therapy practices. Most of the research has focused on the adult population. These research findings must be applied cautiously with the pediatric population; it must be remembered that children are not small adults.

PHYSIOLOGIC DIFFERENCES

Respiratory Differences

Most respiratory problems in children can be related to a single cause, such as a genetic predisposition, known defects, or an infection.[1] Because of the smaller cross-sectional area of the airway in children, small obstructions have the potential to create serious airway obstructions. This smaller cross-sectional area also creates higher resistance to airflow and increases the work of breathing for children. Respiratory rates decrease in childhood as lung volumes increase, from an average of 28 breaths/min at 1 year to 18 breaths/min at 10 years. Children have less ventilatory reserve than adults with less efficient ventilation.[2] In children, the number of alveoli continues to increase from approximately 25 million at birth to approximately 300 million in adults. Chronic disease can interfere with this normal growth process and affect the child's pulmonary reserve later in life.

Other factors related to diminished respiratory function in children include the following:

1. Fatigue-resistant fibers present in the adult diaphragm and other ventilatory muscles are not present until 8 months of age. Many children with neurologic

impairments continue to use primarily chest-type breathing patterns that require more energy. In addition, children have 65% to 70% of adult values for glycogen stores available to sustain anaerobic metabolism.[3]
2. Infants and children lacking good antigravity extension in the prone position and having poorly developed abdominal muscles, are at risk for potential airway obstruction by mucus plugs. Also, children usually lack good, effective coughing mechanisms.
3. In children using insufficient spinal extension in the prone position, the normal, adult rectangular-shaped rib cage may not develop.[4] The development of normal postural tone and alignment of the spine contributes to rib cage descent and an elliptical-shaped anterior-posterior chest diameter.[3,5] Many children with developmental disabilities have muscles of respiration that remain shortened and mechanically inefficient.

Cardiac Differences

As with adults, the most common index of maximal aerobic power in children is maximal oxygen uptake ($\dot{V}O_{2max}$), or the highest rate of oxygen that can be consumed per unit time.[6] This measure is an indication of the overall competence of the cardiovascular and pulmonary systems responsible for the transport of oxygen to tissues. Lean body mass highly correlates with lower $\dot{V}O_2$ values. Because of smaller lung capacities and body size, children have lower absolute $\dot{V}O_2$ values. $\dot{V}O_{2max}$ increases throughout childhood to meet increasing demands. Children's heart rates are higher than those of adults because of lower stroke volume. Stroke volume increases as the total heart volume increases. Cardiac index is similar to that in adults because of the increased heart rates seen in children.[6] After exercise, children also have higher blood flow to muscles and lower exercise blood pressures.[7]

The energy cost of walking ($\dot{V}O_2$ expressed as milligram per kilogram per meter) at a given speed is higher in children because of greater muscle co-contraction, less efficient muscle recruitment, greater stride frequency, ventilatory inefficiency, and soft tissue elasticity.[3] Exercise recovery rates are shorter for children presumably because of lower lactate accumulation and lower rates of perceived exertion.

Fitness Levels of Children with Disabilities

Effective training programs for children should adhere to the same guidelines as those for adults, with individual prescriptions for specificity, intensity, frequency, and duration of exercise.[6] Aquatic programs for children with disabilities are often designed to have training effects, with exercise specifically designed to enhance performance of targeted skills. However, there remains some controversy as to whether $\dot{V}O_{2max}$ can increase in nondisabled, preadolescent children by cardiorespiratory training because many factors, including normal growth and development, confound research results.[2]

A large portion of the children receiving PAT services have chronic conditions and poor fitness levels. Aerobic capacities of children and adolescents with cerebral palsy are 10% to 30% less than those of control subjects.[8,9] During ambulation, children between 6 and 12 years of age with cerebral palsy were found to have $\dot{V}O_2$ values more than twice those of their nondisabled peers.[10] Participation in daily physical activity, even with physical education classes, has not been shown to induce conditioning changes in children with cerebral palsy.[8, 11] Improved training effects for children with cerebral palsy are reported with programs of longer than 6 weeks duration in which heart rates were maintained for 15 to 30 minutes.[12] Swimming was specified as part of the training regimen used in this research.[12]

Although swimming programs are often included as part of the comprehensive physical activity program for children with cerebral palsy, there is only one study documenting the positive effects of a 6-month program of combined swimming and land programs.[13] In this study, baseline vital capacity improved by 65% in the 23 children (aged 5 to 7 years) in the treatment group, whereas in the control group it improved by 23%.

Sherman and associates[14] reported that reduced forced vital capacity, restrictive disease, and respiratory and upper extremity muscle weakness were present in a majority of subjects with myelomeningocele.[14] These children have also been found to be at risk for obesity.[15] Young adults with mental retardation, including Down syndrome, can benefit from cardiovascular training programs when aerobic and strength programs are combined at optimum intensities and frequencies.[3]

In children with asthma, swimming programs have been found to be superior to running for providing cardiovascular training. Swimming programs tailored to the needs of children with asthma have also been shown to improve exercise tolerance and control breathing.[17, 18]

Response to Temperature

Core body temperatures are higher before children begin to sweat, a primary means of heat dissipation not available in the water. With hypohydration in children, core temperatures rise even more sharply. In cooler temperatures, an increased surface area to body mass ratio contributes to increased loss of body heat at much faster rates than in adults.

As Campion states, "When considering water temperature, the things to bear in mind are the type and severity of the exercise in addition to the duration of the activity."[19] Despite the fact that children have a narrower range of comfort in water with less ability to dissipate heat, adult-generated temperature standards are still applied to children. Comfortable, therapeutic temperatures for children vary, depending on the child's impairment(s), portion of the body exposed to air, relative amount of body fat, level of active mobility, duration of activity, and perception of comfort. It should be noted that children generally prefer cooler bath water than adults and will tolerate cooler pool temperatures after an initial warm up. Children playing in water are generally more active than adults. It is recommended that water temperatures between 82 and 86°F (28 to 30°C) be used for adults participating in aerobic activities.[20] Although activity levels of children might be less than aerobic, increased levels are frequently achieved. For this reason, water temperatures for children should be considered in relation to desired activity levels.

Care should be exercised when children are immersed in very warm (>94°F) or very cool (<83°F) water for extended periods because children often ignore the signs of thermal intolerance. Shivering and bluing of the lips are signs of hypothermia. Hypotonia, lethargy, and blushing of the cheeks are signs of hyperthermia.

James McMillan preferred to work with children in cooler pool temperatures (<84°F [29°C]). He claimed that the reduction in muscle tone seen in warmer water is not due solely to warmer water temperatures but rather to proprioceptive input provided by gravity.[21] Aerospace research supports this association between decreased gravitational force and lowered muscle tone. After 15 minutes of submersion at or above T11 or when lying supine, muscle tone drops. Children with the tendency to initiate few movements in the water may cool quickly. It is therefore important that they perform highly energetic, repetitious activity. This increase in activity will elevate the child's core temperature. Core temperature may also be maintained by use of a wetsuit or vest.

The majority of children participating in PAT programs generally have problems with muscular weakness, often combined with high muscle tone and spasticity. Warm water helps to decrease muscle tone associated with spasticity, but its effects are nonselective so that tone in all muscle groups will be reduced.[19, 20] There is a tendency to focus attention primarily on reduction of tone in spastic musculature. However, weakness is frequently present where abnormally increased muscle tone is found.[22] Working with children in very warm pools for extended periods of time can produce undesirable levels of fatigue and diminished muscle tone, which is counterproductive for functional activities.[19]

In summary, whereas therapeutic pool temperatures for adults can range between 92 and 98°F,[20] these temperatures are often too warm for pediatric patients. The exception to this might be children with inflammatory conditions or pain, or children receiving therapy after surgery. Depending on the outside temperature and with the use of wetsuits and vests, pool temperatures between 85 and 92°F can be used successfully for PAT. When warmer temperatures are needed to increase warming or for tone reduction, partial immersion in a whirlpool hot tub can be used judiciously.

PROGRAM PLANNING DIFFERENCES

Functional Task Differences

The PAT program should complement developmental, play, self-help, and impairment-related goals identified in the land-based assessment. PAT is not simply land skills performed in the water. On the other hand, at times it is appropriate to learn land-based skills in the water. Given the mechanical advantages water offers the child, tasks such as rolling, standing, running, jumping, and reaching are often executed with increased success in the water.

Current understanding of motor skill acquisition suggests selection of activities to permit active learning of functional tasks.[23, 24] The term *functional task* for children has a distinctly different meaning than that for adults. Young children acquire motor skills primarily by interacting with their environment and engaging in play.[25] The therapist must learn to incorporate creative strategies to adapt therapeutic applications to resemble play.[26]

Children engaged in PAT must learn a new style of play, involving neuromuscular and sensory adaptations novel to the aquatic experience. For some children with movement limitations, more sophisticated play experiences are possible in the water. For instance, "exercise play" begins at the end of the first year and includes running, chasing, and climbing.[25] "Rough and tumble play" such as wrestling, kicking, and tumbling in a social context is used during preschool and primary years, and continues through adolescence.[25] For some children, the water is often the only environment in which performance of such critical play skills is possible.

Emphasis on Mobility and Swim Skills in Water

Inclusion of appropriate swim skill instruction in the PAT program will promote safe lifetime fitness, mobility, and recreational skills. Aquatic programming for children with long-term disabilities must include swim skill acquisition and an awareness of water safety considerations for both children and family members.

Safe, purposeful mobility (with or without assistance) extended to appropriate aquatic peer programming is the ultimate goal of most PAT programs. The community pool offers the ideal environment for blending both therapeutic and recreational programs, and the skilled aquatic therapist is often the sole professional with the requisite skills to adapt typical swim programming for the child with special needs.

Team Members Providing PAT

There are currently a host of disciplines providing PAT, with each contributing its own reservoir of professional skills. In keeping with the principle of service provision within the continuum of care, the Lyton model for interdisciplinary service delivery within the aquatic setting provides a useful framework for children receiving aquatic therapy services.[27] Figure 12-1[27] depicts modification of the Lyton model for application to the pediatric patient.

Often the needs of the child may change so that aquatic therapy and training may pass from one provider to another. It may also be useful to engage the child in two programs simultaneously. For example, a trained swim instructor will save valuable therapy time by teaching improved water adjustment skills before initiation of PAT programs. Inclusion in typical swim lessons, using an aide as needed, is also recommended to enhance the child's swimming and socialization skills.

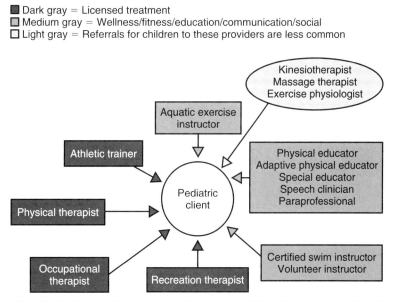

Figure 12-1. Pediatric aquatic therapy providers, adapted from the Lyton model for the aquatic continuum of care.

Collaborative, Family-Centered Care

The pediatric aquatic therapist must address the needs of both the child and family when determining therapeutic goals. For pediatric patients involved in long-term programs involving multiple team members, the pediatric aquatic therapist has the added responsibility of actively participating in a collaborative teaching experience (Fig. 12-2).

The multidisciplinary team works across traditional role boundaries, imparting shared training and skills to all team members.[28] Integrated models of team interaction include opportunities for learning with appropriate peer integration and with flexible expression of new skills into the "natural" environment. The emerging standard for effective team interaction combines the multidisciplinary and integrated models to create the collaborative model, in which service provision is shared across discipline boundaries within naturally occurring contexts.[28, 29] Although the pool may be considered a natural environment, aquatic programming tends to be the responsibility of a select few. Every effort should be made to enlist team members with an interest in aquatics to participate in the therapy program, because those coerced into service rarely achieve optimal outcomes.[30, 31]

Ideally, the aquatic therapist will participate in designing the individualized family service plan for infants, toddlers, and sometimes preschoolers and the individualized

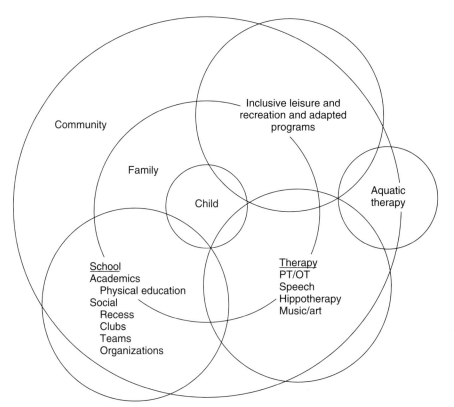

Figure 12-2. Children referred for long-term PAT programs are often served by several members of the inter- or multidisciplinary team. Aquatic therapy for children should relate to meaningful goals needed to improve function in the home, school, and community.

education plan for those 5 to 21 years of age. Consistent with provision of family-centered, multidisciplinary service, the aquatic therapist should recognize and take responsibility for inclusion of educational, social, and communication goals relevant to the aquatic environment.[32]

COMMON PRACTICE SETTINGS FOR PAT

Table 12-1 describes the most common practice settings for delivery of PAT services. PAT may be delivered across a variety of practice settings, including private, educational, community, and within hospitals and rehabilitation facilities. Group aquatic therapy programming, based on Halliwick principles, is well known in the United Kingdom (see Chapter 4).

COMBINING LAND AND WATER THERAPIES

Improved land-based function is a primary goal of PAT, and it is recommended that therapists provide a combination of land and water interventions. This might involve alternating land and water therapy sessions or assigning blocks of time dedicated to one or the other.

Within the framework of direct, individualized delivery of aquatic therapy, frequency of service varies with the needs of the child and family and with availability of service. There are a limited number of pools available for therapeutic use and fewer trained professionals, so it may be necessary to train family members, certified or noncertified assistants, volunteers, or other team members to implement the aquatic program to achieve the desired frequency. Direct, individualized aquatic therapy is the most costly model for service, and long-term family financial considerations should be evaluated when determining the extent of such programming. When long-term care is provided, the aquatic therapist should consider the more cost-effective use of consultative and episodic plans of care.

Table 12-1. Common Practice Settings for Delivery of PAT Services

Setting	Service Provider
Hospital, in- and outpatient facilities	PT, OT, CTRS, ATC, AEI, certified and noncertified aides
Rehabilitation facility, in- and outpatient facilities	Same as above
Educational, including private and public programs, preschool and school-aged	PT, OT, RT, ATC, PE, APE, speech therapist; special educators, certified and noncertified aides and paraprofessionals
Private practice/community facility	Red Cross WSI or any of the above might provide service in this setting

PT, physical therapist; OT, occupational therapist; CTRS, certified therapeutic recreation specialist; ATC, certified athletic trainer; PE/APE, physical educator, adaptive physical educator; AEI, aquatic exercise instructor; WSI, water safety instructor.

POOL LOCATION

PAT can be provided in schools, community centers, health clubs, hospitals, rehabilitation centers, outpatient facilities, and homes. Some therapists have used pools in hotels, apartment buildings, and facilities for the elderly. Of primary concern when a pool is selected for PAT programs is that the pool water and deck be meticulously maintained (as discussed in Chapter 3) because children tend to have more contact with deck surfaces and often ingest pool water. Pool temperature, accessibility, changing facilities, and the availability of a lifeguard are also important considerations. Aquatic therapists may be employed by the facility in which the service is provided or may seek an appropriate pool facility. Therapists generally contract with a facility to use the pool for a rental fee or, occasionally, it may be provided at no cost.

Therapeutic aquatics should not be limited to so-called "therapeutic" pools, usually located in specialized schools, learning centers, hospitals, elder-care facilities, or rehabilitation centers. Although warmer pool temperatures (90 to 98°F) may be the norm in some settings, these temperatures may not be ideal for all children. Again, the exception may be the child with chronic inflammation or pain. These so-called therapeutic pools sometimes promote increased levels of fatigue in children and do not provide appropriate social and peer interaction. Long-term aquatic programs should prepare the child with a disabling condition for use of more typical aquatic facilities and should not create dependence on the use of more isolated therapeutic pools.

Therapists look for alternatives to therapeutic pool environments in an effort to provide optimal, more affordable settings for PAT. Any pool at which there is the opportunity for interaction with nondisabled peers and adults is generally considered more appropriate for PAT programs. Some third-party payers recognize these therapeutic pool alternatives as "natural" environments and pay those who use these pools at an increased rate. Some consider these pools ideal environments to deliver PAT because they are considered the most desirable for functional integration of both land and aquatic skills within the child's natural environment.[28]

Another advantage of the alternative pool environment is the opportunity to involve the entire family in the therapeutic process.[33] Siblings often view aquatic therapy as an unfair privilege bestowed on the child with a disability. Regular visits to the pool, including one or more family members, increase the likelihood of additional family pool outings. A request that a parent or caregiver be present and in the water during therapy sessions promotes "hands-on" therapeutic instruction. This should give the caregiver increased confidence with both appropriate aquatic handling and home programming. When possible, it is recommended that other family members be permitted to swim before, during, or after the therapy session. Generally, caregivers provide additional motivation for both movement-related activities and for enhanced cognitive, communication, and social skill development. Families of children with special needs are often experiencing additional family stressors and are at risk for maladaptation.[34] When given the option to participate, families often report that the family pool experience has positive effects for both parents and children. Siblings are often able to gain new water skills, and parents engage in playful recreational and therapeutic activities perceived as fun for all.

REFERRAL POPULATION SERVED

Participation in the PAT program should be based on review of the pertinent medical history provided by parents and confirmed by the referral for aquatic therapy from the child's physician. Although the referral may not be deemed necessary for purposes of reimbursement, it helps foster communication with the primary care physician. The referral also heightens physician awareness of aquatic therapy programming while protecting the therapist from complications arising from not having the child's complete history. When compared with traditional land therapies, there are additional risks involved in bringing children into the aquatic setting. Each child should be considered individually, and potential risks should be weighed against expected gains from aquatic therapy.

PRECAUTIONS AND CONTRAINDICATIONS TO PAT

Specific precautions and contraindications for PAT are similar to those for aquatic therapy adults.[35]

Precautions

- History of aspiration of liquids and/or aspiratory pneumonia precautions
- Infectious respiratory event (cold, flu, or allergy symptoms) other than very minimal symptoms often experienced by children
- Elevated temperature, at or above 100°F
- Parental report that child does not seem "well": Childhood illness often emerges quickly and is preceded by subtle behavioral changes, such as lethargy and/or irritability.
- Bowel incontinence: This can usually be managed by an effective stool program and appropriate swim undergarments.
- Bladder incontinence: Until approximately age 3, it is accepted that children may be incontinent in the pool; older children, with or without problems or incontinence, should be routinely expected to urinate before aquatic therapy sessions. Immersion in water will increase the child's need to urinate.[36]
- Severe cardiovascular disease where symptoms are exacerbated by immersion
- Severe respiratory compromise with vital capacity less than 1 L[37]: Respiratory symptoms are exacerbated by immersion.
- Infectious skin conditions and open wounds: This does not include typical cuts, abrasions, and insect bites often seen with children unless these are judged to be very deep, raw, weeping, or encrusted with infection. With children, open sores present the possibility of impetigo, a bacterial infection highly contagious to others who come in contact with the child.
- Nasogastric tubes, unless kept completely out of the water
- Gastrostomy tubes
- Colostomy, urostomy, or ileostomy bags
- Percutaneous endoscopic gastrostomy (PEG) tube (permanent feeding port): Avoid prone positioning with weight bearing over the PEG tube site; check for signs of infection surrounding the PEG site.
- Acute orthopedic injury with pain and instability present: The exception may be if the injury (with cast or splint) can be protected from water so that aquatic activities may still be performed.
- Controlled seizure activity: The therapist should know the seizure history and the protocol to follow when seizures occur.

- Controlled diabetes: The therapist must have appropriate intervention (e.g., food or injection) available with a trained staff person or caregiver to offer assistance.
- Chlorine sensitivity
- Latex allergies: These are particularly problematic for children with spina bifida[38, 39]; use caution with swim goggles, inner tubes, toys, and other commonly used aquatic equipment containing this natural rubber.
- Active joint inflammation (juvenile rheumatoid arthritis or hemophilia): Aquatic interventions must be applied with specific goals that do not increase painful symptoms (see Chapter 10).

Contraindications

- Uncontrolled seizure activity
- Persistent diarrhea: All children have episodes of diarrhea, and the pool should be avoided at these times.
- Ineffective stool program
- Open wounds, without bioocclusive dressing
- Menstruation without internal protection
- Tracheostomies: These must be healed with no submersion.
- Burns in acute stage of healing

POPULATION SERVED

Pediatric aquatic services should be available to all children with special needs who have no identified contraindications. It is particularly useful for children with acute and chronic, painful, inflammatory conditions. Children at risk for or having developmental delays, long- and short-term orthopedic conditions, traumatic brain injuries, neurologic/movement impairments, coordination disorders, musculoskeletal conditions, cardiac and respiratory conditions, burns, and genetic and metabolic disorders may also be appropriate candidates for aquatic therapy services.

DEVELOPMENT/FUNCTIONAL SKILL EVALUATION

Land Evaluation

The aquatic therapist should not limit the evaluation of motor skills to the aquatic environment. Every attempt should be made to observe the child in the home, school, or community settings where meaningful motor tasks can be evaluated. Because the aquatic therapist attempts to blend land-based skill development with that in the water, knowledge of a child's land movement repertoire is fundamental. Consultation with the land-based physical and occupational therapists is often helpful because they usually have performed informal or formal standardized fine or gross motor testing. They have assessed primary and secondary musculoskeletal impairments and have identified related functional, land-based treatment goals. In addition, there is usually some measure of a child's feeding, self-care, and play/recreation skills. Additional information concerning sensory and behavioral considerations is frequently offered. Consultation with other team members may appear to be an unnecessary, time-consuming portion of the evaluation process, yet when an aquatic therapist is involved in long-term programming for a child with a disability, information sharing is critical to ensure a well-functioning team.[28]

Water Evaluation

At times it may be necessary to perform water evaluations without the benefit of land evaluation findings. To complete the aquatic therapy evaluation, the aquatic therapist must seek additional information generated by previous land- and water-based testing. Table 12-2 lists items to be considered in the complete, water-based evaluation.

HANDLING CONSIDERATIONS

Alterations in muscle tone can affect the way caregivers carry, position, and handle children for daily activities. Both in water and on land, it is of primary importance that the therapist train caregivers in effective handling techniques to ensure that the child can successfully and comfortably interact with caregivers, the environment, and peers.[40] Prevention of caregiver injuries related to the physical demands of caring for a child with physical impairments should also be addressed. There is no research evidence to support direct, therapist handling making a difference in the ultimate therapeutic outcome.[41] Campbell states the following:

> The principles guiding these methods (of handling) are (1) to use a variety of movements and postures to promote sensory variety, (2) to frequently include positions that promote the full lengthening of spastic or hypoextensible muscle (Figs. 12-3 and 12-4), and (3) to use positions that promote functional voluntary movement of limbs.[26]

Initial handling of children in the water is important because a poor first experience can set the therapeutic process back weeks or even months. Holds will vary, depending on the child's level of confidence in the water, age, size, and level of disability.[42] Initially, the therapist should err on the side of providing too much support, then gradually disengage (see the Halliwick method, Chapter 8) and permit more active movement.[42]

BEGINNING HOLDS IN WATER

Vertical

Generally speaking, the comfort level of the child is enhanced with more vertical, upright positioning while firm contact with the therapist is maintained. Figure 12-5 depicts one possible position from which the child has pelvic and trunk support and visual and communication skills are optimized. From this position, the therapist is able to guide the pelvis by holding the child at about the level of T11 while altering weight-bearing and weight-shifting opportunities in the sitting position. For the child with increased extensor tone in the lower extremities (hips in extension, adduction, and internal rotation), the therapist can facilitate the necessary anterior pelvic mobility to increase control in sitting. This position has the additional advantage of allowing free, yet buoyancy-supported, upper extremity movements. It may be used in standing, but therapists find that greater stability and control are possible by beginning in a seated position.[42]

Table 12-2. Aquatic Therapy Evaluation *(list specific discipline)*

Name :_____Parent(s)/caregivers; other children_____
Other required ID numbers _____
D.O.B.:_____
Diagnosis/problem(s): _____
Phone: _____
Referral source: _____
Date of evaluation:_____
Current therapies/educational program:
_____

History (include pre-, peri-, postnatal complications; adjust chronologic age for prematurity; note chronic upper respiratory infections, chronic otitis media, presence of ear tubes; heart and/or lung disease; surgeries; seizures; major developmental milestones; previous therapies, including speech, PT, OT, hippotherapy, music, other; relevant family history): _____
_____

Precautions (specified by parent and/or physician and those noted from history): _____
_____

Medications (Will it be necessary to provide any emergency medications during aquatic therapy?): _____
Orthotics/other equipment (description of orthosis[es] and recommended use; wheelchair, adaptive stroller, positioning equipment, walkers, mobility toys, self-help aids, augmentative communication): _____
Land-based evaluations (You need not recreate the entire land-based assessment, but *select information that will assist with writing integrated land-aquatic goals* from information reported in fine and gross motor developmental assessments; active and passive range of motion [joint play]; strength and endurance for daily activities; description of muscle tone, patterns/synergies, and aberrant or absent reflexes; movement quality [timing, efficiency], motor planning and coordination; joint contractures and deformities; postural control and mobility [including gait, transitional movements, and transfers]; sensory and pain assessments; dressing, feeding, communication, and cognitive skills; play skills; behavior problems):
_____

Aquatic Skills

Previous therapy or lessons (Consider whether or not the child is a candidate for supplemental swim instruction.): _____
Entry/exit (Specify method of entry and degree of assistance needed for safe performance of skills; see p. 254): _____
Mental adjustment (see p. 256):_____
Breath control (see p. 259):_____
Muscle tone (How is tone influenced by water properties [temperature, turbulence, depth, etc.]? How is tone influenced by changes in type of movement performed, velocity [active or assisted], and position in the water?):_____
Muscle strength and range of motion (Are there differences in water compared with land? Consider influence of pain and sensory limitations; see p. 274):_____
Developmental skill (see Fig. 12-29): _____
Transitional movements (Consider land deficits. Can training occur in water?): _____
Flotation (see p. 279): _____
Swimming skills (see p. 278): _____
Safety awareness (Does child/family need additional training from water safety instructor?):
_____

Treatment outcomes/goals and activities: _____

_____   _____
(Therapist Signature)   (Date)

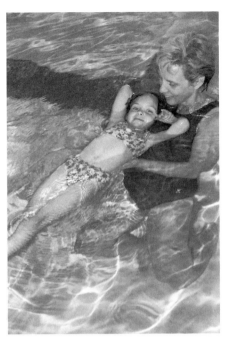

Figure 12-3. Supine-lying position using buoyancy assistance to increase symmetry and elongate trunk and upper extremity structures.

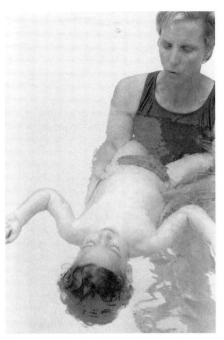

Figure 12-4. Supine-lying position using buoyancy assistance to activate midthoracic and hip extensor musculature, elongate hip flexors, and maintain chin tuck position.

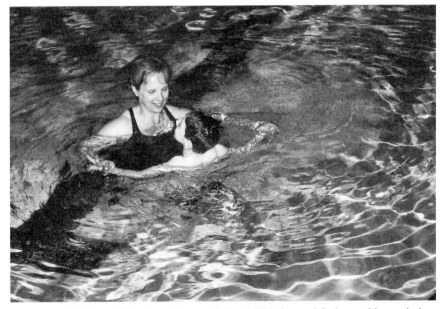

Figure 12-5. Child straddles therapist at waist level. This forward-facing position optimizes visual and communication skills and permits guided pelvic mobility.

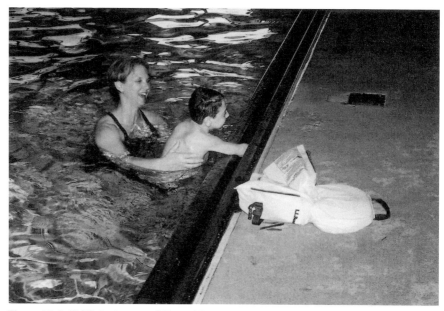

Figure 12-6. Child sits in a straddle position on therapist's flexed lower extremity. Upper extremity and trunk movements are easily assisted without possible grabbing for therapist's neck.

Figure 12-6 offers another choice for securely holding the child during adjustment to the water. This position is especially effective for children who attempt to grab the therapist around the neck. The child has considerable contact with the therapist from head to pelvis, yet the upper extremities are free to move with buoyancy support. Gradual disengagement is possible, especially with smaller children, when weight shift can be moved away from the therapist and weight bearing limited to the therapist's forearm or balanced on the therapist's knee. Because the child faces away from the therapist, there is the opportunity to interact with the caregiver, another child, or a toy.

Prone

Control in the prone position can have a host of benefits for improved postural control against gravity and provides a foundation for increasing mobility skills in the water. The prone position (Fig. 12-7) permits buoyancy-supported antigravity work of the head, neck, and thoracic and lumbar spine. Lower extremity buoyancy-assisted movements are easily accomplished in prone positions. Poor postural strength and control against gravity are often treatment priorities, making this position particularly important. Although work in the prone position is used sparingly in Halliwick methodology, many Halliwick variations in prone positions are possible to encourage combined rotational control (see Chapter 4). Support at the inferior border of the rib cage (to assist in alignment and stability of the rib cage) enables the therapist to facilitate rotation as needed for rolling. A useful modification of prone positioning is seen when the child is supported in a side-lying position in which rotational control of the trunk with facilitation of abdominal musculature is possible (Fig. 12-8). Guided dissociation of the lower extremities

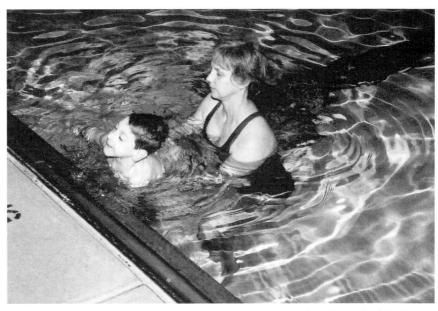

Figure 12-7. Prone positioning permits buoyancy-supported antigravity work of the head, neck, and thoracic and lumbar spine.

and reciprocal kicking occur with buoyancy support. Like prone, this position permits bubble blowing with chin tuck while the upper extremities are free for paddling or stroking.

When work in the prone position is too difficult, use of a semiprone position (Fig. 12-9) is recommended. Whenever the prone position is used, careful attention should be focused on the lumbar spine because there can be an exaggeration of

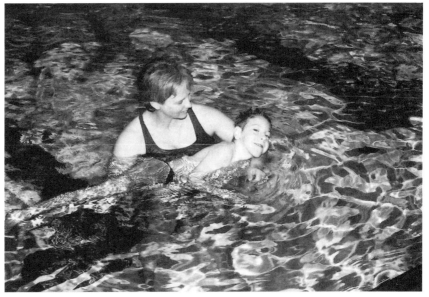

Figure 12-8. Side-lying permits active and assisted rotational control at the trunk with facilitation of abdominal musculature.

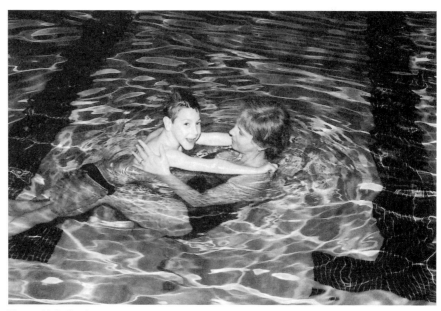

Figure 12-9. Semiprone postioning often promotes better spinal alignment with buoyancy-assisted hip extension and less resisted hip flexion.

undesirable lumbar lordosis as a result of excessive buoyancy. Semiprone positioning often promotes better spinal alignment with more work in assisted hip extension and less resisted hip flexion.

Supine

Many adult aquatic interventions rely on comfortable supine positioning (see Bad Ragaz Ring Method, Chapter 8). For most children, this position provides the least degree of comfort. Considering that postural control to the rear (in vertical) on land is developmentally more difficult to master than to the front or sides, one should not be surprised that the same is true in water. Figure 12-10 suggests that the head and neck be supported initially by resting of the child's head on the therapist's shoulder that is submerged to the appropriate level to maintain the child's optimal cervical spinal alignment. From this position, the child should be instructed to maintain a slight chin tuck while facilitation of the paraspinal and/or gluteal muscles is provided. Control in the supine position aids in lengthening musculature, which typically shortens from the effects of gravity (e.g., capital extensors, pectorals, and hip flexors) while activating short neck flexors, scapular adductors, and thoracic and hip extensor muscles. Supine is often the only position in which a child with severe impairments may function independently. Figure 12-11 depicts the semisupine position from which the child may gain control in coming to sit using buoyancy-assisted trunk flexion with rotation. Because of excessive movement in the sagittal plane, there is often decreased spinal rotation and limited function of the oblique abdominal muscles.[41] This position promotes activation of oblique abdominal muscles, which is a desirable activity for many children with postural control problems.

Pediatric Aquatic Therapy 255

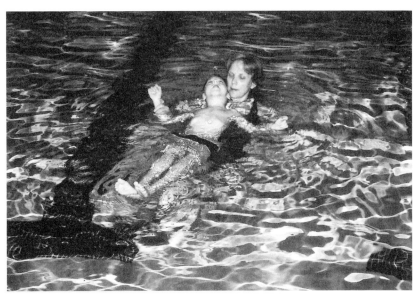

Figure 12-10. Supine positioning begins with the head supported on therapist's submerged shoulder. A slight chin tuck is optimal as paraspinal and gluteal muscles are facilitated.

SAFETY CONSIDERATIONS

When children participate in pool activity, attention to safety is critical. There are considerable health and environmental risks that must be brought to the attention of the child and family. For some families, aquatic therapy may be the first exposure to water activity with their child other than at bath time. Competence in the aquatic

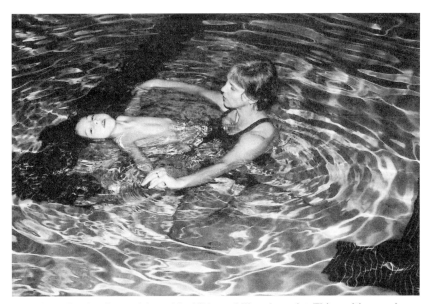

Figure 12-11. Semisupine position with child straddling therapist. This position can be used to gain increased trunk control with buoyancy-assisted trunk flexion/rotation in coming to sit.

therapy session should *never* be extended to recreational swim opportunities without specific limitations delineated by the therapist. The therapist should not assume that caregivers are competent in water and knowledgeable about potential risks. Parents must understand the limitations of any floatation devices recommended for children. Because many children seen for aquatic therapy lack the judgment necessary to assess potential risks, they may never be fully independent in the aquatic environment. In addition to the aquatic therapy program, it is recommended that children be enrolled in swim programs because most of these provide pool safety instruction as part of the training. The aquatic therapist should offer assistance to help adapt activities and train personnel to include children with special needs in swim programs. An aquatic therapist lacking a thorough knowledge of water safety guidelines should consider additional certification offered through the Red Cross, the Aquatic Therapy and Rehab Institute, Inc., or other recognized programs.

AQUATIC THERAPY OUTCOMES/GOALS

Aquatic therapists often comment that aquatic therapy goal writing is the most challenging aspect of service provision. Aquatic therapy goals must meet the same rigorous standard as land-based goals. Aquatic therapists have the added challenge of blending land- and water-based goals.[43]

Development of appropriate goals begins with identification of desired outcomes. Outcome statements need not be measurable, but should have functional, land-based implications.[28] Goals develop as the therapist breaks down aquatic motor learning into logical movement progressions. The following must be included in every aquatic therapy goal[44]:

1. Subject
2. An observable action verb
3. An observable functional performance with a beginning and an end point
4. Conditions under which the performance will be met (conditions describe the circumstances and environment)
5. Criteria for how well the client performs this function

Here is an example of a desired land-based outcome with associated aquatic goals.

Task (Outcome): Parent (of Ryan) has expressed desire to have 4-year-old child with spastic diplegia sit alone and play with toys on floor independently.
Functional Long-Term Land Goal (accomplish in 6 to 12 months): Ryan will be able to assume straddle sit on 10-inch roll, reaching and playing with toys placed in basket at side of roll, independently for 10 minutes, in 6 to 12 months.
Associated Short-Term Aquatic Goals (accomplish in 1 to 6 months):

1. Ryan will straddle 5-inch noodle facing therapist, with water to mid thorax, accepting weight shift to trunk in all directions with no falls for 2 to 3 minutes.
2. Ryan will roll from supine to prone, leading with upper extremities, head, and then shoulders, following with top leg dissociated from lower leg, with minimal assistance, five times in each direction.
3. Ryan will sit alone on 5-inch step (feet supported on lower step), with water to xiphoid process and facilitation to midthoracic spine to increase thoracic extension with slight anterior pelvic tilt, and play with toy independently for 5 minutes.

4. Ryan will climb onto edge of pool, leading with one flexed lower extremity, shift weight to opposite hip, turn, and sit on pool edge, with moderate assistance to pull up and minimal assistance to turn.
5. Ryan will sit on edge of pool, lean forward, and enter pool with upper extremities leading, head and neck in flexion, anterior pelvic tilt with trunk flexion so that lower extremities follow with minimal assistance.

PEDIATRIC AQUATIC THERAPY INTERVENTIONS

From the array of adult-based aquatic therapy interventions arises a handful of interventions deemed suitable for application with children. Halliwick programming is sometimes referred to as neurodevelopmental treatment[45] in the water because of similarities between both approaches. Currently, Halliwick principles are recognized as fundamental to pediatric aquatic therapeutic and recreational programs. Other interventions sometimes used with children include Bad Ragaz, Watsu, spinal mobilization, myofascial release, and Ai Chi.

Halliwick

The Halliwick Concept, devised by the late James McMillan in 1949, is a method of teaching water adjustment, balanced mobility, and swimming skills and is particularly suited to the needs of children with developmental disabilities (see Chapter 4). This method was developed in London using small groups of children, primarily those with cerebral palsy. Halliwick programs use a multidisciplinary model.[21] The activities are geared to interest children, and the program teaches logical movement progressions.

The method is still used worldwide, with both children and adults, and although the principles of therapy remain true, many therapists are modifying the program to suit their client base. Halliwick programs include group format instruction guided by a group leader. Campion described many well-documented, therapeutic group activities suitable for children of a wide age range and with a wide degree of disability.[42] She also suggests that Halliwick methods are complementary with those of conductive education.[46]

Dr. Andras Peto, a physician and educator, is credited with first using conductive education (CE) principles in Hungary in the 1950s. The basic philosophy of CE is that children and adults can learn optimal independence with functional motor tasks performed *intensively* throughout the day with the guidance of a trained "conductor."[47] Motor dysfunction is believed to be strongly influenced by learned strategies.[26] There is a holistic approach to the child, combining both therapeutic and educational programs. In light of the philosophical similarities the two methods share, it is not surprising that Halliwick-based aquatic programming has become central to CE. The reported effectiveness of CE is gaining international attention, and several programs are currently operating in the United States.

Other

Pediatric aquatic therapists currently "borrow" from a range of therapeutic interventions used in adult-based aquatic programs. Therapists also try blend land-based pediatric and adult interventions with PAT programs. The information in Table 12-3

Table 12-3. Aquatic Therapeutic Interventions

Intervention	Advantages	Disadvantages
Bad Ragaz Ring Method (see Chapter 8)	May be appropriate for painful conditions or preparatory activities needed to gain muscular elongation and relaxation, and for use of more desirable patterns of movement	Children often resist supine lying position May not relate strongly to land-based functional needs Requires level of cognition absent in many children Use of flotation interrupts water adjustment training
Watsu, water shiatsu (see Chapter 5)	May be applied for painful conditions or for specific goals related in increasing joint mobility, muscular elongation, and decreasing undesirable muscular stiffness	Considered passive; supine position predominates May not relate strongly to land-based functional needs Requires dependence on therapist May not be the best use of child's limited therapeutic time
Passive manual mobilization[48, 49]; passive mobilization using turbulent drag[50]	Useful during treatment to address periarticular and muscular impairments (in particular, joint range of motion) due to limited active mobility; may provide generalized relaxation	Should be used only by trained professionals Not used for acutely painful conditions May be difficult to find adequate point of stability from which to perform mobilization in water Comfort in supine positions often difficult; may require flotation
Myofascial release[51]	Useful as preparatory activities or during cool-down to improve structural alignment and muscular function by altering fascial restrictions	Passive technique May not be best use of aquatic therapy time unless performed by caregiver May be difficult to find stable working position
Ai chi[52]	Useful with adolescents and young adults to increase overall coordination, balance, flexibility, and breathing effectiveness; may contribute to long-term functional gains and health benefits	May need to simplify for children Requires active participant with ability to follow instructions

is offered as a working tool to guide the therapist's clinical decision making when selecting appropriate PAT interventions.

CLINICAL APPLICATIONS

Pool Entry and Exit

Therapists should teach children and caregivers to enter and exit the pool area with as much independence as possible. Unfortunately, pool decks, changing facilities, and pool surfaces are often slick and present increased risk of falls. Injuries are more likely because the supporting surfaces are often concrete or tile, and many children with motor impairments are without footwear and lack effective protective responses.

Steps/Ramps

Fortunately, many newer pools now have accessible entries, including ramps, steps, and zero-depth designs. Still, children and their caregivers need safe entry and exit strategies suitable for any pool. Ideally, the child will enter the pool standing, using a ramp or steps, with stand-by assistance of the therapist. Most children should be encouraged to use a handrail when entering the pool for added safety. When a child descends stairs to enter the pool, the therapist should be positioned at the side, opposite the handrail, and slightly to the rear of the child because falling forward into the water poses less danger than falls to the rear (Fig. 12-12). When greater assistance is necessary, the therapist may permit the child to lean to the rear while standing, allowing the therapist to support and guide the entry. If the child is larger and unable to assist the therapist, one person should be on either side of the child to negotiate steps. When the child exits the pool, the therapist is again positioned at the side and slightly to the rear of the child, because greater control is possible from this position (Fig. 12-13). The therapist may hold a smaller, nonambulatory child to enter and exit the pool.

Sitting Entry

Entering the pool from a sitting position on the pool deck is an important skill for children to learn because it teaches safety and skilled entry and leads to more

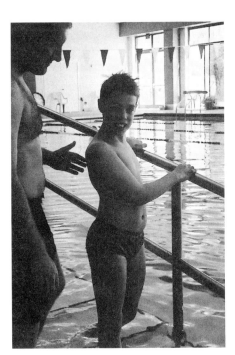

Figure 12-12. When a child descends stairs to enter the pool, the therapist should be positioned to the side and slightly to the rear of the child.

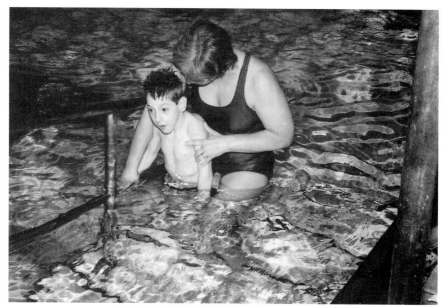

Figure 12-13. For the child to exit the pool using steps, the therapist should be positioned to the nonrailing side and rear of the child for optimum safety and control.

complex progressions in the water. Every child should have experience in guided "falls" into the water, both while sitting and standing.

Wheelchair Entry

Children may be transported in typical or adapted strollers or use wheelchairs, with or without assistance. Transfers from the wheelchair to the pool deck should be performed as near the point of pool entry as possible. The chair should then be removed from the pool area to avoid its becoming an obstacle to other swimmers. Once at poolside, the child should be assisted to enter the pool with as much independence as possible.

Ladders

Whenever possible, children should be taught to use the pool ladder to exit the pool. In some areas of the pool, especially in deep water, the ladder may be the only means of exit from the pool area. Use of the ladder requires climbing skills related to increased upper and lower extremity strength, motor planning, and transitional skill development. When teaching the child to safely exit using the ladder, the therapist remains in the water, providing support as needed from the rear. As the child ascends, the therapist follows one rung behind to prevent a fall backwards.

MENTAL ADJUSTMENT

Mental adjustment of children to water is a necessary prerequisite for higher-level skill acquisition and is often overlooked and misunderstood. Regardless of the level of functioning of the child, the aquatic therapist must make every attempt to maximize comfort in the pool environment, which is rich in sensory input. Although adults may meet aquatic therapy goals without accepting water to the face or submerging, these are important activities in a child's program.

Mental adjustment includes the following considerations:

1. Movement in water (either assisted or independent) should not elicit fearful behavior such as clinging to the therapist, dependence, or contact with support surfaces, sides, or railings.
2. The child should be able to move (with or without support) freely into positions other than vertical (prone, side-lying, and especially supine) without exhibiting fear (Fig. 12-14).
3. Transitional movements (e.g., sit to stand, sit to all fours, or sit to prone on step) and postural adjustments should be experienced without fear.
4. There should be comfort with a variety of movement experiences, including bouncing and jumping (with or without support), changing directions with varied velocities, rolling, and spinning.
5. Movement (with or without assistance) should not elicit startle reactions, undesirable increases in muscle tone, spasticity, or aberrant movement patterns.
6. The child should not avoid water to the face, submersion, splashing, bubble-blowing, or spontaneous play in water.

If the child has difficulty with any of these activities, the therapist should look at land-based motor skills and determine if there is a relationship between land- and water-based fear of movement. Further probing should explore whether fear is related to poor motor skill competency, weakness and influence of altered muscle tone, lack of postural stability and righting mechanisms, ineffective sensory processing, limited motor planning skills, poor motivation, or a combination of several problems. It is usually not appropriate to dedicate large portions of the therapeutic

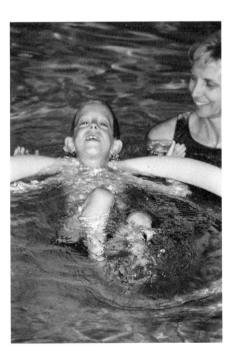

Figure 12-14. Complete water adjustment requires the child to move freely into positions other than vertical.

session to mental adjustment activities, especially if the child continues to cry or exhibit other resistive behavior. If the child continues to display fearful, anxious behavior during therapy, it can be helpful to enlist the assistance of a swim instructor or train the caregiver to increase the child's exposure to the aquatic environment.

Opportunities to increase the child's comfort level in the water start with bathing activities. The aquatic therapist should review positioning in the bathtub, ensuring stable, secure positioning for the child. This may require the use of an adapted bathing chair (Fig. 12-15) or, when funds are limited, might require modification of a typical, plastic booster seat. Caregivers may find reclining positions most effective for performing bathing tasks, yet when encouraging water play, every attempt should be made to position the child in sitting as vertically as possible. Sitting in more upright positions promotes effective head, neck, and upper body postural control against gravity. Positioning children in reclining positions does not require postural adaptations and does not promote optimal use of the visual and upper extremity skills needed for play. At times, it is recommended that the caregiver work in the bathtub with the child because secure handling is facilitated, and therapy activities can be practiced. Water should be at waist level or higher, thereby increasing comfort and ease of movement for the child. Children who are permitted to play in the water during bath time often perceive the larger pool experience in a more positive light. However, caregivers must be aware of the danger inherent in filling the bathtub to higher levels and in allowing longer play periods. Because the child might appear to be very content in the bathtub, the caregiver is sometimes inclined to leave the child alone for brief periods. Regardless of how obvious this may seem, caregivers should be reminded about the heightened risks that occur with bath time activities.

The aquatic therapist should help the family find a suitable pool to help increase the child's comfort level and experience in water, while enabling the child to learn to play and practice functional, therapeutic activities. The first choice for a pool is usually in the community setting, but considering family finances, time constraints,

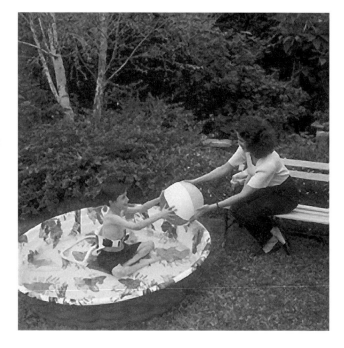

Figure 12-15. Bathing chair permits stable positioning for bathing and water play.

and transportation limitations, a small, plastic backyard pool can be used to help extend therapeutic goals to the home environment.

Breath Control

Breath control is particularly important for the pediatric patient because many water adjustment and higher-level aquatic skill training activities require effective breathing with submersion (Figs. 12-16 and 12-17). Mental adjustment is not complete without competent breath control skills (Fig. 12-18). For children with poor motor control and weakness in postural musculature, proper respiratory support and breathing are probably impaired. Airway control and effective breathing patterns are related to successful oral motor skill development and will have an impact on feeding and expressive speech. Learning to perform controlled inspiration and expiration is important for improvements in respiratory vital capacity, speech production, and lung volume, and for development of effective coughing.[5] Blowing bubbles aids by improving lip approximation and closure[53] and is considered a critical starting point in the progression to water submersion activities.[54] Most children, even those with very limited cognitive and motor abilities who may not be candidates for underwater activities, can learn to accept water to the face and mouth.

Breath Control Skills

A suggested progression of breath control skills in water is the following:

1. Accepts water to face, splashing when bouncing, etc.
2. Quick blowing on face elicits momentary closure of eyes and airway as child is submerged (may be used elsewhere in sequence).
3. Imitates or initiates lip closure with bilabial "m" sounds; uses "b" or "p."[53]

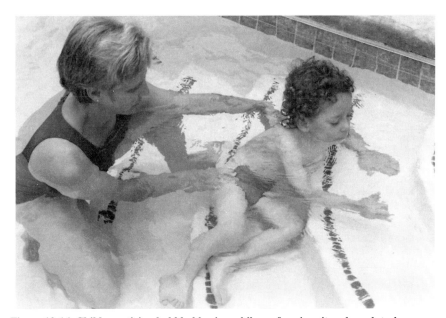

Figure 12-16. Child practicing bubble-blowing while performing sit and reach tasks.

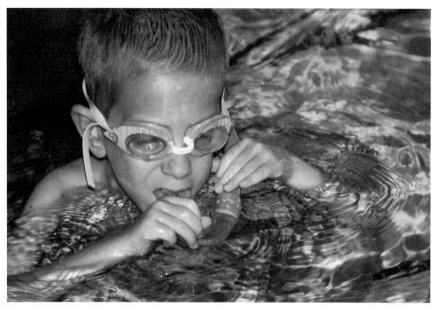

Figure 12-17. Use of snorkel can increase respiratory support musculature and eliminates the need to surface for air.

4. Accepts or initiates mouth submersion; plays with bilabial sounds in water.
5. Blows bubbles imitatively.
6. Uses toy to blow bubbles (plastic eggs or bubble pipe). The therapist may want to avoid use of straw in pool because this might create confusion during feeding.
7. Blows bubbles through nose and mouth.

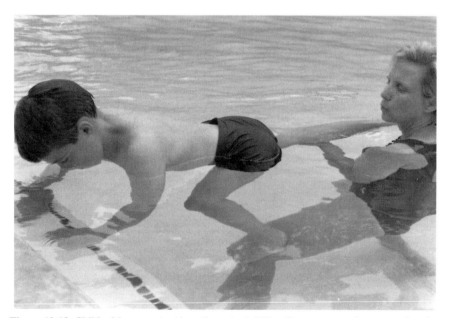

Figure 12-18. Child with competent breath control skills will spontaneously assume face-in position during therapeutic training.

8. Maintains breath control during progressively longer prone glides.
9. Performs rhythmic bobbing, with or without assistance.
10. Performs underwater activity for increased periods; reaches for diving rings and other toys.
11. Maintains breath control during rolling, jumping, or diving in pool and backward roll.
12. Performs rhythmic breathing necessary for stroke development. (Rhythmic breathing can be introduced at other points in the progression but tends to be more difficult for children with motor control problems.)

Underwater Activity

The therapist must carefully assess the child's potential for participation in safe underwater activity and determine whether the child can either close the airway (hold breath) or use an expiratory effort (blow bubbles) to initiate or accept submersion. The overall work of breathing with submersion to the neck increases by approximately 60%.[55] Poor postural alignment, muscular weakness, and altered muscle tone further compromise breathing. Because many children in aquatic programs have decreased respiratory function,[14, 56] the therapist's task is to determine the appropriate intensity and frequency of underwater activity. If the child has a tendency for aspiration of liquids, underwater activities are contraindicated. Any question relating to the safety of underwater submersion should be relayed to the child's physician and speech or occupational therapist.

If the child is a candidate for underwater submersion activities, the therapist should follow typical developmental guidelines for breath control. Attention should be focused on providing optimal positioning to enhance motor performance. Children with poor motor control often require skills to be broken down into several components before they can master the entire skill. The skilled aquatic therapist will recognize necessary adaptations to the typical progression while providing effective positioning and guided breath control activities.

PAT PROGRESSION

The typical PAT program should flow logically from (1) preparatory and warm up activities to (2) impairment-related, component skill training with (3) functional skill training, and conclude with (4) cool-down activities.

Preparatory/Warm up Activities in Water

Many pediatric patients coming to the PAT session have sedentary lifestyles and muscles that have been held in shortened positions. In addition, adjustment to cool water temperatures may warrant the need for a brief warm up. Clear-cut, scientific evidence for the necessity of a warm up before exercise is lacking, yet it is widely recommended as a means of preventing injury and increasing performance.[2, 20, 57] Warm ups should last about 5 to 10 minutes and include activities performed at a slower pace, including active range of motion for the trunk and extremities. The warm up should increase gradually in intensity, raising muscle temperatures to optimal levels.[57]

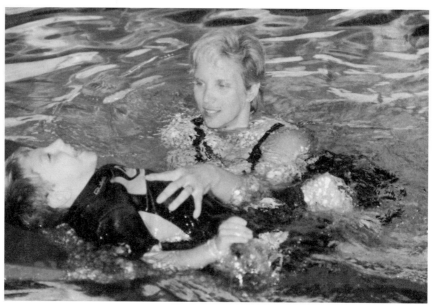

Figure 12-19. Child warms up using flutter kicking in supine position or on therapy mat.

Suggested warm up activities for children are the following:

1. Bouncing, active and assisted, in sitting on large noodle for support or in standing
2. Kicking, usually flutter or frog kick, with or without flotation aids, prone or supine, with emphasis on movements through the entire available range of motion (Fig. 12-19)[58]
3. Bobbing while holding side of pool or with hands held while facing therapist, with feet in contact with pool floor[58]

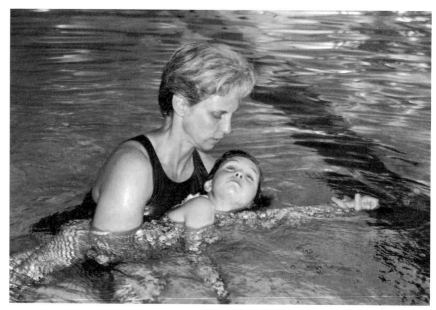

Figure 12-20. Overhead reaching with buoyancy support while rolling over the involved extremity elongates trunk and shoulder structures.

4. Prone and supine glides, with attention to skeletal alignment and transitions in and out of glide position[58]
5. Active and active-assisted reaches in prone, side-lying, supine, or sitting positions with facilitation to elongate and activate targeted muscular structures (Figs. 12-20 and 12-21)
6. Assisted rolling, which is particularly useful to modify high muscle tone, elongate and activate trunk and extremity musculature, and increase active spinal rotation (Fig. 12-22)

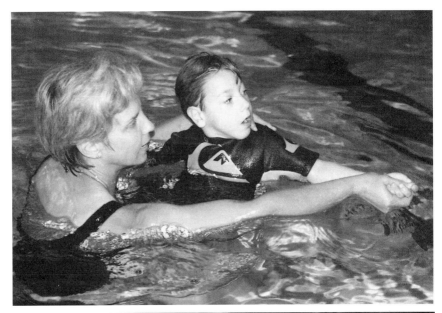

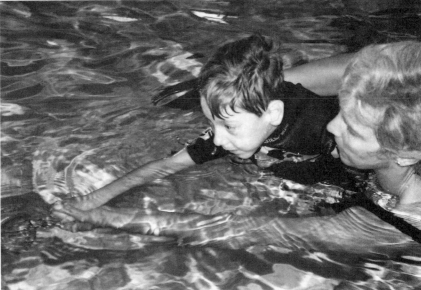

Figure 12-21. Active-assisted reaches in sitting position progressing to prone position elongates trunk and upper extremities and prepares child for higher-level skills.

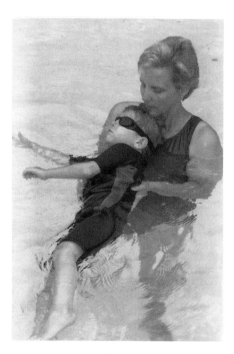

Figure 12-22. Assisted rolling can modify high muscle tone, elongate and activate trunk and extremities, and increase spinal rotation.

The choice of warm up activities will depend on the desired treatment goal. For example, bouncing while sitting astride a large noodle may decrease undesirable extremity tone and increase alertness (via the reticular activating system) and muscle activation in the postural antigravity musculature (Fig. 12-23). Slow, controlled movements may also prepare the child by increasing the available joint range

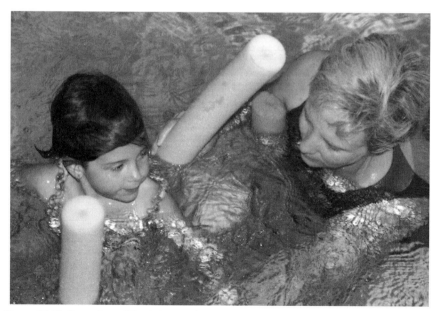

Figure 12-23. Bouncing while sitting astride a large noodle may decrease undesirable extremity tone while increasing postural antigravity musculature activity.

of motion with elongation of muscular structures before more skilled movement. The skilled therapist will continuously focus attention on effective handling holds, positioning, and velocity of movement because they may alter muscle tone.

Functional Motor Skills Training

The task of the aquatic therapist is to identify meaningful, developmental skill training that relates to functional land-based goals. Essential to effective aquatic therapy programming is the promotion of meaningful, active movement. The gravity-friendly aquatic environment promotes enhanced opportunities for movement activity, enabling children to learn desired motor skills with increased range of motion, fluidity, and motor control. Children often experience success with motor skills in the water first and then later generalize those skills to land (Fig. 12-24). Use of the task-type training approach has been documented with adults surviving a stroke.[24] In this approach, aquatic work is performed in functional positions with functional tasks and the participant engages in active problem solving. In response to current research related to learning of purposeful tasks, it is suggested that the pediatric aquatic therapist promote practice of relevant, functional, purposeful tasks, spatial and temporal anticipation strategies, and routine rather than random activities (Fig. 12-25).[59]

Teaching motor skills in water can be superior to land training because children experience constantly changing postural challenges due to the relative lack of postural stability combined with the effects of water turbulence (Fig. 12-26). This opportunity for repetition results in increased exercise intensity, which is often more difficult to achieve with land-based activities. When children respond to postural perturbations in water, there is increased reaction time and little fear of injury from falls. Guided functional activity in water permits hundreds of possible postural shifts and generally encourages increased active pelvic and spinal rotation.

Cool-Down Activities

Cool-down activities lasting 5 to 10 minutes might include active or assisted movements similar to those used at the beginning of the session.[60] If available, a warmer pool in which the child should achieve maximum benefit from guided stretching activities could be used.

CASE STUDIES

Using case format, two patients with common conditions frequently referred for aquatic therapy are described. Examples of treatment activities are offered with impairment-related rationale. These programs represent a range of therapeutic interventions used with these children. For each child, a sampling of treatment activities is presented with measurable goals identified. This information is presented in a format conducive to guiding clinical reasoning and is not necessarily the format suggested for treatment program documentation.

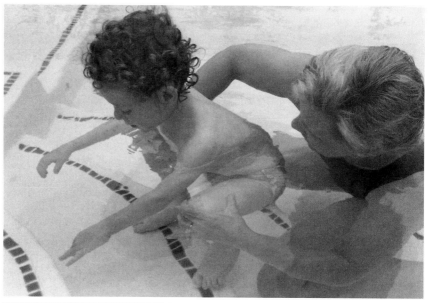

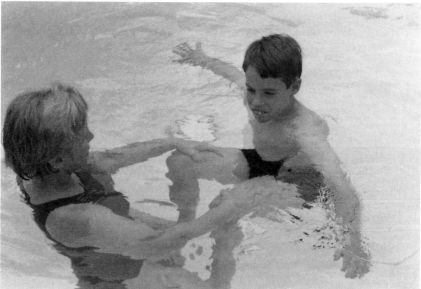

Figure 12-24. Motor skills often emerge initially in water and later generalize to land.

Cerebral Palsy

Background Information

One of the most common conditions of patients referred for PAT is cerebral palsy, a nonprogressive defect or lesion that occurs in utero, during birth, or shortly after birth that is manifested by motor impairment and sensory deficits that are usually evident in early infancy.[26] This diagnosis can be confusing and makes the task of evaluation and treatment more difficult. There are usually a host of related impairments associated with cerebral palsy, with aberrant muscle tone being among the most problematic. Children's conditions are typically classified as spastic,

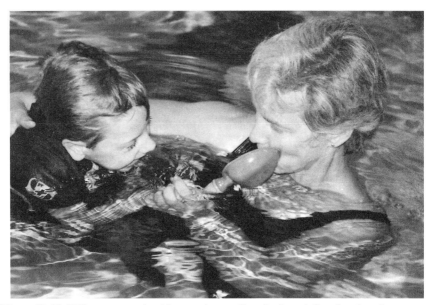

Figure 12-25. PAT programs should promote practice of relevant, functional, and purposeful tasks.

dyskinetic or athetoid, and ataxic and are further identified by the area of the body affected (e.g., monoplegia, diplegia, hemiplegia, or quadriplegia).

Problems Relevant to Aquatic Therapy Programming

- Altered shape and density (see Halliwick Concept, Chapter 4)
- Generalized weakness in postural musculature with ineffective responses to gravity

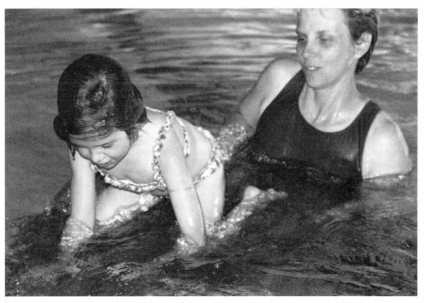

Figure 12-26. Motor skill training in water can be superior to land training due to constantly changing postural challenges.

- Presence of spasticity (high muscle tone), especially prevalent in extremities, with stereotypical patterns of movement
- Interfering reflexes, especially tonic neck reflexes and hyperactive startle
- Asymmetries leading to skeletal deformities such as hip subluxations, dislocations, and scoliosis
- Movement in partial arcs of motion leading to compensatory weakness, poor spinal rotation, and shortening of muscles and soft tissues
- Diminished vital capacity and poor fitness[13]
- Paucity of movement; lack of selective control of muscles
- Inefficient movement patterns demanding high energy expenditure
- Poor sensory processing
- Poor motor planning and coordination
- Communication, vision, hearing, and cognition deficits

Case 1: Long-term PAT Program for Child with Cerebral Palsy

Brent is 6½ years old and has severe spastic quadriplegic cerebral palsy.

Birth History. The birth history includes full-term gestation with vaginal delivery. Perinatal acidosis and fetal distress during labor were reported with seizures occurring within the first 15 hours after delivery. Seizures were well managed with medication until Brent was approximately 3 years old when they occurred more often, necessitating an increase in medication.

Health Problems and Family. Seizures continue to occur sporadically and have been associated with illness. Brent is generally judged to be in good health, with the exception of problems with self-feeding and esophageal reflux. Because of poor weight gain, Brent received a gastric feeding tube at 4 years of age. Since that time, weight gain and endurance have improved markedly. Brent has one brother, 4 years old, and a sister, 2 years old. He lives with his mother and father who provide a loving, supportive home. Brent's mother is present for most aquatic therapy sessions.

Referral and Early Aquatic Therapy. Brent was referred for PAT at 8 months of age by his developmental pediatrician. He generally received weekly, individualized PAT sessions from the physical therapist. His program was complemented by participation in center-based early intervention programs including special education, speech, physical, occupational, hippo, and music therapies.

During the first few sessions in the water, the therapist noted that Brent preferred vertical positioning because he had poor head, neck, and trunk control against gravity. When placed in the supine position, he was unable to roll for more than a few degrees in either direction. He logrolled to his back from the prone position. Tailor sitting required maximum assistance and long periods of sitting proved difficult, even with assistance. Brent was unable to maintain a four-point creeping position for more than a few seconds.

Increased lower extremity tone, especially in the hamstring and gastrocnemius musculature, was apparent as Brent attempted to engage in voluntary movements of almost any kind. Scissoring (hip extension and adduction with internal rotation) was observed with his attempts to bear weight in standing. In the supine position, increased tone with intentional movement was apparent in cervical and spinal extensors, upper trapezius, and triceps musculature. Over time, there was the tendency to use patterns of wrist flexion, with forearm pronation; his hands were often fisted. Voluntary reach and grasp were not present, yet Brent attended visually to people and toys and attempted to bat and bring the upper extremities to the midline. Brent was hypersensitive to many textures and withdrew from light touch.

Brent could be described as generally "fussy" at home and in therapy and required almost constant handling and attention from his caregiver. It was noted that Brent became increasingly fearful of movement during land-based therapy and had periods of resistive behavior during aquatic therapy as well. Permitting Brent's mother to perform portions of the aquatic program usually increased Brent's adherence to therapy activities.

By 22 Months. Direct aquatic therapy continued three to four times monthly and by 22 months of age, Brent had limited independent floor mobility and tended to play in the supine position with partial arc rolling to either side. Sitting required maximum support or use of assistive equipment, such as a corner chair. Botulism toxin (Boxon) injections were administered beginning at 22 months until 6 years of age. One to three muscle groups were targeted, every 4 to 6 months, with primary emphasis on the medial hamstrings, gastrocnemius, soleus, iliopsoas, and pectoral muscles. Upper trapezius and left thumb adductor pollicus muscles were also injected on occasion. Botox injections were judged to markedly improve Brent's overall comfort and function by all involved team members and his family. After Botox injections, both carrying and positioning Brent were performed with less effort on the part of the caregiver. Brent required less support in the preferred tailor sitting position on the floor and used his upper extremities to reach, grasp, and play with toys and other children with more success.

Aquatic Treatment Programs

Three Years of Age
Task (Outcome): Parents have expressed desire to have Brent use Rifton gait trainer to independently ambulate at home and at preschool (Table 12-4).
Functional Long-Term Land Goal: Brent will use Rifton gait trainer walker to exit pool facility, a distance of approximately 100 feet, with three to four rests of 30 to 60 seconds, with stand-by assistance, within 10 minutes in 6 to 9 months.

Five Years of Age
Task (Outcome): Parents and child have expressed desire for improved function of right upper extremity in preparation for school-related demands (Table 12-5).
Functional Long-Term Land Goal: Brent will make clockwise, circular movement of 10 to 12 inches in diameter with large crayon (using crayon holder) with wrist in near neutral position in preparation for face-drawing acitivity.
Summary of Progress: Brent is currently entering the first grade and recently began receiving intrathecal baclofen infusion therapy. He continues to receive weekly, direct, individualized PAT treatment. His progress with PAT is slow, yet gains are measurable and continuous. Brent enjoys independent play (with stand-by assistance) in the water assisted by arm floats or a life jacket. He self-submerges for 2 to 3 seconds, changes positions by rolling with assistance, floats in supine position for 3 to 5 seconds independently, plays successfully in supported standing position, and flutter kicks using a reciprocal pattern in

Table 12-4. PAT at 3 Years of Age

Impairments (Primary and Secondary)	Associated Aquatic Activities
1. Decreased active control of pelvis in anterior/posterior direction with poor transfer of weight during ambulation	1. Brent will straddle therapist's knee in face-forward direction, accepting rocking movements in an anterior/posterior direction without falls (15 to 20 repetitions).
2. Decreased dissociation of lower extremities with shortened stride length	2. Brent will roll with moderate assistance from supine to side with top leg flexed at hip and knee, maintaining lower leg hip and knee extension (5 repetitions in each direction).
3. Limited spinal rotation with decreased lateral weight shift and single leg support	3. Brent will sit on pool step with water to the xiphoid process, reaching for toys placed at his side and moving to midline (5 repetitions to each side). Facilitation given alternatively to gluteal, paraspinal, and lower abdominal muscles to increase weight shift to one hip with spinal rotation in the opposite direction.
4. Increased tone in spastic musculature (hamstring and gastrocsoleus), limiting full range of motion and fluidity of gait	4. Brent will short sit on bench with support at knees in hot tub (98°F) with water to waist; facilitation given to midthoracic spinal extensor muscles (5 to 7 minutes).
5. Poor endurance for sustained activity due to changes in rib cage and altered respiratory patterns	5. Brent will assume supine float from tall kneel with shoulders flexed to approximately 90 degrees with slight chin tuck and moderate assistance to hold position for 15 seconds (3 repetitions).

Table 12-5. PAT at 5 Years of Age

Impairments	Related Aquatic Goals
1. Increased spasticity and shortened pectorals and upper trapezius muscles; limits active and passive mobility in shoulder flexion with scapular depression needed for reaching tasks	1. Brent will assume supine float from tall kneel, positioning upper extremities from side of body to 90-degree shoulder flexion/abduction; facilitation at paraspinal muscles in midthoracic spine[48] (60 seconds, 3 repetitions).
2. Lack of active, upper thoracic spinal extension with rotation and decreased weight shift (especially to left upper extremity); limits control and endurance for sitting and for fine motor tasks	2. Brent will accept weight shift to left upper extremity (flexed elbow) while in supported prone position on therapy mat (10 to 12 repetitions and then repeat on the right side).
3. Use of synergistic extensor patterning of the right upper extremity with tendency to use trunk extension (initiated at hips) to substitute for shoulder flexion, with locking of the elbow in extension, forearm in pronation, wrist flexed; prevents optimal oculomotor function and selective control of upper extremity; limits self-feeding	3. Brent will use small sand shovel (½-inch diameter handle) to scoop water from right side to bucket held just above water at midline, using elbow flexion, forearm to neutral, when carrying water to bucket (8 to 10 repetitions).
4. Poor graded control of right upper extremity leads to decreased precision and adaptability for fine motor tasks with diminished sensory feedback; limits sensory feedback necessary for higher order motor learning[61]	4. Brent will hold upper extremities of soft-body water toy (buoyancy-supported position of upper extremities) and "dance" side to side, use circular and underwater movements, and accompany movement by singing "Row, Row, Row Your Boat" (2 repetitions).

semiprone position for up to 25 yards. Brent ambulates at school and at home with the use of the Rifton Pacer walker with stand-by assistance. Community ambulation is possible for 15- to 20-minute periods traversing distances of up to 500 feet. Upper extremity function is improved with self-feeding of finger foods, use of writing utensils with increased accuracy, and activation of switches for computer technology.

Childhood Rheumatic Diseases

Background Information

Rheumatic diseases involve inflammation of connective tissue, with juvenile rheumatoid arthritis (JRA) occurring most often.[62, 63] JRA is classified by clinical symptoms presenting in the first 6 months after onset. Pauciarticular disease occurs in 40% of patients and involves arthritis in four or fewer joints. Polyarticular disease is present in 50% of patients and affects five or more joints. Systemic disease is marked by the presence of fever and rash, with various joints involved over the course of the disease. Approximately 10% of children with JRA present with systemic JRA; 25% of this group continue to have severe systemic disease.[63] A variety of drugs have proved effective in the management of chronic synovitis associated with JRA.[62]

Chronic inflammation of synovial membranes leads to invasive overgrowth into adjacent cartilaginous and bony structures and results in joint destruction.[63] Secondary impairments include pain and stiffness, both at rest and with movement, limited joint range of motion with contractures, muscular weakness, and postural and gait deviations. Research in children with JRA indicates that decreased levels of exercise performance and workload capacities also are seen.[64] Functional limitations vary with the course and extent of the disease, from little or no functional limitations to wheelchair and caregiver dependence.

Problems Relevant to Aquatic Therapeutic Interventions

- Tendency for morning stiffness and joint pain
- Joint effusion
- Articular tenderness; loss of joint play
- Limited range of motion (active and passive); tendency toward shortened flexor musculature due to antigravity muscular weakness
- Ligamentous laxity may develop as a compensation for movements lacking terminal extension
- Reduced aerobic capacity ($\dot{V}O_{2max}$) and endurance[65]
- Limited self-care skills
- Gait and mobility impairments with secondary decline in gross and fine motor developmental skill acquisition
- Limited play and/or recreation skills

Case 2: Short-Term/Episodic PAT Program for Child with JRA

History and Referral. Ashley is a 5-year-old girl with a diagnosis of polyarticular JRA who was referred for PAT by her rheumatologist. She is slender and of small stature, and is initially shy. She ambulates independently but prefers to hold her mother's hand. Her mother indicates that she requests to be carried for all but household ambulation.

Ashley is the only adoptive child in a family with three other siblings. All children are home-schooled. At birth, a congenital dislocation of the right hip was reported. Recurrent ear infections during her first year resulted in placement of ear tubes bilaterally. The primary care physician has judged them to be no longer in place. Gross and fine motor developmental skills are reported as being delayed by her mother, and early intervention services, including occupational and speech therapies, have been provided in the home since age 3. Her mother reports overall skill development to be more like that of a 3-year-old child.

Current Level of Function. Ashley currently depends on her parents and siblings for most of her self-care and mobility needs. In all active movements, Ashley works in limited ranges of motion, keeping her upper extremities close to the trunk. Little spinal rotation is used for activities. Ashley uses no more than 5 to 10 degrees of active cervical flexion/extension for function. Active-assisted range of motion measures indicate limitations in shoulder flexion (-20 degrees) and abduction (-25 degrees), wrist flexion (-50 degrees) and extension (-45 degrees left, -60 degrees right), hip abduction (-10 degrees), knee extension (-25 degrees), and ankle dorsiflexion (-15 degrees right, -20 degrees left), and plantar flexion (-25 degrees right, -30 degrees left). Parents report that she walks with assistance for 10 to 12 feet, then she requests to be held. Ashley ambulates with one hand held using a crouched gait, decreased step length, shortened stance phase, and lack of reciprocal arm swing and trunk rotation. Asymmetry is apparent with lower extremity weight bearing because Ashley avoids weight shifting onto the left hip during standing and walking tasks.

She has a tendency to stay in one position for extended periods, usually sitting at a small chair and table, playing with manipulative toys and making simple art projects. Ashley self-feeds, preferring the left hand, but requires food that is easily chewed and requests finger foods to avoid use of utensils.

Ashley began a drug therapy program within 4 weeks of referral to aquatic therapy. There was regular, effective communication between the aquatic physical therapist, physician, and occupational therapist to address pain management and coordinate treatment interventions.

Aquatic therapy was initiated twice monthly with intensive parent instruction and home programming. The family purchased a pre-owned hot tub, which was used frequently when Ashley was experiencing acute symptoms. One month after initiation of aquatic therapy programming, sessions were increased to once weekly. Within the first few aquatic therapy sessions, it was determined that Ashley had very poor mental adjustment skills, and she was referred for private swim instruction for 6 weeks. This weekly instruction proved valuable and was provided in addition to weekly aquatic therapy.

Aquatic Treatment Programs

Outcome (Task): Parents have expressed desire to decrease how often Ashley is carried and increase ambulation without complaints of pain (Table 12-6).
Short-Term (1 to 6 Months) Land-Based Function Goal: Ashley will ambulate independently in household and backyard, using wagon or stroller support for longer distances, with no carrying required.

Table 12-6. Short-Term PAT Program

Impairments (Primary and Secondary)	Related Aquatic Goals
1. Poor mental adjustment (Ashley tends to cling to the therapist, is fearful of unsupported movements, and does not accept water to face); limits therapeutic program and active mobility in water	1. Straddled on two noodles with therapist support from the rear, Ashley will accept gentle "snaking" movements, side to side in the water, upper extremities holding noodle for 60 sec, in first 2–3 weeks; referral to private swim instructor
2. Limited active spinal rotation; restricts active range of motion and mobility, leading to postural deformity, weakness, and loss of functional skills	2. Modified Bad Ragaz Ring Method, beginning with isometric patterns, progressing to isotonic patters; position in semisupine with slight chin tuck, support at rib case, ask Ashley to roll slightly bringing one hip to the surface; progressing to holding position as child is moved in circle around therapist
3. Limited range of motion in active movements of spinal, shoulder, wrist, hip, knee, and ankle extension in vertical (against gravity); leads to increased weakness, joint changes, contractures, and limits movements necessary for daily skills	3. Ashley will begin in short sit (on step), support with one hand on step; reaching with the opposing upper extremity for toys placed at end point ranges to the front and sides to increase active upper extremity movement for play, therapist guiding weight shift and spinal rotation (5 repetitions), repeat with opposite extremity, increase as tolerated (ongoing activity); same activity may be performed in tall kneel, half kneel, and standing positions
4. Weakness in antigravity musculature; utilizes inefficient, high-energy muscle groups, leads to limitations in joint strength and range of motion, compromises gait fluidity and skilled gross motor task performance	4. Prone position, with support at lower rib cage, alternate support to increase spinal rotation, Ashley will flutter kick 15–20 times (3 repetitions); repeat with frog kick
5. Poor standing balance; limits stance during ambulation, leads to falls with risk of injury, and limits gross motor skill acquisition and play	5. Water walk with support from barbell; water to chest height; use marching songs and encourage increasing hip flexion while holding stance phase with opposite extremity (gluteus medius activity); teach taking "giant steps" and move in all directions; gait training activity up to 10 minutes, as pain permits
6. Painful, limited active range of motion in positions where joint loading occurs; leads to poor postural alignment and further limitations in active movement, decreased motor skills, and decreased quality of life	6. Ashley will hold balanced supine float with facilitation at gluteal and rhomboid muscles for 30 seconds (5 repetitions) in 6 months

Summary of Progress. Ashley continued with weekly, individualized, aquatic therapy programs for 6 months. Her painful symptoms were dramatically reduced with both the aquatic program and an effective drug therapy regimen. Swimming skills continued to improve with good mental adjustment, and other skills continued to emerge. The occurrence of joint contractures was minimized, and good, active range of motion was available for functional activities. Ashley continues attending a follow-up clinic for children with JRA; she swims regularly and has good endurance for daily mobility needs and play.

SPORTS INJURIES

In the United States, there is a trend to push the training of children to and beyond their physical limits. This training begins at an earlier age and often includes repetitive, high-impact activities. Young, prepubescent athletes often lack the joint stability and muscular strength to withstand such intense training without injury. Many coaches, teachers, and trainers lack adequate time or the educational background necessary to design sports training programs for children. Proper training requires careful attention to avoid training errors leading to repetitive trauma or "overuse" injuries. In addition, children are at risk for injury when coaches fail to attend to individual differences in anatomic alignment, musculotendinous strength, flexibility, or bulk, as well as proper footwear, old injuries, or disease states.[66]

Aquatic therapy has been used successfully for many years in the rehabilitation of college and professional athletes. The use of aquatic therapy for rehabilitation of children with sports injuries is becoming more widespread.[67,68] As for adults, water can often be the most effective environment for retraining activities.[69] Non-disabled children with sports injuries often have had previous swimming experience and have access to a swimming facility. Assuming that they perceive pool activity as enjoyable, there is increased likelihood of adherence to the home (water) exercise program.[70]

Well-structured water therapy sessions provide the opportunity for maintenance of cardiovascular fitness, mobility, and flexibility, while aiding in the prevention of chronic problems. Water protects the young athlete from sports-related forces including ground reaction, repetitive shock, shearing, compression, and distraction.[67] Appropriate aquatic exercise can unload articular cartilage and bones while protecting ligaments, tendons, and muscles from excessive torque and vibration forces.[67] The "10% rule" for land-based retraining suggests that no weekly increases in training intensity greater than 10% are considered safe.[71] Additional studies are needed to determine whether the 10% rule can be modified for aquatic programs to help return young athletes earlier to full, safe activity levels.

WEIGHT TRAINING

Weight training for children, with or without disabilities, has been a subject of considerable controversy. The concern is primarily with the potential for injury of growing bones in prepubescent children by overloading them with heavy, repetitive stress forces. Research supports the use of well-supervised weight training in the prepubescent athlete, noting that there will be definite increases in muscular strength, but little change in muscle bulk will occur.[72] Strength training programs in children with cerebral palsy have been shown to produce increases in muscular strength. In one such program, gains in quadriceps and hamstring muscle strength were seen, yet these gains were not related to alterations in gait velocity and efficiency.[73] Another study by Damiano and associates,[74] found increased muscle strength in hamstring and quadriceps muscle groups after training, and related these changes to improvement in the degree of crouch at initial floor contact and increased stride lengths at slow and fast speeds.

Application of resistance to selected muscle groups during aquatic therapy is common practice with adults.[75] Velcro weights, gloves, paddles, kickboards, and barbells are sometimes used in aquatic programs for children and are frequently used with adult aquatic programs. Because therapy for children relies heavily on play activities, the list of resistive equipment is different from that for adults.

Adding Resistance

The following can be used to add resistance to movement in water with children:

- Tennis shoes during ambulation: Use inexpensive Velcro-closing canvas shoes to increase full foot contact and stability and decrease effects of buoyancy.
- DAFOs, AFOs: Cover with tennis shoes and use when stability for standing, transitions, and gait is desired.
- Fins: Fins can also provide lower extremity flotation and are often trimmed to provide less resistance for the child.
- Balls: Increased size is related to increased resistance; multiplane resistance is possible with pushes forward, backward, sideways, and underwater.
- Barbell floats: Use single handle or one per upper extremity.
- Noodles: These range in size from 2½ to 4 inches in diameter and can be configured in a variety of shapes. A larger size provides greater resistance and offers more support.
- Kickboards: Consider shape and size; smaller, lighter-weight, softer boards, with rounded edges are usually better suited to children.
- Buckets and pails: Filling these with water can increase resistance considerably (Fig. 12-27).
- Squeeze toys: Sometimes these are too difficult for children with severe impairments; seek out dog toys and softer, more lightweight toys.
- Squirt toys: These can require considerable strength and motor skill; look at toys with pumping action (soaker-type guns) rather than trigger mechanisms.
- Pushing activities and games (Fig. 12-28): Push with upper extremities against the therapist (e.g., "King of the Mountain" game).

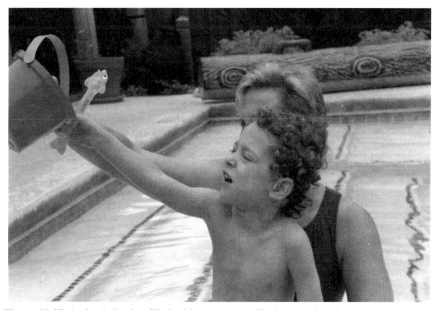

Figure 12-27. A plastic bucket filled with water can offer increased resistance to movement and provide weight-training effects.

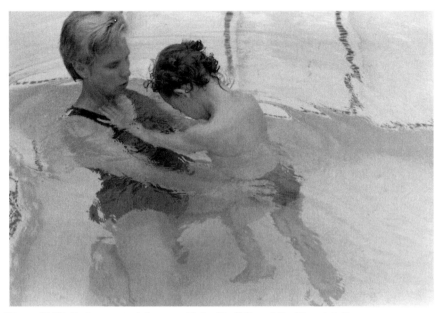

Figure 12-28. Resistance training provided with "King of the Mountain" game.

- Weighted rings and sticks: Rings are generally safer and easier to retrieve.
- Watering cans: Look for a variety of sizes; these can be difficult to use if they are too large.
- Any object that floats: Taken under water, this offers resistance to movement.

Because of the range of toys and equipment available for children, it is usually not necessary to use cuff-style weights in the water.

Training for Activities of Daily Living

The aquatic therapy session provides an ideal opportunity to train children to improve independence with self-help skills. Increased independence in the aquatic environment can lead to improved functional land-based goals.

The aquatic therapist should be available to assist in evaluation of dressing skills, showering, toileting, and related grooming. Caregivers should be instructed in safe transfer and assistance procedures.

Water can be used to strengthen necessary movement patterns such as hand to mouth, hand to foot, and hand to face and head. Buoyancy-assisted movements, performed in a vertical position, often provide the assistance to shoulder and hip flexion necessary to teach these skills. In the child with more severe motor impairment, supported semi–side-lying can also be used teach these critical, self-care movements (Fig. 12-29).

SENSORY PROCESSING PROBLEMS

Many children who present with poor motor skills, with or without aberrant muscle tone, will demonstrate problems with adaptive processing of sensory information.

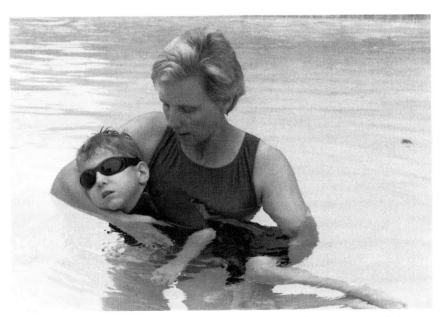

Figure 12-29. Supported semilying position can be used to teach movements needed to perform self-care skills.

Central to the principles of sensory integration treatment are the following:

1. Provide a variety of controlled sensory inputs targeted at the production of an *adaptive response* that includes motor behaviors, social interactions, or cognitive skills.
2. Promote the child's *intrinsic motivation* (Fig. 12-30).
3. Look for *purposeful behaviors* within a meaningful activity.[76]

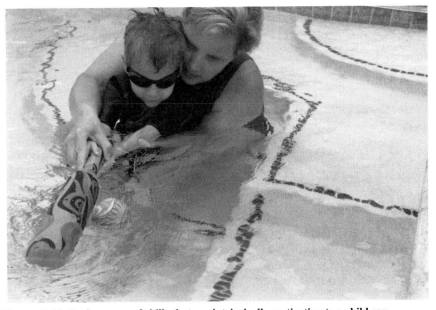

Figure 12-30. Performance of skills that are intrinsically motivating to a child can contribute to improved sensory processing and motor skill acquisition.

Table 12-7. Examples of Sensory Variables and Their Possible Effects in the Aquatic Environment

Increasing Sensory Information	Decreasing Sensory Information
Bright lights, loud noises	Minimized lighting and noise (calming music)
Increased water turbulence	Calm water
Cluttered deck, many people	Limited equipment, few people
Colder water temperature	Warmer temperature (88 to 90°F); highly variable with child
Barefoot (may trigger unwanted tone in lower extremities)	Water shoes (may also increase sensory input by adding weight, resistance, and stability)
Vertical position requires least postural adaptation and often feels most stable	Prone and supine positions may feel destabilizing
Deep pressure through joint surfaces (often prefer 4-point position, sitting, or standing—wherever the most contact with the support surface is achieved)	Unstable, unsupported positions
Fast, jerky movements (splashing, jumping, falling)	Slow, rhythmical movements (rocking, gentle bouncing, gliding, rolling)
Firm contact with skin—swimsuit, vest, or wetsuit (needs to fit snugly)	Light touch (may be interpreted as aversive); flapping garments can be disorganizing
Familiar, organized program; clear behavioral expectations and feedback	Lack of program structure and appropriate feedback

Children need to organize sensory information from the body and the environment to effectively execute desired motor skills.[77] Sensory modulation occurs when the child scans available sensory information and responds with the requisite level of arousal and activity.[78] There are abundant opportunities to increase the amount of sensory information in the aquatic environment, and careful assessment by the therapist is required to determine proper manipulation of the available vestibular, tactile, and proprioceptive variables (Table 12-7).

AQUATIC AND SWIMMING SKILL TRAINING

The teaching of aquatic and swimming skills within the context of an aquatic therapy program is the subject of much discussion among aquatic professionals. There appears to be confusion about the appropriateness of including these skills in the context of a therapeutic program. The teaching of swimming and safety skills is particularly important for the child with a lifelong developmental disability because the aquatic environment may offer the most appropriate opportunity to engage in self-directed, meaningful exercise, swim skill, fitness, and recreation.

The aquatic therapist should ask the following questions when considering the inclusion of swimming skills in an aquatic therapy program:

- It this skill necessary for further progression of this child's therapeutic goals?
- Could the parent (caregiver) or swim instructor teach this skill, or does it require the training of a therapist?
- Does this skill have impairment-related implications that contribute to functional land goals?
- Is acquisition of this skill the best use of my limited, therapeutic time?
- Do I understand the typical components necessary for the acquisition of this skill?
- Is an adaptation required, and do I know how to provide it?

Consider the example of the child with spastic diplegia, learning to dive into the pool from a half-kneel position.

Target skill	*Dive into deep water from half-kneel position*
Components	***Relationship to land function***
Child assumes balanced, half-kneel position on deck (dissociation of lower extremities)	Required for floor to standing transition
Trunk forward with chin tuck, weight transferred from back to front leg, center of gravity moves forward	Necessary for effective transfer of weight during ambulation
Concentrically contract quadriceps of front leg to rise from floor while pushing off with back leg ankle plantar flexors	Controller terminal extension at the knee with graded plantar flexion needed during push-off phase of gait[79]; also relates to improved unilateral support for hopping

Flotation

Ideally, children should learn to perform movements in the water without use of flotation aids. Flotation provides altered feedback between a moving body and water. For this reason, flotation is generally not used with Halliwick training programs.[21] Increased reliance on flotation aids may create a false sense of security.[80] Still, when young children are taught competency in water, flotation aids can provide added support. Flotation aids have limited application during the therapeutic session but may often be used to assist parents during recreational swim sessions. The aquatic therapist should know the relative benefits of potential flotation devices and be able to match them to client needs (Fig. 12-31).

The following are flotation aids are frequently used for children with motor impairments:

Attached to body

- Life jackets: For children with severe motor impairments, the use of a life jacket may be the most appropriate aid to permit "independent" supine mobility in the water (stand-by assistance is always necessary).
- Inflatable or foam arm bands: These usually require the use of shoulder flexion with adduction, which may not be a desirable movement in some children; children tend to stay more vertical and often avoid a face-in experience. However, they can be useful with performance of lower extremity "deep-water" exercise.
- Suits, vests, with adjustable flotation: Suits with built-in flotation panels can be dangerous in that they often provide too much flotation and can trap children in face-down positions; suits such as Swimfree allow adjustable inflation and can sometimes provide needed trunk support; adjustable flotation vests (e.g., Safe T. Seal) fit snugly against the torso and can aid in optimal alignment and support of the trunk.
- Collars: Collars should be adjustable and small enough to prevent undue stress to posterior neck structures.

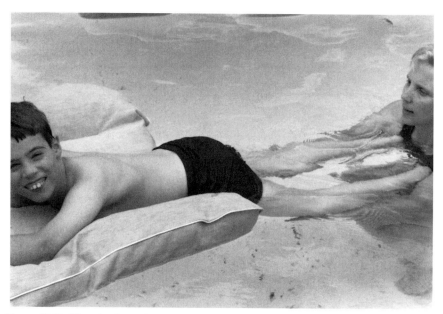

Figure 12-31. Flotation is used to support the upper body and trunk while lower extremity skill training is performed.

- Deep-water belt (e.g., AquaJogger Jr.): This assists in deep-water exercise programs and is also used to promote better balance and alignment of the trunk in horizontal positions. It is particularly useful for encouraging longer distance swimming for a child with trunk or lower extremity weakness.
- Cubes or oval-shaped flotation strapped to back: These can sometimes be useful in helping to support and align weakened trunk and lower extremities. Use with caution because there is the tendency to push the child with weak head and neck extensors into a head-down position.
- Inflatable baby floats or inner tubes: Baby floats might be useful to provide caregiver relief and increase head control with upper extremity weight bearing; they are potentially dangerous because tipping forward occurs frequently. Small inner tubes can be use sparingly to perform deep-water exercise and teach circular/rotational patterns of movement in water.

Held by child

- Kickboards: These come in many shapes and sizes that are better suited to small hands and bodies. A higher-functioning child is required to control the board.
- Single-bar barbell floats: These may assist with ambulation but often provide too much force to the shoulder when used in prone and supine positions. Note that flexion/abduction range of motion is more limited in children than in adults.[48]
- Barbell floats, one for each upper extremity: Careful attention should be focused on the shoulder to prevent subluxation of the glenohumeral joint from forceful upward buoyancy forces.
- Therapy mats, in foam, sometimes with cushion support: These provide excellent support from which to elicit postural stability over a movable base.

- Noodles: Although they come in various sizes, larger (4-inch) noodles have the advantage of increasing stability, for example, straddle-sitting, but they may provide too much upward force into the child's shoulder joint to be used effectively in the prone position. One or more smaller noodles (2½-inch) can be used creatively to support the head, neck, trunk, and extremities, bringing the child in more favorable alignment for activity.
- Blow up toys, boats, and other larger water toys: Large turtles, sharks, etc., can be used to provide fun, movable bases of support from which the child can accept dynamic postural changes. Small paddle boats (powered by lower extremities) can provide strong motivation while strengthening lower extremities, particularly at the ankle. Refer to Chapter 6 for more details regarding toys and flotation.

CONCLUSION

Aquatic programming should be part of *every* child's life experience, and children with disabilities are no exception. The aquatic environment is often the least restrictive environment from which to accomplish a multitude of patient- and family-centered goals. Aquatic therapists have barely touched the surface of the almost limitless possibilities available to clinicians when guiding children with disabilities through an aquatic therapeutic program.

While moving ahead with the development of solid, scientific bases for pediatric aquatic interventions, our highest priority is to respond with sensitivity to the needs of the child and family. Campbell advises the following:

> Recognition of the immediate family and larger sociocultural environments for the developing child supports effective intervention for children of all ages.... Therapists who search for family-oriented outcomes related to the child's movement and collaborate with families on the process of care, are engaging in best practice for children and their families.[34]

REFERENCES

1. Waring WW: Respiratory diseases in children: an overview. Respir Care 20:1138–1145, 1978.
2. Bar-Or O: Physiologic responses to exercise in healthy children. In Bar-Or O (ed): Pediatric Sports Medicine for the Practitioner. New York: Springer-Verlag, 1983, pp 1–65.
3. Lewis CL: Physiologic response to exercise in the child: considerations for the typically and atypically developing child. Paper presented at the Combined Sections Conference of the American Physical Therapy Association, February 2001, San Antonio, Tex.
4. Nelson CA: Cerebral palsy. In Umphred DA (ed): Neurological, 4th ed. St Louis: Mosby, 2001, p 272.
5. Massery M: Chapters 20–22. In Frownfelter D (ed): Chest Physical Therapy and Pulmonary Rehabilitation, 2nd ed. St Louis: Mosby, 1987.
6. Stout JL: Physical fitness during childhood and adolescence. In Campbell SK, Linden DV, Palisnao RJ (eds): Physical Therapy for Children. 2nd ed. Philadelphia: WB Saunders, 2000, pp 141–169.
7. Koch G: Muscle blood flow after ischemic work during bicycle ergometer work in boys aged 12. Acta Pediatrica Belg Suppl 28:29–39, 1974.
8. Bar-Or O, Inbar O, Spira R: Physiological effects of a sports rehabilitation program on cerebral palsied and poliomyelitic adolescents. Med Sci Sports 8:157–161, 1976.

9. Lundberg A: Maximal aerobic capacity in young people with spastic cerebral palsy. Dev Med Child Neurol 20:205–210, 1978.
10. Koop SE, Stout JL, Drinken WH, et al: Energy cost of walking in children with cerebral palsy [abstract]. Phys Ther 69:386, 1989.
11. Berg K: Effect of physical training of school children with cerebral palsy. Acta Paediatr Suppl 204:27–33, 1970.
12. Ekblom B, Lundberg A: Effect of training on adolescents with severe motor handicaps. Acta Paediatr Scand 57:17–23, 1968.
13. Hutzler Y, Chacham A, Bergman U, et al: Effects of a movement and swimming program on vital capacity and water orientation skills of children with cerebral palsy. Dev Med Child Neurol 40:176–181, 1998.
14. Sherman MS, Kaplan JM, Effgen S, et al: Pulmonary dysfunction and reduced exercise capacity in patients with myelomeningocele. J Pediatr 131:423–418, 1997.
15. Hayes-Allen MC, Tring FC: Obesity: another hazard for spina bifida children. Br J Prevent Soc Med 27:192–196, 1973.
16. Tecklin JS: Pulmonary disorders in infants and children and their physical therapy management. In Tecklin JS (ed): Pediatric Physical Therapy, 3rd ed. Philadelphia: Lippincott Williams & Wilkins, 1999, p 537.
17. Fitch KD: Swimming, medicine and asthma. In Erikson B, Furburg B (eds): Swimming Medicine. Baltimore, Md: University Park Press, 1978, Vol IV, pp 16–31.
18. Carlsen KH, Oseid S, Odden H, et al: The response of children with and without bronchial asthma to heavy swimming exercise. In Oseid S, Carlsen KH (eds): Children and Exercise XIII. Champaign, Ill: Human Kinetics, 1989. Vol 19, p 351.
19. Campion MR: The physiological, therapeutic and psychological effects of activity in water. In Campion MR (ed): Hydrotherapy: Principles and Practice. Oxford, UK: Butterworth-Heinemann, 2000, pp 7–8.
20. Bates A, Hanson N: Aquatic Exercise Therapy. Philadelphia: WB Saunders, 1996.
21. Cunningham J: Halliwick method. In Ruoti RG, Morris DM, Cole AJ (eds): Aquatic Rehabilitation. Philadelphia: Lippincott, 1997, pp 305–331.
22. Carmick J: Managing equinus in children with cerebral palsy: electrical stimulation to strengthen the triceps surae muscle. Dev Med Child Neurol 37:965–975, 1995.
23. Goldberg C, Van Sant A: Normal motor development. In Tecklin JS (ed): Pediatric Physical Therapy, 3rd ed. Philadelphia: Lippincott Williams & Wilkins, 1999, p 26.
24. Morris DM: Aquatic rehabilitation for the treatment of neurologic disorders. In Becker BE, Cole AJ (eds): Comprehensive Aquatic Therapy. Boston: Butterworth-Heinemann, 1997, pp 49–71.
25. Campbell SK: The child's development of functional movement. In Campbell SK, Linden DV, Palisnao RJ (eds): Physical Therapy for Children, 2nd ed. Philadelphia: WB Saunders, 2000, p 34.
26. Olney SJ, Wright MJ: Cerebral palsy. In Cambell SK, Linden DV, Palisnao RJ (eds): Physical Therapy for Children, 2nd ed. Philadelphia: WB Saunders, 2000, pp 533–570.
27. Norton CO, Jamison LJ: The Lyton model for the acquatic continuum of care. In Norton CO, jamison LJ (eds): A Team Approach to the Aquatic Continuum of Care. Boston: Butterworth-Heinemann, 2000, p 8.
28. Effgen SK: The education environment. In Cambell SK, Linden DV, Palisnao RJ (eds): Physical Therapy for Children, 2nd ed. Philadelphia: WB Saunders, 2000, p 919.
29. Dunn W: Integrated related services. In Meyer LH, Peck CA, Brown L (eds): Critical Issues in the Lives of People with Severe Disabilities. Baltimore, Md: Paul H Brookes, 1991, pp 353–378.
30. Carter MJ, Dolan MA, LeConey SP: Designing Instructional Swim Programs for Individuals with Disabilities. Reston, Va: American Alliance for Health, Physical Education, Recreation and Dance, 1994, pp 38, 45–46.
31. Dulcy T: An integrated program for children with autism. Nat Aquat J 8(2):7–10, 1992.
32. Lunnen KY: Physical therapy in the public schools. In Tecklin JS (ed): Pediatric Physical Therapy, 3rd ed. Philadelphia: Lippincott Williams & Wilkins, 1999, p 566.
33. Rosenbaum P, King S, Law M, et al: Family-centered service: a conceptual framework and research review. Phys Occup Ther Pediatr 18:1–20, 1998.

34. Kolobe T, Sparling J, Daniels LE: Family-centered intervention. In Campbell SK, Linden DV, Palisnao RJ (eds): Physical Therapy for Children, 2nd ed. Philadelphia: WB Saunders, 2000, p 887.
35. Salzman A: Available at Aquaticnet@yahoogroups.com.
36. Becker BE: Biophysiology aspects of hydrotherapy. In Becker BE, Cole AJ (eds): Comprehensive Aquatic Therapy. Boston: Butterworth-Heinemann, 1997, p 43.
37. Skinner AT, Thomson AM: Duffield's Exercise in Water, 3rd ed. London: Bailliere Tindall, 1983, p 46.
38. Tappit-Emas E: Spina bifida. In Tecklin JS (ed): Pediatric Physical Therapy, 3rd ed. Philadelphia: Lippincott Williams & Wilkins, 1999, p 211.
39. Scoggin AE, Parks KM: Latex sensitivity in children with spina bifida: implications for occupational therapy practitioners. Am J Occup Ther 51(7):608–611, 1997.
40. Barrera ME, Rosenbaum PL, Cunningham CE: Early home intervention with low birthweight infants and their parents. Child Dev 57:20–33, 1986.
41. Meade V: Partners in Movement. San Antonio, Tex: Therapy Skill Builders, 1998.
42. Campion MR: Practice of paediatric hydrotherapy. In Campion MR (ed): Hydrotherapy: Principles and Practice. Oxford, UK: Butterworth-Heinemann, 2000, pp 31–134.
43. Styer-Acevedo J, Cirullo JA: Integrating land and aquatic approaches with a functional emphasis. Orthop Phys Ther Clin North Am 3:177, 1994.
44. Styer-Acevedo J: Physical therapy for the child with cerebral palsy. In Tecklin JS (ed): Pediatric Physical Therapy, 3rd ed. Philadelphia: Lippincott Williams & Wilkins, 1999, pp 107–162.
45. Harris SR: Neurodevelopmental treatment approach for teaching swimming to cerebral palsied children. Phys Ther 58:979–983, 1978.
46. Campion MR: The Halliwick method and conductive education. In Campion MR (ed): Hydrotherapy: Principles and Practice. Oxford, UK: Butterworth-Heinemann, 2000, pp 169–174.
47. Kozman I, Balogh E: A brief introduction to conductive education and its application at an early age. Infants Young Chil 8:68–74, 1995.
48. Brooks-Scott S: Mobilization for the Neurologically Involved Child. San Antonio, Tex: Therapy Skill Builders, 1997.
49. Corrigan B, Maitland GD: Practical Orthopaedic Medicine. Sydney, Australia: Butterworth, 1983.
50. Hill J: Spinal mobilizations. In Campion MR (ed): Hydrotherapy: Principles and Practice. Oxford, UK: Butterworth-Heinemann, 2000, pp 226–241.
51. Barnes JF: Pediatric myofascial release, 1991. Modified from Myofascial Release I Seminar Workbook 1999, pp 1–21.
52. Konno J, Sova R: Ai chi. Paper presented at the Aquatic Therapy & Rehab Institute Symposium, August 2000, Orlando, Fla, pp H13–H24.
53. Styer-Acevedo J: Aquatic rehabilitation of the pediatric client. In Ruoti RG, Morris DM, Cole AJ (eds): Aquatic Rehabilitation. Philadelphia: Lippincott, 1997, pp 151–171.
54. Bullock K: Waterproofing Your Child. Sydney, Australia: Rigby, 1982.
55. Agostoni E, Gurtner G, Torri G, et al: Respiratory mechanics during submersion and negative pressure breathing. J Appl Physiol 21:251–258, 1966.
56. Unnithan VB, Clifford C, Bar-O O: Evaluation by exercise testing of the child with cerebral palsy. Sports Med 26:239–251, 1998.
57. Pollock ML, Wilmore JH: Exercise in Health and Disease, 2nd ed. Philadelphia: WB Saunders, 1990.
58. American Red Cross Staff: Swimming & Diving. St Louis: Mosby Lifeline, 1992, p 131.
59. Schmidt RA: Motor Learning and Performance. Champaign, Ill: Human Kinetics, 1991.
60. Payton O: Manual of Physical Therapy. New York: Churchill Livingstone, 1989.
61. Newton RA: Contemporary issue and theories of motor control: assessment of movement and posture. In Umphred DA (ed): Neurological Rehabilitation, 4th ed. St Louis: Mosby, 2001.
62. Klepper SE, Scull SA: Juvenile rheumatoid arthritis. In Tecklin JS (ed): Pediatric Physical Therapy, 3rd ed. Philadelphia: Lippincott Williams & Wilkins, 1999, pp 429–467.
63. Albinson Scull S: Juvenile rheumatoid arthritis. In Campbell SK, Linden DV, Palisnao RJ (eds): Physical Therapy for Children, 2nd ed. Philadelphia: WB Saunders, 2000, pp 227–246.

64. Jasso MS, Protas EJ, Giannini EH: Assessment of physical work capacity in juvenile rheumatoid arthritis patients and healthy children [abstract]. Arthritis Rheum 29(suppl 75, no 86): S158, 1986.
65. Giannini MJ, Protas EJ: Aerobic capacity in juvenile rheumatoid arthritis patients and healthy children. Arthritis Care Res 4:131–135, 1992.
66. Maffulli N: Intensive training in young athletes. Sports Med 9:229–243, 1990.
67. Tierney T: Aquatic rehabilitation of the athlete. In Ruoti RG, Morris DM, Cole AJ (eds): Aquatic Rehabilitation. Philadelphia: Lippincott, 1997, pp 211–225.
68. Bernhardt-Bainbridge D: Sports injuries in children. In Campbell SK, Linden DV, Palisnao RJ (eds): Physical Therapy for Children, 2nd ed. Philadelphia: WB Saunders, 2000, pp 429–464.
69. Collman C: Aquatic sports rehab and conditioning. Paper presented at the Aquatic Therapy & Rehab Institute Symposium, August 2000, Orlando, Fla, pp H371–H376.
70. Martin JE, Dubbert PM: Adherence to exercise. In Terjung R (ed): Exercise in Sports Science Review. New York: Macmillan, 1985, pp 137–167.
71. Trepman E, Micheli LJ: Overuse injuries in sports. Semin Orthop 3:217–222, 1988.
72. Ramsey JA, Blunkie C, Smith K, et al: Strength training effects in prepubescent boys. Med Sci Sports Exerc 22:605–614, 1990.
73. MacPhail HE, Kramer JF: Effect of isokinetic strength-training on functional ability and walking efficiency in adolescents with cerebral palsy. Dev Med Child Neurol 37:763–775, 1995.
74. Damiano DL, Kelly LE, Vaughn CL: Effects of quadriceps femoris muscle strengthening on crouch gait in children with spastic diplegia. Phys Ther 75:658–667, 1995.
75. Thorpe DE, Reilly M, Case L: The effects of aquatic resistive exercise on strength, balance, energy expenditure, functional mobility and perceived competence in an adult with cerebral palsy. Paper presented at the Combined Sections Meeting of the American Physical Therapy Association, February 2001, San Antonio, Tex.
76. Blanche EI, Botticelli TM, Hallway MK: Combining Neurodevelopment Treatment and Sensory Integration Principles: An Approach to Pediatric Therapy. Tucson, Ariz: Therapy Skill Builders, 1995.
77. Fisher A: Sensory Integration—Theory and Practice. Philadelphia: FA Davis, 1991.
78. Szklut SE, Breath DM: Learning disabilities. In Umphred DA (ed): Neurological Rehabilitation, 4th ed. St Louis: Mosby, 2001, pp 308–350.
79. Gage JR: Gait analysis in cerebral palsy. Clin Dev Med 121:92–93, 1991.
80. American Red Cross Staff: Water Safety Instructor's Manual. St Louis: Mosby Lifeline, 1992, pp 111–113.

Chapter 13
Aquatic Therapy: From Acute Care to Lifestyle

Bruce E. Becker, MD, and Juliana Larson, BS, LMT

One of the most important qualities of aquatic therapy is its utility across the full spectrum of health care, from the acute management of musculoskeletal injuries to its use as a health-maintaining, physically preserving activity. The physical properties of water provide a margin of therapeutic safety unequaled by most other treatment methods as described earlier in this book. The opportunity to create a single environment that facilitates both health restoration and maintenance has been left largely undeveloped, however, and most aquatic facilities have specialized in serving either diseased or healthy populations, but not both. This fragmentation of care divorces disease management from health restoration and rehabilitation as well as from healthy living. As a consequence, the health of the population continues to be impaired by an increasingly sedentary lifestyle, while aquatic facilities continue to be underused and rehabilitative efforts continue to be disconnected and inefficient. We hope to offer a solution in this chapter.

During the late 1800s, preventive and therapeutic health care took place in several distinct venues: hospitals, asylums, sanitaria, and health spas. Patients generally spent little time in hospitals because they were viewed as frightening places generally reserved for the very ill or dying, and convalescence often occurred at home or in sanitaria, which usually specialized in a single disease, such as tuberculosis.[1] The healthier segment of the affluent population often used spas for extended recovery and for health maintenance. However, during the post–Civil War era, changes in transportation and communication facilitated the development of the general hospital as the primary site of health care, so that from 1873 to 1920, the number of hospitals in America grew from 200 to 6000.[1]

With the increase in the number of hospitals, the spa was thought of less as a treatment facility than as a health resort, largely for the affluent. With the advent of widespread antibiotic use, sanitaria began to close. Hospitals occasionally housed pools, but the field of physical therapy was in its infancy. Fear of disease precluded widespread use of pools in most hospitals. Many spas had resident physicians, most of whom were trained in European aquatic techniques, but as hospitals became the focus of health care, the spas became more centers of a diverse social life, with promenades, clubs, cotillion, masked balls, and other balls.[2] From the mid-1800s until the early 1900s, hydropathic facilities were built in the major American cities, serving the needs of the public who had chronic illness but rarely those with acute illness. However, both spas and urban water cure establishments experienced a significant decline in the early part of this century.[2]

The modern whirlpool was developed in Germany at the turn of the century and was used extensively by the French army in World War I. The first whirlpool in the United States was installed at Walter Reed Hospital, the U.S. Army facility in Washington, DC. As Sidney Licht described, the whirlpool was gradually accepted, so that by the end of World War II, nearly every hospital with a therapy department had one. The modern Hubbard tank was first described in 1928 as a device permitting a broader range of exercises, useful particularly for patients with arthritis.[2]

In these facilities, patients were almost always treated individually, treatment sessions were short, and the (authorized!) recreational use of these facilities was nonexistent. During the latter half of this century, fewer general hospitals included pools in new construction because of construction and maintenance expenses. Freestanding rehabilitation hospitals nearly always included a therapeutic pool, often using these pools for group classes and activities and sometimes for recreational events for disabled populations but rarely for the general public. At the same time, the community pool was developed, largely with the able-bodied individual in mind. Many pools were built with no feasible access for the disabled and had no programs to encourage disabled individuals to use the facility. There was little crossover between the community and the therapeutic aquatic world.

Today, aquatic therapy occurs in many venues. Most aquatic therapy still happens in small facility-based pools, under therapist supervision, in one-on-one settings. Many facilities with moderate-sized pools conduct group sessions, often for disease-based populations, such as those with adult or juvenile arthritis. Occasionally, these facilities serve as a site for community groups but often in a mission-based way, such as a program for elderly persons.

Community pools have rarely had significant linkage with the formal health care system. YMCA pools usually offer the program for persons with arthritis that they codeveloped with the Arthritis Foundation. School-based pools frequently offer some group exercise programs, but because of school scheduling, they rarely allow the public to use pools during school hours. Programming is fragmented, facilities are underused, and there is poor coordination of programs.

The message that we hope to communicate is that much is to be gained through interfacility coordination and communication. The underpinning value is that a healthy lifestyle needs to combine prevention, occasional rehabilitation, exercise, and education, and this can happen easily in the aquatic environment.

AQUATIC THERAPY FACILITIES

The range of facilities currently used to provide aquatic therapy is broad. Table 13-1 lists the most frequently used types of facilities, their options, their designs, their advantages and disadvantages, and typical programs offered.

Many communities have facilities with all these options, and among them there is an aquatic therapeutic venue to suit most patient populations. However, the coordination between facilities is often suboptimal, and even awareness of program options elsewhere in the community is poor. With coordination and communication, a patient could move seamlessly from acute management through subacute recovery into lifestyle maintenance using each facility at an appropriate time. This is an aquatic therapy ideal, achieved too infrequently.

Table 13-1. Aquatic Therapy Facilities

Health facility pools
  Design
    Typically warm water, 88–94°F (31–34°C)
    Typically 2.5–4.0 feet deep, even bottom or gradual slope
    Often ground level, with access difficult for groups
    Usually small, preventing large group treatment
    Expensive staff (high salaries and wages, trained worker shortage)
    Sling or ramp access most common
  Advantages
    Staff usually medically knowledgeable
    Access to health facilities makes acute patient treatment safer
    Warm water more comfortable for low-level activities and prolonged staff immersion
    Ease of access for even severely disabled patients
  Limitations
    Limited depth options
    Shortage of trained and experienced staff nationally
    Lack of temperature adjustability precludes some populations, such as patients with multiple sclerosis
    Liability requires high level of supervision, typically individual
    Restricted public access is typical
    Ground level makes transfers to and from the water labor intensive
    High temperature restricts use for advanced conditioning activities
  Suitable populations
    Hospital-based acute rehabilitation
      Joint replacement, other orthopedic populations
      Neurologic rehabilitation
    Early outpatient
      Arthritis and arthroplasty rehabilitation
      Neurologic rehabilitation
      Rehabilitation programs for deconditioned people
  Program and technique options
    Bad Ragaz Ring Method
    Halliwick Concept
    Aquatic massage
    Low-level conditioning activities
    Red Cross arthritis classes
    Conventional physical therapy, usually 78–82°F (26–28°C)

Community pools
  Design
    Ground level
    Cool water
    Usually ladder or stair access
    Varying depths, typically 3–9 feet
    Heavy occupancy
  Advantages
    Public access
    Varying depths make broad range of program options feasible
    Ideal for high-level conditioning programs
    Vertical and horizontal exercise options feasible
    Extended hours often available
  Disadvantages
    Staff size limited
    Medical expertise lacking
    Cool water makes low-level activities (e.g., passive aquatic therapies) difficult
    Difficult environment for the severely disabled

(continued)

Table 13-1. Aquatic Therapy Facilities—*Continued*

　Program and technique options
　　Community open swim programs
　　Lap swim programs, including swim teams
　　Swim classes
　　Limited special population programs usually offered

Hot tubs, spas, and therapeutic tanks
　Design
　　Small, low volume
　　Single depth, shallow to very shallow
　　Hot water, usually ≥101°F (38°C)
　　Added turbulence often featured
　Advantages
　　High heat level makes low-level activities comfortable
　　Heat level therapeutically useful for joint rehabilitation
　　Turbulence diminishes pain, may reduce swelling
　Disadvantages
　　High heat limits patient populations, treatment length
　　Shallow depth limits activity range
　　Small size limits activity range
　　Essentially individual treatment modality
　Technique options
　　Simple range-of-motion exercises
　　Joint mobilization

Deep-water environments
　Design: Variable, from diving sections to custom-built facilities
　Advantages
　　Permit full gravity off-loading
　　Broad range of vertical exercises available
　　May range from acute rehabilitation to high-level conditioning
　　Swimming skill not required
　Disadvantages
　　Require close supervision
　　Usually require flotation apparatus
　　Fewer staff familiar with possibilities
　　Difficult with hydrophobic population
　Technique options
　　Aquajogging and water running
　　Aqua-dance or ballet movements
　　Wide range of aerobic movement options
　　Gravity-eliminated range-of-motion exercise

CASE STUDY: PROTOTYPE OF AN IDEA

Eugene, Ore, is a community of approximately 150,000 served by two major hospitals and an active Department of Parks and Recreation. In 1987, neither hospital had a therapeutic pool, and although the parks and recreation system had a number of pools, they were not coordinated with the health care system. The Easter Seals program built a large therapeutic pool with philanthropic dollars, largely for the use of the pediatric disabled population. The authors saw a need for an adult therapeutic pool and approached both hospitals, but at the time neither was interested in investing money and energy in the project. In the autumn of 1987, we decided to begin a program on our own, under the business name of SciEx, Inc.

Space was secured in a medical office building adjacent to the larger of the two hospitals, and facility planning began. The facility was built to include two large, deep-water tanks. These tanks were manufactured by Therapeutic Systems, Inc. (Philadelphia, Pa) and were prototypes of the current Aqua-Ark systems. Each tank, 6.5 feet × 5 feet × 6 feet deep, had its own heating system, so that pool temperatures could rapidly be adjusted up or down, depending on the patient being treated and the activity. We typically heated the pools to 88 to 92°F. Each had its own filtration and chlorinating system. The water treatment and high-turnover filtration were considerably greater than conventional swimming pool standards. To facilitate transfers into and out of the tanks, they were built partially above ground to a lip height equal to that of a seated patient in a wheelchair (Fig. 13-1). The tanks were large enough to accommodate vertical suspension of patients, who were tethered in one to four directions and supported by flotation devices. The facility included a reception/waiting area, adjacent showering and bathroom facilities, a storage room for pool supplies, and a pool manager's office with full-length sliding glass doors onto the pool area. We negotiated with the hospital for acquisition of a part-time physical therapist, and the facility employed a full-time aquatic therapist in addition to a part-time exercise physiologist (Fig. 13-2).

A thorough evaluation of each patient was made before entry into a program, including an evaluation by a physician, a presentation of functional capabilities, and a statement of patient expectations and outcomes sought. The program incorporated education, attitude adjustments, and motivation. The patient was able to exercise from the first session in a gentle protected motion (depending on ability level) and progress to vigorous movement in a gravity off-loaded environment. Individual programs were developed for specific musculoskeletal dysfunctions, and individuals were directly supervised during exercise. Constant repetition demonstrated the patient's retention level and skill in maintaining appropriate body posture to the

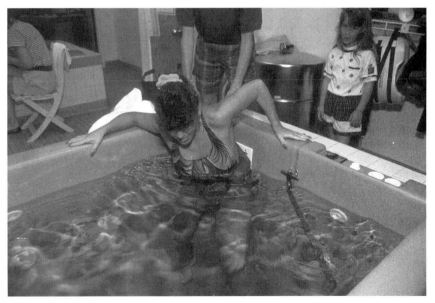

Figure 13-1. Pool entry via wheelchair transfer.

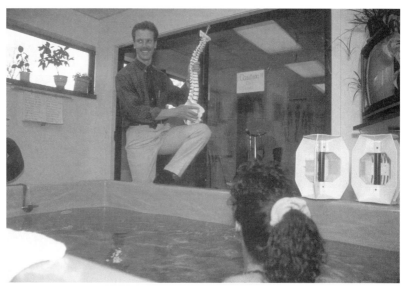

Figure 13-2. Poolside patient education.

physiatrist and the therapist. This required a coordinated team effort, and communication occurred on a daily basis. The close coordination allowed for modification of goals and treatment plans as necessary.

Patient referrals came with prescriptions that contained the diagnosis, hydrorehabilitation modalities desired, and duration and frequency of treatment. This standard referral was then translated into fluid mechanics, considering the individual's needs and the desired functional outcome. The translation process often required a significant amount of creativity in the choice of specific exercises, equipment, and program of activities. Our services were most commonly requested when the patient had failed to achieve the desired functional outcome with conventional physical therapy.

The facility rapidly attracted a broad range of clients, from those with acute athletic injuries, including fractures and stress fractures, to hospital inpatients. Patients with chronic neurologic disease were treated next to elite athletes (Fig. 13-3). Workers injured on the job were treated beside Olympic competitors. An aquatic specialist provided clinical oversight under the direct supervision of a physical therapist and a physiatrist. We found through experiment that the ideal treatment length was 45 minutes, and we began to design a structured set of deep-water exercises that could be adapted to the needs of a broad range of populations. Normal tank temperature was set at 88°F, but we frequently lowered the temperature to 78°F or lower for some patients with multiple sclerosis or raised the temperature into the mid-90s for patients in very early treatment phases. Often, we would lower the temperature during the session to prevent an increase in core temperature during strenuous exercise. We found that our most effective marketing tool was word of mouth among the athletic and medical communities. The facility became known within the Department of Parks and Recreation, and we began a series of liaison education sessions with department personnel.

In the beginning, third-party billing was managed in standard fashion, and we typically used the existing pool therapy code, which was at that time CPT 97240 and 97241. Reimbursement was adequate to cover expenses quite early on, and at the first anniversary, the facility was profitable. We spent considerable time educating

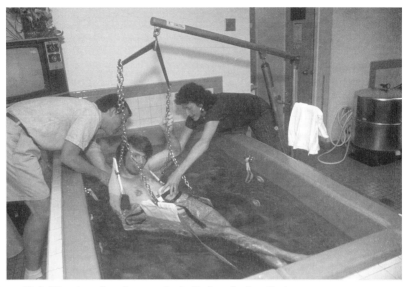

Figure 13-3. Sling transfer of a neurologically impaired patient.

third-party case workers and invited many to the facility to watch treatment sessions for covered patients, generally to the satisfaction of the third-party system.

We found that there was no suitable flotation system for high-intensity, deep-water workouts. Consequently, we began the process of designing a belt that would allow tethering, flotation in the appropriately upright position, and adjustment for a range of girths and flotation needs and that would not bind during strenuous workouts. This design was subsequently acquired by Excel Sports Science, Inc. (Eugene, Ore) and is currently marketed as the Aqua-Jogger. With this device we found that we could keep even the most muscularly dense elite athlete in proper position. Design changes were constant, even when the device was commercially produced, and we cut out and added foam where appropriate to achieve the desired result (Fig. 13-4).

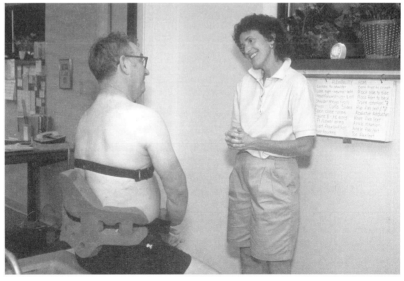

Figure 13-4. Flotation system for vertical exercise.

EVOLUTION OF DOCUMENTATION

One of the key elements in the process of third-party billing is documentation. We found that we had to develop our own systems of accountability for progress. We could not find a useful initial evaluation format that served our needs, so we created one. We evaluated the individual's medical status, preexisting medical problems, medications, swimming background, and exercise habits and included a pain disability scoring sheet. From these data, we built an aquatic therapy plan of care. Trial and error showed that an optimal treatment week was two or three sessions. In an unpublished study completed during 1989, we measured treatment outcomes in terms of pain reduction, flexibility, strength gains, and functional improvement measures in a group of patients with low back pain seen during a 6-week period, and we found no greater objective benefit from four or more sessions per week, whereas there was significant slowing of rate of gain with only one session per week. We listened to the case managers, who expressed a need for refinement of daily visit notes. We began with the system of charting developed by Lawrence Weed with sections on Subjective aspects, Objective aspects, Assessment of progress and goals, and Plan of care (SOAP charting). A formalized protocol was established for each patient treatment session. Programs were structured to generally include at least the following:

- A functional flexibility test before and after treatment
- Monitored perception of pain levels before and after treatment
- Progressive activity levels (1 through 10), organized into interval set format
- Heart rate monitoring and cadenced music or videos
- Stretching and relaxation exercise by the whirlpool jets

These factors were measured and compiled into a daily patient status log.

We developed a formalized daily note that assessed pain after the previous session and progress on a functional status impairment scale, monitored sleep pattern and new symptoms, and measured range of motion and flexibility and response to exercise with respect to both pulse rate in water and relative perceived exertion during exercise (Fig. 13-5). To establish a measurement system for exercise progression and documentation of progress, we developed an endurance workout measurement scale for the program of specific exercises. We asked patients to monitor their early morning pulse rates but with little success. We created a weekly summary report, which was compiled from the day sheets and included objective measurement of progress toward goals, barriers to achievement, range of motion and flexibility, pain levels, endurance testing, and changes in goals and plans. Summaries were sent to referring sources and to insurance carriers for billing purposes.

Next we established a transition program, which we termed *homework*. This usually required that the patient make a visit to one of the community pools and meet with the pool manager to assess program options and times. Early on, we began the process of transferring the patient into the community with a record of his or her program for poolside use and with a log book for review with the patient's treating physician. Our discharge summary format included the initial evaluation with the weekly summaries and outcome data. We attempted to compile a record of patients who continued in pool therapy after discharge to compare with the record of patients who did not continue, but this information proved impossible to collect reliably through phone contact. Several outcome studies compared functional outcome measures before and after therapy.

Hydrorehabilitation Progress Report

SciEx, Inc. Hydrorehabilitation

Name: _____ Date: _____

Session No: 1 2 3 4 5 **6** 7 8 9 10 11 **12** 13 14 15 16 17 **18**
19 20 21 22 23 **24** 25 26 27 28 29 **30** 31 32 33 34 35 **36**
37 38 39 40 41 **42** 43 44 45 46 47 **48** 49 50 51 52 53 **54**

SUBJECTIVE REPORTING

Linear Pain Scale: 1 2 3 4 5 6 7 8 9 10
   Pretreatment   _____
   Posttreatment _____

Response Since Last Session:

Injury Site Tenderness:	Worse	Same	Improved
Muscle Tenderness:	Worse	Same	Improved
Relaxation:	Worse	Same	Improved
Mobility:	Worse	Same	Improved
Energy:	Worse	Same	Improved
Sleep Pattern:	Worse	Same	Improved
Other Therapy:	Worse	Same	Improved
Home Program:	Worse	Same	Improved

Significant complaints/comments:

OBJECTIVE PROGRAM ACTIVITY

	Level	PE	Time	Individual Program
Flexibility/ROM:	____	.__-	____	_____
Strengthening: (Mod. Oxford)	____	.__-	____	_____
Endurance Interval:	____	.__-	____	_____
Relaxation:	____	.__-	____	_____
Pulse Rate:	_ _ _			
Monitored Heart Rate:	____		**Body Wt.:**	**Flexibility:**

Perceived exertion achieved: _____

Starting: [ ]   Pretreatment [ ]
Current: [ ]   Posttreatment [ ]

OVERALL ASSESSMENT:

TREATMENT PLAN:

©1990, Sciex, Inc.

_____   _____
     Supervisor   **Therapist**

Figure 13-5. Hydrorehabilitation progress report. (Copyright 1990, SciEx, Inc., Eugene, Ore.)

There was significant turnover of physical therapists. This led to some inefficiencies because the interest, background, and experience in aquatic therapy varied widely among therapists, and our documentation systems had rapidly become quite specific and rigorous. The exercise physiologist departed, but we had incorporated most of the physiologist's guidance into our core program so that there was no major program impact. The hospitals noticed the success of the facility. The smaller hospital built its own therapy pool, and the hospital adjacent to us negotiated with the Easter Seals program to allow an expanded outpatient adult population to use the facility. Several community-based physical therapists negotiated with local health clubs for pool use time. None of these other programs actively sought linkage with the broader community Parks and Recreation program, though, so we did have an advantage with case managers.

The Parks and Recreation connection had become quite deep by the end of 1991, and as a result, many of our protocols could be readily transferred to the community. We found the relationship with the department personnel to be symbiotic because they could more readily defend their budget by explaining the ties with the health care system, which required slightly higher staffing ratios and more complex programming. In late 1992, SciEx closed its doors as the first author moved to Michigan and the second author joined the Department of Parks and Recreation as Director of Sheldon Pool Programs.

ANOTHER CASE STUDY: THE IDEAL PROCESS

One of the most important lessons learned from our experience is the potential importance of a community support system for hospital-based aquatic therapy activity. Such a program serves the needs of the patient while lowering health care costs, encouraging patient responsibility, and building a base of individuals sufficient to support unique program needs.

Integration of programming into a broad range of population needs is demonstrated in the concept of the Aquatic Hub (Fig. 13-6). The mission of Hub programs is to provide progressive levels and options of aquatic activity in a comfortable, familiar, caring, and educational environment. The Aquatic Hub bridges the gap between hospital-based therapy programs and an active exercising lifestyle. By using the "learning moment" provided by an injury or illness and initiating an aquatic exercise regimen when appropriate, the patient becomes aware of the usefulness of aquatic therapy in recovery. By moving the patient into the community setting early, while the willingness to alter lifestyle is still present, the individual gains familiarity with the community pool environment. Once the patient is involved, the Hub's diverse programming fulfills the patient's expectations of competent instruction through individualized classes and fitness choices. This truly benefits the mission of municipal facilities to provide a range of structured, supervised classes to benefit the broad taxpayer base. The Aquatic Hub is a management and citizenry effort to maximize the use of the facility and staff with the goal of promoting wellness. This concept has achieved great success at Sheldon Pool and Fitness Center in Eugene, Ore.

Sheldon Pool is one of eight year-round pools in the Eugene-Springfield metropolitan area, serving a population of 150,000. Sheldon has two rectangular pools, one a 25-yard, six-lane, graduated-bottom pool and the other a diving well (Fig. 13-7). Both pools are maintained at 85.5°F. The pools are convenient to parking, wheelchair accessible (Fig. 13-8), and attractive.

Aquatic Therapy: From Acute Care to Lifestyle 299

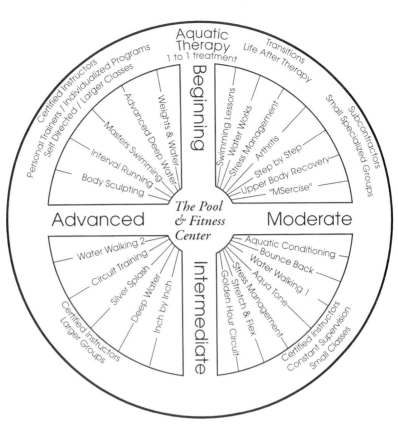

Figure 13-6. The Aquatic Hub: interdisciplinary approaches to progressive aquatic programming. Community pools meeting the continuum of needs from the physically challenged to the physically fit. (Copyright 1993, revised 1995, Juliana Larson, BS, LMT, and Sylvia Schepps, CRT.)

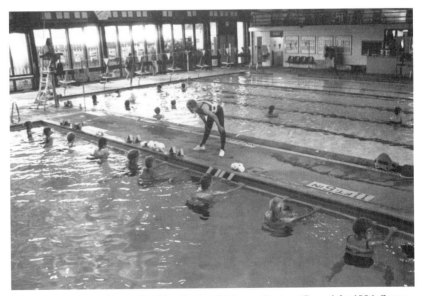

Figure 13-7. Pool overview at Sheldon Pool and Fitness Center. (Copyright 1996, Susan Detroy, Eugene, OR.)

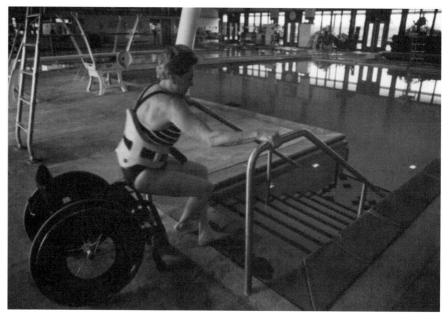
Figure 13-8. Entry access for limited ambulators.

It is the goal of the Sheldon staff to structure a program for any individual to maintain or improve the function he or she has gained from therapy or to continue to enhance recreational opportunities the individual wants to pursue. In this facility's programming, a patron can receive the continuum of care needed after therapy to continue on a recovery pathway. The staff works with the individual to assist in achieving the skill and knowledge to continue life after therapy to a fitness level that meets his or her daily and recreational needs. It is a challenge to the staff to design a sufficient variety of classes to meet the needs of all patients, from top athletes to those who are severely physically challenged. Experts from many disciplines participate, including a massage therapist who teaches back conditioning classes, athletic trainers and marathoners who teach deep-water running classes, a midwife teaching pre- and postnatal classes, a movement therapist teaching stress-release stretching classes, and an oncology nurse or mastectomy patient teaching upper body recovery classes. The pool encourages community therapists to contract pool time to run small group or individual sessions with patients next to swim classes or water fitness classes to which a patient may move when ready. Programs beget more programs, and teachers emerge from the group of pupils, so the process is a dynamic, vital one. The challenge is to have a director with the skills to recruit teachers, schedule programs, plan with the general and health communities, and negotiate the tricky waters of the municipal budget process. All the classes mentioned previously began on paper, were presented to the public, and are being well attended at Sheldon Pool, along with more traditional classes for patients with arthritis and multiple sclerosis, or for elderly persons, aquatoning, and beginning through advanced deep-water classes. At present, the pool runs 72 water fitness classes per week and 148 swim lessons, including all American Red Cross levels plus infant, adult, and adapted programs (Fig. 13-9). Every day, the facility hosts 12 hours of child care, 4 hours of after-school activity, and 4 hours of recreational swimming; each week there are two to four community meetings and 4 to 10 hours of massage therapy. Temporary employees account for 87% of personnel, which lowers staffing costs.

Aquatic Therapy: From Acute Care to Lifestyle 301

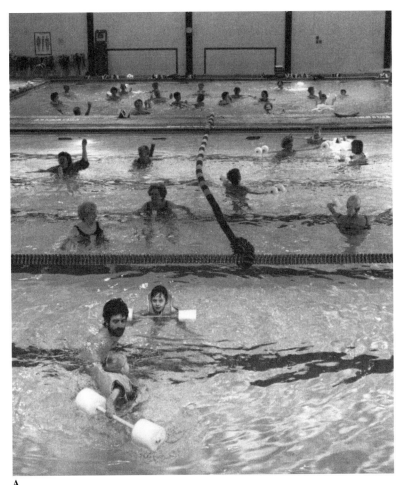

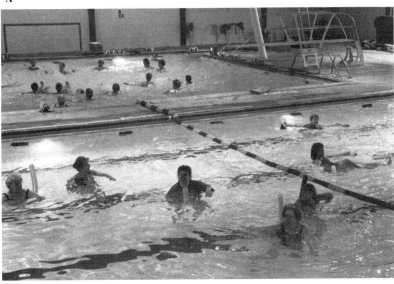

Figure 13-9. *A*, Simultaneous classes in operation. *B*, Different generations performing different activities simultaneously. (Copyright 1996, Susan Detroy, Eugene, OR.)

It is important that the community pool, as the center of the Aquatic Hub activities, be a drawing point for persons of all ages and ability levels, serving as a learning facility for swimming as a life skill, a meeting place for support groups as well as team sports, and a satellite for physical, occupational, and recreational therapy. The Hub should promote an intergenerational approach to lifelong fitness. The patrons, clients, patients, health care providers, and insurance companies that refer should trust the facility management to be responsive to their needs. The communication and educational processes should go both ways.

The intent of the program is to provide sufficient options so that no reasonable need is unmet. The availability of on-site child care removes one major obstacle. The wealth of class opportunities removes another. Physical accessibility removes an important obstacle to the transition process for disabled people. There should be no screening for acceptability, as is the case in many health clubs. Ideally, an interdisciplinary program of this type promotes multigenerational usage for a diverse community. Within the same block of time, a grandmother, a daughter, and a grandson should be able to participate in different enjoyable and therapeutic activities under the same roof. The results of this creative programming include staff loyalty and enthusiasm, high levels of customer service and satisfaction, increased attendance, and community support.

It is significant that the Eugene-Springfield area is one of the most penetrated areas in the nation with respect to managed care. Consequently, area physicians are constantly searching for practical methods of decreasing health care costs without compromising health care quality. Sheldon Pool plays an increasingly important role in this effort: It is often used as a primary therapy resource, either through involvement with a therapist working with one of our programs or by direct recommendation of a patient to one of our programs. Physicians encourage patients to move from formal hospital-based therapy activities into one of our programs, which require fewer therapy sessions and encourage more responsibility on the patient's part. For aquatic therapy to be cost-effective, though, it must be efficient and facility use must be high because maintenance and upkeep costs are great, even for small facilities.

One of the by-products of the Americans with Disabilities Act of 1994 has been the requirement for all public recreational facilities to become fully accessible. Consequently, it is now feasible to develop larger subspecialized programs for disabled Americans with unique needs and to meet these requirements in community facilities. Accessibility creates a larger market opportunity. In the past, the disabled community has had limited access to fitness facilities, and health care consequences related to inactivity are common among those who are disabled. Community facilities such as Sheldon Pool provide the means for healthier lifestyles for this population, but every community facility now has the opportunity to better serve its community as well. Although it is true that accessibility improves life for the disabled, it also benefits parents with children in strollers, older adults with grandchildren in tow, and many others.

BARRIERS AND FACILITATORS

The success of the Sheldon Pool is due largely to the efforts and energies of many people within the Department of Parks and Recreation to gain support to the broad external community, particularly health care providers. It has also taken many years and much dialogue to break down the barriers of suspicion, professional jealousy, and competition over turf. To start, a key barrier was the attitude that a community pool facility was an inappropriate site for health care activities. For physicians to develop trust in the facility, a great deal of communication was necessary. Programs have been developed to respond to suggestions from the provider community, and patient outcomes needed to reflect follow-through. A significant advance in credibility was made when physical therapists began to create programs within the facility. It is difficult to assess the impact that the managed care environment had in building willingness in the health care system to release a patient from a more costly service to a potentially less costly one. Another barrier was the physical distance between the facility and any health care facilities.

The difficulty of finding trained program leaders, especially in new areas, also presented problems. We have found that innovation has enabled us to work our way through this problem: the inclusion of movement therapists, oncology nurses, nurse midwives, and others has actually become a strength. However, not every step along the way has been smooth.

A significant barrier is the complexity of coordinating all these programs. Although multidisciplinary programming sounds ideal, rescheduled or misbooked classes have offended many. Open communication mends some of these wounds, but some participants leave, never to return. The goal is to replace them with flexible, open class leaders.

The traditionalism of the health care community has at times been a barrier. There is almost no substantive outcome research in aquatic therapy, so it is simply impossible to reassure physicians that there is a body of research supporting some of our programs. Here again, the managed care environment has facilitated openness to new and alternate methods. Eugene-Springfield has always had a strong untraditional element in its population, so a traditional attitude has presented more professional concerns than public ones. The public must always know that professionalism prevails, however, and this requires that programs must be clinically solid and respectable. Traditional programs may be created in innovative ways. Nontraditional programs must be created around traditional values: personal responsibility, integrity, and ethical standards of care.

STRATEGIC PLANNING

Sheldon Pool and Fitness Center has adopted the strategic planning process to implement these programs. To do this, four strategic objectives have been chosen, with measurement objectives and work activities to support each. These are the following:

Strategy 1: Offer program to meet customer needs.
   Objective: 90% of customers surveyed are satisfied or very satisfied with program choices offered.
      Work Activities:
         Implement survey.
         Create a user advisory board.
         Attend conferences or pursue other avenues to keep up with trends in programming.

Strategy 2: Market program content and service benefits.
Objective: Increase the number of active participants by 3% per year.
Work Activities:
Identify baseline measure.
Identify new target populations.
Develop and implement a marketing plan.

Strategy 3: Maintain an acceptable level of instructor quality.
Objective: 100% of customer evaluations of staff indicate good or better performance.
Work Activities:
Produce and maintain an annual training calendar that maintains required certifications.
Institute peer evaluations for all staff.
Recruit bilingual staff.
Implement survey.

Strategy 4: Increase maintenance performance in meeting program and customer needs while decreasing costs.
Objectives: 95% of customers surveyed are satisfied or very satisfied with the cleanliness of the facility.
Work Activities:
Clarify duties and responsibilities for maintenance of the facilities between the aquatics program staff and the assigned Public Works Department maintenance staff.
Develop maintenance-related customer satisfaction measures.
Formalize feedback to maintenance custodial staff and measure performance.
Evaluate alternatives for custodial services.

Based upon this strategic plan, an organization system map was created to identify suppliers, inputs, core and supporting processes, outputs, and direct customers. Obviously, organizational activity such as this requires knowledgeable administrative staff in addition to operational staff. System buy-in becomes essential to success of the endeavor.

CONCLUSION

Traditional health care has taken place largely within formal medical environments. Although it serves to isolate the person who is ill, this division from society has not facilitated change. The health care system is now changing radically. Public recognition of the value of exercise is widespread, even if the practice is not. As a society, we are becoming more obese and more sedentary, and we are spending more on health care costs associated with these issues. Yet often, community aquatic facilities are underused, and even more often they are isolated from any contact or involvement with the health care system.

A potential solution may be to move health maintenance and prevention out of the health care facilities and into the community. Lifestyles built around healthy exercise, socialization across generations, and development of a sense of community are likely to improve more than the public health status; they may begin the process of healing society. This may sound like too grand a goal for aquatic therapy, but with a broad regional effort, the creative juices of many individuals, and the collaboration of a diverse group of involved professional and community leaders, it is possible to make a significant start. In so doing, the health and well-being of many and the benefit of the community will be served. We hope that our example may serve as a springboard for many more beneficial facilities.

REFERENCES

1. Starr P: The Social Transformation of American Medicine. New York: Basic Books, 1982, p 76.
2. Kamenetz HL: History of American Spas and Hydrotherapy. In Licht S (ed): Medical Hydrology, Physical Medicine Library. New Haven, CT: Elizabeth Licht, 1963, p 160.

Chapter 14
Hydrotherapy and Pressure Ulcers

Chester H. Ho, MD, and David T. Burke, MD, MA

Ever since the time of Hippocrates (460 to 370 BC), bathing has been used for healing.[1] Asclepiades (124 to 40 BC) was one of the ancient physicians who prescribed water as a treatment regimen and recommended regular bathing for therapy, and Galen (131 to 201 AD) introduced hydrotherapy for the treatment of a variety of specific diseases.[2] These concepts had an influence on European civilization throughout history. Although bathing was discouraged in the Dark Ages, spas were established across Europe during the 16th and 17th centuries, the use of mineral waters became more prevalent, and resorts developed at various springs.[3] More recently, many physicians have addressed various beneficial aspects of hydrotherapy for ongoing wound management.

In current medical practice, hydrotherapy is widely used for a number of conditions, including the management of wound cleansing and wound débridement, pain and musculoskeletal conditions,[4-6] and management of burns.[7-10] Among the more common uses of hydrotherapy is wound management in individuals suffering from pressure ulcers.

Pressure ulcers are a prevalent, expensive, and burdensome medical problem. There are many reports on the incidence of pressure ulcers, varying from 15% in hemiplegic patients to as high as 60% in a population with spinal cord injuries.[11] The cost of treatment ranges from $2000 to $30,000 per pressure ulcer in acute care settings.[12] Some have estimated that the cost of pressure ulcer treatment in all health care settings, including acute care facilities, nursing homes, and home health, may exceed $10 billion annually.[13] Although the magnitude of this problem has long been recognized, it is interesting to note that, despite efforts, the Fourth National Pressure Ulcer Prevalence Survey in 1997[14] found that the prevalence of pressure ulcers was not decreasing. It is particularly important for those in the field of rehabilitation that, beyond the costs of treating these ulcers, there are unique problems that these ulcers create in the course of delivering quality rehabilitative care. The restrictions of weight bearing on ulcerated surfaces place severe limitations on therapists and nurses, who must minimize the risk of further trauma while still trying to engage the patient in an aggressive and active rehabilitation program. The prompt and effective treatment of pressure ulcers therefore demands our thorough scrutiny.

The use of hydrotherapy for the treatment of pressure ulcers is currently part of the United States Department of Health and Human Services Agency for Health

Care Policy and Research (AHCPR) Pressure Ulcer Treatment Clinical Practice Guideline.[15] Although not often listed as an essential element of the standard of care for these wounds, hydrotherapy is often used as an adjuvant treatment coinciding with regular dressing changes, pressure relief, and the identification and treatment of underlying medical conditions. Other adjuvant treatments such as ultrasound, laser, electrical stimulation, various growth factors, and hyperbaric oxygen therapy have not had the widespread acceptance that hydrotherapy has enjoyed.

There are two ways by which hydrotherapy can be applied in pressure ulcer treatment: whirlpool or pulsatile lavage. Whirlpool therapy is the more conventional form of hydrotherapy. Currently no data on the prevalence of the use of either treatment in the United States are available, but use probably varies significantly from one institution to another, with notable regional variations.

Both whirlpool and pulsatile lavage treatments have been used for the treatment of pressure ulcers that contain exudate, slough, or necrotic tissue. However, the rationale behind the use of these treatments and the research supporting their use come from very different sources, and scientific data specifically addressing these treatments are lacking.[16] Much of the evidence on the effects of whirlpool treatment has been extrapolated from the literature on burn care, whereas that for pulsatile lavage treatment has come largely from military dental research from the late 1960s and early 1970s. Regardless of the source of scientific research, it has been theorized that both whirlpool and pulsatile lavage therapies exert their effects during the inflammatory phase of wound healing.[17]

Despite the lack of data on the prevalence of hydrotherapy in the treatment of pressure ulcers, 92%[8] to 94.8%[7] of North American burn units routinely incorporate hydrotherapy as part of their routine wound treatment regimen.[9, 10, 18] In the following sections, we shall discuss the use of each of these treatments separately.

WHIRLPOOL THERAPY

Whirlpool therapy for the treatment of pressure ulcers consists of the immersion of the wound in a tank filled with clean, heated, and often agitated water. Temperatures between 33.5 and 35.5°C are usually prescribed. The treatment is often performed by physical therapists and nursing staff.

Currently, the AHCPR Clinical Practice Guideline for Pressure Ulcer Treatment[15] recommends that whirlpool therapy be considered for "cleansing pressure ulcers that contain thick exudate, slough, or necrotic tissue." These guidelines suggest that the use of whirlpool therapy should be discontinued when the ulcer is clean. Otherwise, there is no official guideline on contraindications. In practice, pressure ulcers that are clean with granulating tissues are often not addressed by whirlpool therapy, perhaps because they are viewed as fragile and easily damaged by the agitated water.

The theories and benefits of whirlpool therapy include the following[17]:

- Physical débridement of the wound
- Improvement of local tissue perfusion
- Analgesic effects

Physical Débridement of the Wound

Many variables affecting the débridement property of the whirlpool have been reviewed. These include the following:

- Bacterial load
- Agitation of whirlpool water and rinsing of the wound
- Water temperature
- Duration of immersion
- Frequency of whirlpool treatment
- Use of antiseptic agents in the water

The often-quoted study of Niederhuber and associates[19] compared several of these variables. This study involved 76 subjects who had no open wounds in their feet. The subjects were divided into different treatment groups. They were then treated with the following regimens:

1. The use of three different whirlpool water temperatures (32.2, 37.7, and 43.3°C) with immersion and agitation of the water.
2. The water agitation (30 minutes), spraying (30 minutes from a distance of 15 cm), and soaking (30 seconds) of the feet were compared at a water temperature of 37.7°C.
3. The use of water agitation (30 minutes) alone was compared with agitation (30 minutes) followed by spraying (30 seconds).
4. The effects of the whirlpool treatment with water agitation were compared at immersion times of 5, 10, 20, and 30 minutes. The water temperature was kept constant at 37.7°C.

Outcome of the treatment was measured by the bacterial load on the skin of the plantar surface of the feet. The bacterial load was measured before and after whirlpool treatment. The results were then compared. The many conclusions of the Niederhuber and associates study will be discussed in the relevant sections below.

Bacterial Load

Bacterial load is the area of whirlpool treatment of wounds in which most research has been done. It has been shown that hydrotherapy decreases the number of bacteria in the wound. Niederhuber and associates[19] showed that whirlpool treatment with water agitation decreased bacterial load by a mean reduction of 81.9% in the non–open skin area in the plantar surface of the feet, as measured by skin swabs. The overall reduction in bacterial load was further increased to 94.6% if the whirlpool treatment was followed by spraying, demonstrating the effectiveness of the combined technique.

Bohannon[20] reported a case study on the use of whirlpool treatment of a chronic venous ulcer. In this study, the bacterial load in the whirlpool water after treatment that was sampled daily was found to increase with time. This was attributed to the whirlpool's effectiveness for bacterial débridement from the wounds. Neither study mentioned the type of bacteria isolated.

Other studies have shown a positive correlation between lower bacterial load in the wound and a faster healing rate[21] and an association between a lower bacterial load ($<10^5$) in the wound and the process of healing.[22, 23]

One may then conclude that one of the mechanisms by which hydrotherapy helps to increase the healing rate of pressure ulcers is by the reduction of bacterial load. However, to date, there is only one randomized, controlled study that attempted to verify this relationship.[24] Therefore, more randomized, controlled trials with larger number of subjects are required.

Agitation of the Whirlpool Water and Rinsing of the Wound

Agitation of the whirlpool water is useful in decreasing bacterial load. This is usually achieved by an electrical agitator in the whirlpool tank. Niederhuber and associates[19] demonstrated that agitation was more effective than spraying or soaking of the skin surface for removing bacteria. They found that with agitation alone, the mean reduction of bacterial load was 81.9%, whereas the figures were 16.2% with only spraying and 3.8% with soaking alone. As discussed earlier, Niederhuber and associates also showed that agitation followed by spraying was the most effective method, removing up to 94.6% of the bacterial load. This latter observation was supported by studies carried out by Bohannon[20] and Rodeheaver and colleagues.[25]

Water agitation is commonly used in whirlpool therapy now, and hydrotherapy tanks are equipped with a standard agitator. Although the amount of direct pressure on the wound generated by the agitated water has not been stated in the medical literature, elements that have been measured with accuracy include the pressures generated by irrigation devices such as syringe and needle or pulsatile lavage devices. Obviously, the pressure caused by water agitation will not be easily measured or be consistent because it depends on the design of the whirlpool tank, the location of the wound in relation to the agitator, and the direction of the water current.

Water Temperature

The results of the experiments of Niederhuber and associates[19] showed that there was no significant difference in the bacterial load reduction, even with the large variations in temperatures used (32.2, 37.7, and 43.3°C). No other published trial has looked specifically at the effect of temperature in whirlpool therapy. The current AHCPR Clinical Practice Guideline for Pressure Ulcer Treatment does not have a recommended temperature for whirlpool therapy. The following temperature choices have been recommended by Sussman[17]:

- Nonthermal/tepid: 27 to 33.5°C (80 to 92°F)
- Neutral: 33.5 to 35.5°C (92 to 96°F)
- Thermal: 35.5 to 40°C (96 to 104°F)

The choice of water temperature is influenced by the patient's comfort level, local perfusion, body surface area to be treated, and concurrent medical conditions. Tepid temperature is suggested for the use on patients with venous disease and neutral temperature for treatment with larger body surface area. The use of higher temperature has been reported to be associated with swelling of the lower extremity in the dependent position.[26] Vascular congestion was felt to be the cause of this increase in lower extremity volume.[17] However, in their study, McCulloch and Boyd[26] used a temperature as high as 40°C (104°F), which is not recommended for the use in pressure ulcer treatment. It would also have been useful to know the length of time it took for the lower extremity to return to its previous volume after whirlpool therapy; if the volume effects were only transient, there may be fewer clinical concerns. Moreover, though the authors discussed the possible scenario of an increased lower extremity compartmental pressure after whirlpool therapy with higher water temperature, the pressure was not measured.

Although the above study expressed concerns regarding the use of high water temperature in hydrotherapy, it is also often theorized that local circulation may be improved by whirlpool therapy. This theory has yet to be formally tested.

Duration of Immersion

The duration of whirlpool treatment was assessed by Niederhuber and associates[19] too. They found that as the duration of the immersion time increased, there was a steady increase in the number of bacteria removed from the foot. This effect lasted for up to 20 minutes' immersion time. At 30 minutes, there was no additional benefit. This evidence supports the current practice of immersion lasting for 20 minutes.

Frequency of Whirlpool Therapy

This aspect has not been widely researched. Burke and associates[24] found that whirlpool therapy once a day would produce beneficial effects for the healing of pressure ulcers. There is otherwise no clinical trial suggesting that other whirlpool treatment frequencies would be more beneficial. In practice, the frequency of whirlpool therapy is probably determined by the availability of therapy personnel and of the whirlpool. Until further research clarifies this issue, the study of Burke et al serves as the only published parameter.

Use of Antiseptic Agents in the Water

The AHCPR[15] specifically recommends the avoidance of topical skin cleansers or antiseptics for the direct cleaning of pressure ulcers because these agents may be harmful to wound tissues. Agents to avoid include sodium hypochlorite solution (Dakin's solution), hydrogen peroxide, povidone-iodine, iodophor, and acetic acid.[27]

However, there is no guideline on the addition of antiseptic agents in the whirlpool water. These agents are added to the whirlpool water for two purposes: (1) to reduce the number of wound organisms and (2) to sterilize whirlpool tanks and equipment.

Various antiseptic agents have been used as additives to the whirlpool water. Sussman[17] and Walter[9] listed four such agents that have been commonly used at low concentrations:

- Povidone-iodine (Betadine)
- Sodium hypochlorite (Dakin's solution, Clorox)
- Chlorhexidine (Hibiclens)
- Chloramine-T (Chlorazene)

In the 1990 survey by Thomson and colleagues[8] sodium hypochlorite was the most commonly used agent in hydrotherapy (used in 33% of the burn programs surveyed), followed by chlorhexidine (20%) and povidone-iodine (14%).

The use of antibiotics and cytotoxic agents in the whirlpool water is consistent with the theory that the rate of wound healing increases with the reduction of bacterial load. Moreover, nosocomial wound infection as a result of contaminated hydrotherapy equipment has been one of the biggest concerns with the use of hydrotherapy. Therefore, the use of various antiseptic agents as a procedure to decontaminate hydrotherapy equipment has been examined. This issue will be discussed in greater detail in the section on the potential side effects of hydrotherapy.

Ideally, antimicrobial agents used in hydrotherapy should be effective against a broad spectrum of bacteria (both Gram-positive and Gram-negative) and fungi. At the same time, they need to be nonirritating and nonsensitizing to either intact skin or open wounds.[28] Interestingly, the use of antibiotics has been more extensively studied with pulsatile lavage irrigation, which will be discussed in subsequent sections. The addition of antiseptic agents in the water has been studied mainly with whirlpool therapy.

Henderson and associates[29] found that with 300 ppm of chloramine-T solution in the whirlpool water, there was a significantly reduced number of cultured *Pseudomonas aeruginosa* colonies from the full-thickness cutaneous wounds of guinea pigs compared with whirlpool treatment without the addition of chloramine-T. Despite the bactericidal effectiveness of chloramine-T, there was no difference in the rate of epithelialization in either the water- or chloramine-T–treated animals. The authors therefore concluded that water containing 300 ppm of chloramine-T was effective as a bactericidal agent but did not affect the rate of wound healing.

The use of povidone-iodine was studied by Simonetti and colleagues.[28] They used a concentrate of povidone-iodine to yield 4 ppm of available iodine in the whirlpool water. This reduced the number of cultured bacterial colonies in the whirlpool water by as much as 92%.

Simonetti and colleagues[28] also attempted to indirectly determine the amount of iodine absorbed through the skin by measuring the protein-bound iodine levels and the thyroxine levels in six randomly selected subjects. These levels were measured before and after a 5-day course of 30-minute hydrotherapy sessions. They did not find any significant change in these measurements after treatment, suggesting that there was no significant absorption of povidone-iodine through the skin. However, the study did not examine the effect of the povidone-iodine on wound healing.

Therefore, there is some scientific evidence to support the addition of certain antiseptic agents to the whirlpool water. However, no consensus or guidelines for their use exist, and thus judicious use is recommended.

Improvement of Local Tissue Perfusion

It has been postulated that the use of whirlpool treatment may be a way to enhance local perfusion, hence improving the delivery of oxygen, nutrients, antibiotics, leukocytes, and systemic antibiotics to the wound tissues.[17] Although this is a very attractive theory, there has been little scientific verification.

Cohen and associates[30] attempted to examine this theory. They studied the effects of whirlpool therapy on blood flow in the forearm, with and without agitation of the water. Other variables were also considered, including the temperature of the water (at 38.6, 41.0, and 42.5°C) and the flaccidity (normal versus flaccid) and trophic state of the extremity.

Of the 20 subjects enrolled in this study, 11 had a normal extremity, 5 had flaccid upper extremities, and 4 had atrophy from disuse. Each subject would be given two treatments, with and without water agitation. The blood flow in the forearm was measured by plethysmography. The results demonstrated that when compared with whirlpool therapy without agitation, whirlpool therapy with agitation did not significantly increase the blood flow in the treated extremities. There was no difference between normal, flaccid, or atrophic upper extremities. Despite the apparent erythema seen in the skin after treatment, there was only a slight increase in the total circulating blood volume of the limb; at 38.6°C, the effect lasted for about 45 minutes. At 41.0 to 42.5°C, there was a significant increase in blood flow, but this was only maintained for about 15 minutes. Furthermore, these temperatures were too high and not recommended for whirlpool therapy for wound care. Exactly how these findings would correlate with the healing of pressure ulcers was beyond the scope of the study.

In a more recent study, McCulloch and Boyd[26] looked at the effect of temperature on the volume of the lower extremity after whirlpool therapy in the dependent position. The results showed that there was an increase (3.7% mean) in the volume of the lower extremity after whirlpool therapy at 40°C (104°F). When the lower extremity was left in the whirlpool for the same time (20 minutes) without whirlpool therapy, the increase in volume was only 1.85%. No causative factor for the swelling was identified in this study. How this change in the volume of the extremity would actually affect the local tissue perfusion, especially with regard to the healing of pressure ulcers, is again not known.

From these studies, we have evidence that at water temperatures higher than the commonly used temperatures of 33.5 to 35.5°C, there is an increase in the blood flow and also swelling of the treated extremities. Although increased blood flow may improve healing of the wounds, tissue swelling may not. There is also concern that raised temperature may produce a demand for oxygen, and because this is not met, local tissue necrosis may occur.[31] We have not yet found the best temperature range at which tissue healing, swelling, and oxygen demand will be optimally balanced.

Analgesic Effects

The soothing, analgesic effects of whirlpool treatment are well known to therapists. However, the exact physiologic mechanisms of the analgesic effects are not well understood. Certainly hydrotherapy has been used for relaxation and for the treatment of pain in other conditions, such as rheumatic diseases.[5] Its use in postoperative wound pain management has also been explored.[32] However, until further studies are completed to examine this issue more closely, the analgesic effects of whirlpool treatment remain anecdotal.

Side Effects of Whirlpool Therapy

Most of the side effects of whirlpool therapy in the medical literature are extrapolated from the burn literature because hydrotherapy has been an important treatment for burns.[7, 8] There are potential adverse effects for both patients and the operator of the whirlpool.

Adverse Effects for Patients

Infections. This is the main concern with the use of whirlpool therapy. There have been numerous reports about nosocomial infections from the use of whirlpool therapy, ranging from local infection such as otitis externa, folliculitis,[33] and wound infection,[34] to bacteremia and sepsis.[35-37] The organism most frequently reported as being responsible is *P. aeruginosa*.[7, 33, 37] Other reported organisms include *Legionella pneumophila*,[34] *Staphylococcus aureus*, and *Enterobacter cloacae*.[36]

This is clearly a serious issue because wound infections may affect healing, for reasons discussed earlier. Furthermore, bacteremia and sepsis may have even more devastating consequences. However, one must bear in mind that these reports were done on patients with burns, whose wounds may have a much larger surface area than those of patients with pressure ulcers and thus are more prone to infection. Nevertheless, rigorous decontamination techniques of the whirlpool should be performed, regardless of the patient population.

There is no governmental regulation on the decontamination of whirlpool equipment for pressure ulcer treatment. Various procedures for the decontamination of hydrotherapy tanks and equipment have been proposed.[38, 39] The Centers for Disease Control and Prevention together with the American Physical Therapy Association have produced the following guidelines[40, 41]:

- Pools should be drained and cleaned every week or two and after each treatment session.
- Pools, pumps, and other equipment used should be scrubbed with a phenolic germicidal detergent.
- All scrubbed equipment should be rinsed thoroughly before refilling.
- Chlorination of water is recommended when organic matter is removed by a filtering system or, when continuous filtering is not possible, iodine should be used instead.

The addition of antiseptic agents to the whirlpool water may decrease the number of bacterial colonies in the water, but their effects on the healing of the wounds must also be considered (see the section on use of antiseptic agents in water).

There has also been a report on febrile response to whirlpool therapy without bacteremia by blood culture.[42] The authors theorized that transient bacteremia not documented by blood culture or the release of toxin from necrotic tissue driven into the systemic circulation by the mechanical action of the whirlpool could be the cause. Otherwise there have not been any further reports on febrile response in the medical literature.

Burn Injury. The use of whirlpool water to treat a patient with a burn injury may be potentially dangerous, especially if the patient has sensory impairment in the treated body part. Hwang and coworkers[43] reported a case of bilateral amputation after burn injury of the lower extremities from whirlpool therapy in a paraplegic patient with sensory deficits. The use of appropriate, monitored temperature is therefore very important. Whirlpool therapy must be used with extra caution for patients with sensory impairment, such as those with peripheral neuropathy and spinal cord injury or for patients whose cognitive impairment prevents appropriate feedback of the water temperature.

Hypothermia. Hypothermia is possible, especially when a large surface area is treated. Both the ambient and water temperatures must be kept to an appropriate level to prevent hypothermia. A hydrotherapy treatment time of 20 minutes is suggested to avoid chilling in patients with burns.[9] Devices such as heat shields/lamps may be used.[18] Once again, patients with burns are probably more susceptible to hypothermia because of the much larger open wound surface area involved.

Cardiovascular Effects. Raising the body temperature may increase the metabolic rate and hence oxygen demands. This may increase the burden on the cardiovascular system. Therefore, precautions must be taken for patients with problems such as coronary artery disease, peripheral vascular disease, and stroke.

Adverse Effects to the Whirlpool Operator

There are reports of folliculitis and contact dermatitis in health care workers who operate whirlpools.[44] These can be caused by the additives in the whirlpool water such as bromine or by bacteria such as *P. aeruginosa*. These are issues that need to be addressed in the future protocol design for whirlpool therapy.

PULSATILE LAVAGE THERAPY

Pulsatile lavage therapy is a newer and less common choice of hydrotherapy for pressure ulcers. For patients who may benefit from hydrotherapy for pressure ulcer care, but for whom the whirlpool is inaccessible due to concurrent medical problems or immobility of the patients, pulsatile lavage therapy offers a convenient alternative. Furthermore, it may be useful for wounds with tunneling and undermining. There are many ways by which pulsatile lavage therapy can be applied: it can be produced by the simple use of an irrigating syringe and needle or by devices specifically designed for such purposes (Fig. 14-1).

Wounds can be cleansed by simple irrigation. This can be done with a rubber-bulb syringe that produces a single pulse of water to clean the wound. Studies comparing the cleansing effects of syringe irrigation and pulsatile lavage therapy have found that the latter is a much more effective way to clean wounds.[45-49]

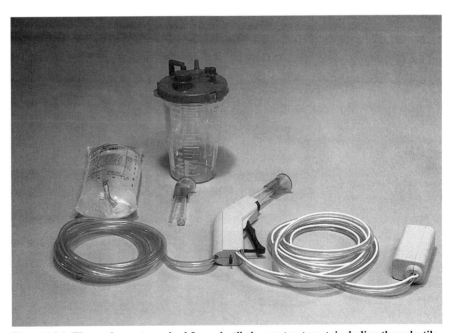

Figure 14-1. The equipment required for pulsatile lavage treatment, including the pulsatile lavage device, suction tubing, suction canister, and normal saline.

Loehne[50] described the theoretical rationales for the use of pulsatile lavage therapy: cleansing via irrigation and débridement, the reduction of bacteria and infection, and the promotion of granulation and epithelialization.

Review of the literature over the last 30 years revealed that, interestingly, most of the research on pulsatile lavage therapy was from dentists in the U.S. military in the 1970s. They studied the effects of pulsatile lavage on wounds obtained during military duty and its use in dental practices. The effects studied included the following:

- Pressures produced by pulsatile lavage
- Effects of pulsatile lavage on the removal of debris and wound infection
- Side effects of pulsatile lavage

Otherwise there has been minimal direct research on the use of pulsatile lavage in the treatment of pressure ulcers, although there have been some anecdotal reports[51] and pilot studies[52, 53] on its use for pressure ulcers (Fig. 14-2).

Pressures Produced by Pulsatile Lavage

The AHCPR of the U.S. Department of Health and Human Services published a clinical practice guideline on the treatment of pressure ulcers in 1994.[15] They recommended that for wound cleansing, one should "use enough irrigation pressure to enhance wound cleansing without causing trauma to the wound bed." The recommended pressures ranged from 4 to 15 pounds per square inch (psi).

The use of different equipment for pulsatile lavage can produce tremendously varying pressures on wounds—8 psi can be delivered by the use of a 35-mL syringe with a 19-gauge needle,[54, 55] whereas the Army medical irrigator can emit water jets from 0 to 200 psi.[56] Different pulsatile lavage pressures have been used in different studies, and the concern is that excessive pressure may damage the treated tissues.[57] The upper limit of 15 psi as recommended by the AHCPR was based on the study by Rodeheaver and colleagues,[25] who found that at 10 to 15 psi, 84.8% of the soil particles placed in the experimental wounds were removed. The same study also found that irrigation pressures between 1 and 5 psi were not as effective. However, other studies have used much higher pressures without any deleterious effects. Bhaskar and associates[58] used as high as 70 psi irrigation pressure in their study and found only transient swelling of the tissue lasting for 2 hours, without any permanent tissue damage. In another study, Bhaskar and associates[59] examined the effect of water jets at 70, 100, 150, and 200 psi on the healthy mucosa of the dog tongue. The results showed that at 70 psi, there were histologic changes consistent with edema and hemorrhages in the tongue. These changes were more severe with higher pressures. A pressure of 70 psi or less was also recommended by Selting and colleagues[60] for the use in water jet devices for oral hygiene procedures.

The many different devices available on the market produce vastly different irrigation pressures. Note that even with the same device, proper use is essential, because how the device is used may affect the irrigation pressure delivered. For instance, the tip to tissue distance and the variations in the shape and size of the tip and orifice may affect the irrigation pressures.[61]

How accurately one can apply the above findings to pressure ulcers is debatable, given that many of these studies were not performed on open wounds. Also, irrigation pressures between 15 and 70 psi have not been as extensively studied.

Hydrotherapy and Pressure Ulcers 317

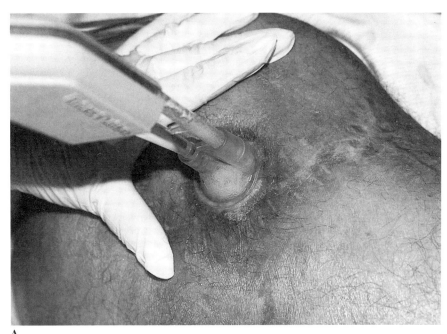

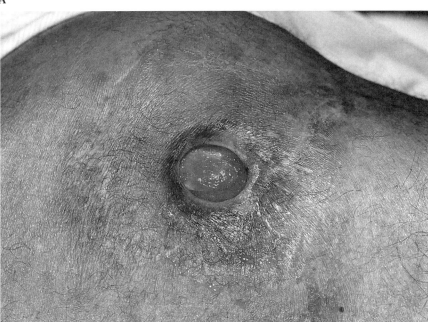

Figure 14-2. A stage IV pressure ulcer being treated with pulsatile lavage. *A*, Pressure ulcer during treatment. *B*, Pressure ulcer after treatment.

Therefore, is the recommended pressure range of 4 to 15 psi the optimal range for pulsatile lavage? Although we know that an irrigation pressure of 15 psi can effectively reduce the amount of soil particles in wounds, could a higher pressure of less than 70 psi be even more effective without causing tissue damage? Obviously one does not want to use unnecessarily high irrigation pressures to cause tissue damage.

Future research needs to be performed to more closely examine the optimal irrigation pressure one should use for pulsatile lavage to maximally clean wounds with minimal tissue damage.

Effects of Pulsatile Lavage on the Removal of Debris and Wound Infection

The effectiveness of pulsatile lavage therapy on wound care has been well documented. Studies have shown that it is useful both for the removal of debris from the wound and for the treatment of wound infections.

Removal of Debris

For the removal of contaminants, Green and associates[45] demonstrated that pulsatile lavage therapy was more effective than rubber-bulb syringe irrigation in the removal of iron filings from avulsive wounds. Grower and Bhaskar[46] assessed the removal of a radioisotope of zinc from facial wounds of rats; they also concluded that pulsatile lavage therapy was more than bulb syringe irrigation. Then, directly from dental research in the military, Selting and colleagues[60] found that pulsatile lavage was three times more efficient in removing debris from experimental pockets in an acrylic dental model than the conventional bulb syringe.

The above studies looked at the removal of nonorganic materials from wounds only. Grower and associates[47] went one step further and carried out a study that examined the removal of nonvital tissue from standardized wounds in rats. Once again, they concluded that pulsatile lavage therapy was much more effective than irrigation alone in the removal of nonviable tissue fragments. Therefore, they recommended it for wound débridement.

Effects on Wound Infection

Wound infection is obviously a major concern in contaminated wounds. The effects of pulsatile lavage therapy on the removal of bacteria from wounds as well as the use of antiseptic agents in pulsatile lavage therapy has been examined in many studies.

As early as 1969, Bhaskar and associates[58] studied the removal of *Klebsiella pneumoniae* and *Proteus mirabilis* from contaminated wounds in rats with the use of water lavage and found it to be effective. Then in the 1970s, Gross and colleagues,[62] Madden and associates,[49] and Stevenson and coworkers[54] all found pulsatile lavage to be efficient in the removal of bacteria from wounds.

In their much-quoted study, Rodeheaver and colleagues[25] not only looked at the effectiveness of decontamination with lavage treatment but also at the rate of infection after such therapy. They concluded that at an irrigation pressure of 10 to 15 psi, the rate of wound infection after treatment was significantly lower than that in wounds subjected to an irrigation pressure of 1 psi.

More recently, Lopez and associates[48] performed a randomized study with 95 postoperative patients who had purulent peritonitis. They compared the effects of pulsatile lavage with manual irrigation on the surgical wounds of these patients, measuring their bacterial counts and infection rate. The results demonstrated a significantly lower rate of wound infection when pulsatile lavage therapy was used.

It is notable that Lopez and associates used lavage pressures as high as 50 and 70 psi. Although tissue damage was not directly measured, the authors assumed that it was not significant because the wounds continued to heal with the use of high-pressure lavage.

Use of Antibiotics and Antiseptic Agents in Pulsatile Lavage

Topical antibiotics and antiseptic agents have been used commonly as part of wound care regimens. Their beneficial effects have also been well studied. Given that pulsatile lavage therapy has been proved to be helpful for the treatment of wound infection, it follows that the use of antibiotics and antiseptic agents in pulsatile lavage may possibly have an additive or synergistic effect, making it even more effective in wound infection control. There have been a few published studies examining the usefulness of this combination treatment.

Gross and colleagues[63] studied the use of penicillin and streptomycin in the standardized wounds contaminated with bacteria that are commonly responsible for wound infections, including *P. mirabilis, P. aeruginosa, K. pneumoniae,* and *S. aureus.* This was a nonblinded, prospective, controlled study comparing the effects on wound bacterial growth by pulsatile lavage with penicillin and streptomycin added and pulsatile lavage with saline alone. In both the experimental and control groups, 110 albino rats were used. The results showed that with just one lavage with antibiotics, the number of positive cultures from the wounds was reduced as high as 4.5 times. However, in this study, the pulsatile lavage therapy was performed only 30 minutes after the wounds were contaminated with the soil particles that contained the four types of bacteria. This is probably very different from real life situations in which pressure ulcers and wounds are more insidiously and chronically infected. Furthermore, effects on healing of the wounds were not studied here.

With a similar experimental design, Cutright and associates[64] looked at the effects of the addition of the combination of vancomycin and streptomycin and tetracycline alone with pulsatile lavage treatment in a nonblinded, prospective, controlled trial. Once again, standardized wounds of albino rats were contaminated with *P. mirabilis, P. aeruginosa, K. pneumoniae* and *S. aureus.* In each of the control, tetracycline, and vancomycin/streptomycin groups, 75 animals were used. Results demonstrated that the combination of vancomycin and streptomycin was the most effective in removing bacteria from contaminated wounds, whereas tetracycline was effective against *K. pneumoniae, S. aureus,* and *P. mirabilis,* but not against *P. aeruginosa.* The above comments made on the experimental design of the study by Gross and colleagues[63] are also applicable here.

Although both studies discussed here showed encouraging results with the use of antibiotics in pulsatile lavage therapy, subsequent studies on this treatment are lacking. It would be useful to have further studies on the effects of antibiotics and pulsatile lavage treatment on wounds with chronic infections. Also, the optimal duration of administration and concentration of antibiotics used will need to be worked out.

Use of Antiseptic Agents in Pulsatile Lavage

As discussed in the section on whirlpool therapy, antiseptic agents can be useful in wound care. Despite the research interest on the use of antiseptic agents in whirlpool therapy, there has been very little research on the use of antiseptic agents in pulsatile lavage therapy.

Gross and colleagues[65] studied this with a nonblinded, controlled, prospective trial on standardized wounds of 480 albino rats contaminated with the same four types of bacteria as in their studies discussed above. The rats were equally divided into control (water) and three experimental groups, using undiluted povidone-iodine, a 20% solution of pHisoHex, and a 0.1% solution of benzalkonium chloride with pulsatile lavage in the experimental groups. They did not find any significant difference in the reduction of wound infection by any of the four types of bacteria among the water, povidone-iodine, and pHisoHex groups. However, the use of benzalkonium chloride significantly reduced the number of wounds infected with colonies of *S. aureus*, although there was no significant difference with the other three types of bacteria.

Side Effects of Pulsatile Lavage

The side effects of pulsatile lavage are fewer than those of whirlpool therapy because it is a local treatment, and the patient will not be required to be submerged in the whirlpool tank. Therefore there are likely to be fewer systemic effects. However, a high-pressure system is being used on open, fragile tissue here. Therefore, the main concerns with pulsatile lavage treatment are damage to healthy tissues and risk of bacteremia.

Because the issue of pressures and potential damage to wound tissues has already been fully discussed in the earlier section on pressures produced by pulsed lavage, we shall focus our discussion here on the risk of bacteremia.

The concern that bacteremia may be a side effect of pulsatile lavage is due to these theoretical problems:

- High-pressure irrigation may damage issue defenses, thus allowing entry of bacteria through the damaged tissues and promoting the risk of wound infection.
- The foreign bodies and bacteria on the wound surface may be disseminated throughout the wound by the high pressure of irrigation.

Wheeler and associates[66] carried out the most comprehensive experiments on these issues. They examined the dissemination of both irrigation fluid and bacteria in their experiments at different irrigation pressures. Standardized wounds in pigs were used in three experiments. In each of the experiments, the wounds were irrigated with either a syringe (producing an irrigating pressure of 8 psi) or a pulsatile lavage device (producing a pressure of 70 psi).

In the first experiment, the wounds were irrigated and the extent of the spread and the depth of the penetration of the irrigated fluids were measured. In the second experiment, the wounds were inoculated with an equivalent dose of *S. marcescens* and the dissemination of bacteria was then measured. In the last experiment, the wounds were pretreated with two different irrigation methods before they were inoculated with *S. aureus* and then closed. Four days later, the extent of infection and the bacterial count from the wounds were assessed.

The results showed that the fluid delivered to the wound by high-pressure irrigation spread more laterally, rather than penetrating deeply in the wound. The dissemination of fluids, although present, was not accompanied by the dissemination of bacteria, even with high-pressure irrigation. Furthermore, high-pressure irrigation significantly reduced the number of bacteria in the wound. However, they also found that high-pressure irrigation produced the highest rate of wound infection, implying that there might have been damage to the tissue defense mechanisms.

Other authors have looked at the risks of bacteremia during high-pressure lavage of wounds. Back in 1971, Gross and colleagues[67] examined the effects of high-pressure (70 psi) pulsatile lavage on standardized wounds of 75 albino rats that were contaminated with equal amounts of *S. aureus, P. aeruginosa, K. pneumoniae,* and *P. mirabilis*. Blood cultures drawn from the rats demonstrated a very low incidence of bacteremia. The authors concluded that the probability of bacteremia from pulsating water jet lavage of wounds was therefore negligible.

More recently, Tabor and colleagues[68] assessed the issue again. They studied standardized wounds of 20 dogs contaminated with equal amounts of *S. aureus*. Pressures of 28 psi and 1 to 2 psi were used in the two experimental groups. Blood cultures were drawn from the animals at set intervals after the lavage. These authors found no bacteremia in any of the blood cultures of the experimental groups.

Therefore, there is evidence that fewer and less serious potential side effects are associated with pulsatile lavage therapy than with whirlpool therapy. The water pressures produced by commercial equipment for pulsatile lavage therapy are often within the irrigation pressure guidelines set by the AHCPR and are much lower than those used in the above studies. This further increases the safety of this treatment modality.

CONCLUSIONS

Despite the medical advances made throughout the decades, pressure ulcers remain a prevalent challenge for clinicians. The huge costs associated with their treatment, in addition to the enormous physical, psychological, and social impact on patients, demand that any potentially efficacious treatment be thoroughly investigated and examined.

Whirlpool therapy has been used for the treatment of pressure ulcers for a long time. It has been accepted by the AHCPR as one of only two modalities recommended for the treatment of pressure ulcers. There has been much anecdotal success, but few scientific studies to examine its benefits. So far, it has been used mostly for mechanical débridement of necrotic tissues in pressure ulcers, and although there is also evidence to suggest that it may accelerate the rate of wound healing, the exact mechanism by which this occurs remains to be discovered.

Pulsatile lavage therapy is a newer form of hydrotherapy. It is already commonly used in trauma care and orthopedic surgery for the débridement and cleansing of wounds. It has many of the benefits of whirlpool therapy without the risks, adverse effects, and labor involved. It is particularly useful in patients with impaired mobility or for whom the use of whirlpool therapy would be particularly cumbersome or even risky. Moreover, unlike whirlpool treatment, it can be used in the home care setting. With its versatility, ease of operation, and potentially lower cost, it is expected to gain popularity among clinicians involved with care of pressure ulcers.

Future research is needed to help us to understand the specific mechanisms by which the efficacy of hydrotherapy is achieved. It is imperative for us to understand the changes that occur in pressure ulcers on a cellular level as a result of hydrotherapy. This knowledge will not only help us use our resources appropriately, but it will also serve as a model for the enhancement of healing of pressure ulcers with other potential treatments.

REFERENCES

1. Kellogg JH: A Manual of Rational Hydrotherapy, 2nd ed. Philadelphia: FA Davis, 1902.
2. Jackson R: Waters and spas in the classical world. Med Hist Suppl 10:1–13, 1990.
3. Routh HR, Bhowmik KRB, Parish LC, Witkowski JA: Balneology, mineral water, and spas in historical perspective. Clin Dermatol 14:551–554, 1996.
4. Resch K-L: Long term effects of spa therapy on OA [guest editor's commentary]. Rehabil Rev 6(2):1, 1998.
5. Hall J, Skevington SM, Maddison PJ, Chapman K: A randomized and controlled trial of hydrotherapy in rheumatoid arthritis. Arthritis Care Res 9:206–215, 1996.
6. Danneskiold-Samsoe B, Lyngberg K, Risum T, Telling M: The effect of water exercise therapy given to patients with rheumatoid arthritis. Scand J Rehabil Med 19:31–35, 1987.
7. Shankowsky HA, Callioux LS, Tredget EE: North American survey of hydrotherapy in modern burn care. J Burn Care Rehabil 15:143–146, 1994.
8. Thomson PD, Bowden ML, McDonald K, et al: A survey of burn hydrotherapy in the United States. J Burn Care Rehabil 11:151–155, 1990.
9. Walter PH: Burn wound management. AACN Clin Issues Crit Care Nurs 4:378–387, 1993.
10. Howell JW: Management of the acutely burned hand for the nonspecialized clinician. Phys Ther 69:1077–1089, 1989.
11. Rodriquez GP, Murphy KP: Current trends in pressure ulcer research. Crit Rev Phys Rehabil Med 8(1&2):1–18, 1996.
12. NPUAP: Pressure ulcers prevalence, cost and risk assessment: consensus development conference statement [review]. Decubitus 2:24–28, 1989.
13. Marwick C: Recommendations seek to prevent pressure sores [news]. JAMA 268:700–701, 1992.
14. Barczak CA, Barnett RI, Childs EJ, Linda MB: Fourth National Pressure Ulcer Prevalence Survey. Adv Wound Care 10:18-26, 1997.
15. Pressure ulcer treatment. Clinical Practice Guideline No 15 (AHCPR Publication No. 95-0652). Rockville, Md: US Department of Health and Human Services, Agency for Health Care Policy and Research, 1994.
16. Ferrell BA: Pressure ulcer products and devices: are they safe, much less effective? J Am Geriatr Soc 46:654–656, 1998.
17. Sussman C: Whirlpool. In Sussman C, Bates-Jensen BM (eds): Wound Care: A Collaborative Practice Manual for Physical Therapists and Nurses. Gaithersburg, Md: Aspen, 1998, pp 447–460.
18. Duncan DJ, Driscoll DM: Burn wound management. Crit Care Nurs Clin North Am 3:199–220, 1991.
19. Niederhuber BS, Stribley RF, Koepke GH: Reduction of skin bacterial load with use of the therapeutic whirlpool. Phys Ther 55:483–486, 1975.
20. Bohannon RW: Whirlpool versus whirlpool and rinse for removal of bacteria from a venous stasis ulcer. Phys Ther 62:304–308, 1982.
21. Lyman IR, Tenery JH, Basson RP: Correlation between decrease in bacterial load and rate of wound healing. Surg Gynecol Obstet 130:616–621, 1970.
22. Sapico FL, Ginunas VJ, Thornhill-Joynes M, et al: Quantitative microbiology of pressure sores in different stages of healing. Diagn Microbial Infect Dis 5:31–38, 1986.
23. Robson MC, Lea CE, Dalton JB, Heggers JP: Quantitative bacteriology and delayed wound closure. Surg Forum 19:501–502, 1968.
24. Burke DT, Ho CH-K, Saucier MA, Stewart G: Effects of hydrotherapy on pressure ulcer healing. Am J Phys Med Rehabil 77:394–398, 1998.
25. Rodeheaver GT, Pettry D, Thacker JG, et al: Wound cleansing by high pressure irrigation. Surg Gynecol Obstet 14:357–362, 1975.
26. McCulloch JM, Boyd VB: The effects of whirlpool and the dependent position on lower extremity volume. J Orthop Sports Phys Ther 16:169, 1992.
27. Phillips I, Lobo AZ, Fernandez R, Gundara NS: Acetic acid in the treatment of superficial wounds infected by *Pseudomonas aeruginosa*. Lancet 1:11–14, 1968.

28. Simonetti A, Miller R, Gristina J: Efficacy of povidone-iodine in the disinfection of whirlpool baths and Hubbard tanks. Phys Ther 52:1277–1282, 1982.
29. Henderson J, James D, Leming JT, Melon-Niksa DB: Chloramine-T solutions: effect on wound healing in guinea pigs. Arch Phys Med Rehabil 70:628–631, 1989.
30. Cohen L, Martin GM, Wakim KG: Effects of whirlpool bath with and without agitation on the circulation in normal and diseased extremities. Arch Phys Med 30:212–219, 1949.
31. McCarthy DJ: Therapeutic considerations in the podiatric care of ulcerations. Clin Podiat Med Surg 3:487–504, 1986.
32. Juve Meeker B: Whirlpool therapy on postoperative pain and surgical wound healing: an exploration. Patient Educ Couns 33:39–48, 1998.
33. Penn C, Kain KC: *Pseudomonas* folliculitis: an outbreak associated with bromine-based disinfectants—British Columbia. Can Dis Wkly Rep 16:31–33, 1990.
34. Brabender W, Hinthorn DR, Asher M, et al: *Legionella pneumophila* wound infection. JAMA 250:3091–3092, 1983.
35. Tredget EE, Shankowsky HA, Joffe AM, et al: Epidemiology of infections with *Pseudomonas aeruginosa* in burn patients: the role of hydrotherapy. Clin Infect Dis 15:941–949, 1992.
36. Mayhall CG, Lamb VA, Gayle WE Jr, Haynes BW Jr: *Enterobacter cloacae* septicemia in a burn center: epidemiology and control of an outbreak. J Infect Dis 139:166–171, 1979.
37. McGuckin MB, Thorpe RJ, Abrutyn E: Hydrotherapy: an outbreak of *Pseudomonas aeruginosa* wound infections related to Hubbard tank treatments. Arch Phys Med Rehabil 62:283–285, 1981.
38. McMillan J, Hargiss C, Nourse A, Williams O: Procedure for decontamination of hydrotherapy equipment. Phys Ther 56:567–570, 1976.
39. Nelson RM, Reed JR, Kenton DM: Microbiological evaluation of decontamination procedures for hydrotherapy tanks. Phys Ther 52:919–924, 1972.
40. Feedar JA, Kloth LC: Conservative management of chronic wounds. In Kloth LC, McCulloch JM, Feedar JA (eds): Wound Healing: Alternatives in Management. Philadelphia: FA Davis, 1990, pp 135–172.
41. American Physical Therapy Association: Hydrotherapy/Therapeutic Pool Infection Control Guidelines. Alexandria, VA: American Physical Therapy Association, 1995.
42. Greenberg MI, Balsamo A, Palmaccio A: Febrile response to whirlpool treatment [letter]. JAMA 238:1912, 1977.
43. Hwang JCF, Himel HN, Edlich RF: Bilateral amputations following hydrotherapy tank burns in a paraplegic patient. Burns 21:70–71, 1995.
44. Penny P: Hydrotherapy pools of the future—the avoidance of health problems. J Hosp Infect 18(Suppl A):535–542, 1991.
45. Green VA, Carlson HC, Briggs RL, Stewart JL: A comparison of the efficacy of pulsed mechanical lavage with that of rubber-bulb syringe irrigation in removal of debris from avulsive wounds. Oral Surg Oral Med Oral Pathol 32:158–164, 1971.
46. Grower MF, Bhaskar SN: Effect of pulsating water jet lavage on radioactive contaminated wounds. J Dent Res 51:536–538, 1972.
47. Grower MF, Bhaskar SN, Horan MJ, Cutright DE: Effect of water lavage on removal of tissue fragments from crush wounds. Oral Surg Oral Med Oral Pathol 33:1031–1036, 1972.
48. Lopez EV, Perez SY, Zuniga PL, Trallero EP: Evaluation of pulsating jet lavage in prevention of surgical wound infection. J Abdom Surg March and April:34–38, 1984.
49. Madden J, Edlich RF, Schauerhamer R, et al: Application of principles of fluid dynamics to surgical wound irrigation. Curr Top Surg Res 3:85–93, 1971.
50. Loehne HB: Pulsatile lavage with concurrent suction. In Sussman C, Bates-Jensen BM (eds): Wound Care: A Collaborative Practice Manual for Physical Therapists and Nurses. Gaithersburg, Md: Aspen, 1998, pp 389–403.
51. Nourse AM, Myers W: Dental water irrigating device used for cleaning decubitus ulcers. Phys Ther 58:1219, 1978.
52. Diekmann JM: Use of a dental irrigating device in the treatment of decubitus ulcers. Nurs Res 33:303–305, 1984.
53. Diekmann JM, Smith JM, Wilk JR: A double life for a dental irrigation device. Am J Nurs 10:1157, 1985.

54. Stevenson TR, Thacker JG, Rodeheaver GT, et al: Cleansing the traumatic wound by high pressure syringe irrigation. JACEP 5:17–21, 1976.
55. Rogness H: High-pressure wound irrigation. J Enterostomal Ther 1985. 12:27–28, 1985.
56. Bhaskar SN, Cutright DE, Gross A, Hunsuck EE: The Army medical irrigator and the hydroscrub device. J Am Dent Assoc 84:854–857, 1972.
57. Cutright DE, Beasley JD III, Bhaskar SN, Larson WJ: Water lavage and tissue calibration study in rats. J Dent Res 52:26–29, 1973.
58. Bhaskar SN, Cutright DE, Gross A: Effect of water lavage on infected wounds in the rat. J Periodontol 40:671–672, 1969.
59. Bhaskar SN, Cutright DE, Frisch J: Effect of high pressure water jet on oral mucosa of varied density. J Periodontol 40:593–598, 1969.
60. Selting WJ, Bhaskar SN, Mueller RP: Water jet direction and periodontal pocket debridement. J Periodontol 43:569–572, 1972.
61. Cutright DE, Bhaskar SN, Larson WJ: Variable tissue forces produced by water jet devices. J Periodontol 43:765–771, 1972.
62. Gross A, Bhaskar SN, Cutright DE, et al: The effect of pulsating water jet lavage on experimental contaminated wounds. Oral Surg Oral Med Oral Pathol 31:32–38, 1971.
63. Gross A, Cutright DE, Bhaskar SN, et al: The effect of antibiotics and pulsating water jet lavage on contaminated wounds. Oral Surg Oral Med Oral Pathol 31:32–39, 1971.
64. Cutright DE, Bhaskar SN, Gross A, et al: Effect of vancomycin, streptomycin and tetracycline pulsating jet lavage on contaminated wounds. Milit Med 136:810–813, 1971.
65. Gross A, Bhaskar SN, Cutright DE, et al: The effect of antiseptic agents and pulsating jet lavage on contaminated wounds. Milit Med 137:145–147, 1972.
66. Wheeler CB, Rodeheaver GT, Thacker JG, et al: Side-effects of high pressure irrigation. Surg Gynecol Obstet 143:775–778, 1976.
67. Gross A, Bhaskar SN, Cutright DE: A study of bacteremia following wound lavage. Oral Surg Oral Med Oral Pathol 31:720–722, 1971.
68. Tabor OB, Bosse MJ, Hudson MC, et al: Does bacteremia occur during high pressure lavage of contaminated wounds. Clin Orthop Relat Res 347:117–121, 1998.

Chapter 15
Staff Training and Development in Aquatic Therapy

Ruth I. Meyer, MEd, RKT

One of the more challenging issues facing managers of rehabilitation facilities is finding staff adequately trained in aquatic therapy. In a verbal self-report survey of therapists attending national aquatic therapy conferences, many therapists stated that they received less than 1 day of exposure to aquatics, whereas a rare few had 1 week of exposure during their course of study in therapy school, and others had exposure during their clinical rotations. Facilities with pools will rethink how they run their pools and staff their aquatic therapy practices after reading this chapter and book. To fully exploit all of the therapeutic advantages that aquatic therapy can offer, it is important that the number of staff be sufficient and that they be trained in the essential elements of therapeutic pool operation: safe pool management, an understanding of the physiologic properties of the aquatic environment, a sufficient range of established treatment techniques to provide for a wide range of patients, and the ability to monitor and document progress. For a comprehensive clinical aquatic therapy program the facilities and staff must be evaluated to determine strengths and weaknesses. Safety issues for staff and clients must be considered.

Typical training in aquatic therapy has been quite minimal. In a survey of Detroit, Mich, therapy training programs in 1999, the physical therapy assistant students at Macomb Community College received 3 hours of training; Oakland University physical therapy students had a 1-hour lecture and a 2-hour laboratory in the pool, in which they practiced using basic pool equipment and the pool lift, discussed transfers, and used various flotation devices to support a client on the surface, and would then practice passive range of motion, active range of motion, and ankle active-assisted range of motion; and Wayne State University physical therapy students had a 1-hour lecture followed by almost 3 hours of pool instruction and practice.

Aquatic therapy is not a core course in the required curriculum of typical therapeutic programs (physical therapy, occupational therapy, kinesiotherapy, therapeutic recreation, and massage therapy). A few schools do have a semester-long course on aquatic therapy and adapted aquatics (e.g., University of Toledo). In the past 3 years, University of North Carolina Greensboro (UNCG) and West Virginia University (WVU) initiated aquatic therapy specialties at the undergraduate level. Because physical therapy and occupational therapy are now graduate-level programs, students now can attain aquatic therapy specialization before their graduate program and apply those skills within the context of their advanced professional training. The University of Alabama, Birmingham, is developing an aquatic physical therapy program as well.

As a result, hiring new graduates is a challenge for the owners of a facility hiring staff for a therapy pool. Generally they will need to train their own staff. Ideally, there is a senior therapist with 5 to 10 years of experience to provide in-service training for new hires. Other options that are often chosen are to send one or more staff members to a 1- to 5-day national or regional conference with expectations for them to come back to train the rest of the staff or to hire a consultant to come to the facility to specifically train staff for the pool design and clientele served.

Another option is for the facility owners to hire one staff person to start an aquatic therapy program, expecting this person to be in the pool all day. Depending upon the age, design, sanitation system, and heating, ventilating, and air conditioning system of the pool, this practice may pose a health risk to that solitary therapist. Safe long-term exposure in the pool requires pristine water and air quality and adequate hydration and nutritional intake by the therapist.

Therefore the initiation of an aquatic therapy program, whether hospital- or community-based, requires understanding of the total picture: the aquatic environment and staff expertise.

EVALUATION OF STAFF

A staff survey to determine interest, understanding, and learning styles will save management time and money. Staff members who understand hydrodynamics will provide concise explanations and demonstrations of techniques and protocols. The survey should include prior experience, prior training, and information on particular interest areas and willingness to pursue independent study. Safety skills are too often neglected in surveys. The end result of the survey should be an understanding of existing resources and training needs. Hiring and training staff can be a major expense. It is best to hire skilled staff, but if that option is not feasible, it is essential to know which type of training is most important for your staff. You may have a very willing staff person whom you send to a conference with expectations that he or she will train the rest of the staff. Matching the learning style of your staff with the teaching style of the consultant trainer will optimize the training. Understanding the learning style of your audience/staff is essential for creating a program that allows your staff to learn and integrate into their daily practice. Understanding that clients have unique learning styles with the challenges of chronic pain, sleeplessness, medication use, and physical and mental changes allows development of varied teaching strategies for aquatic therapy. The use of verbal descriptions, visual demonstration, and sensory feedback as well as a provision of handouts with pictures and verbal descriptions will help clients remember the correct execution of their aquatic therapy program.

Ideally when aquatic therapy methods are learned, equal time in the pool and classroom is provided to allow actual practice and feedback on performance of the techniques. The ability to differentiate aquatic and land therapy by actual application of methods to the environment will assist the therapist in developing evaluation and therapeutic plans. Many aspects of aquatic therapy require a hands-on approach and therefore having the therapist actually perform the activity is essential. Some clients require verbal and visual cues to go along with the kinesthetic activity, so having a repertoire of words to describe a movement or activity and having poolside notes in large print can facilitate learning.

Training is influenced by settings (temperature in the classroom, pool, and locker room, lighting, and audiovisual equipment), logistics (schedule of the day, formats used, and flexibility in the schedule based on student response), and organization (overview of the process, breakdown into lessons, continued review of what has been covered, and use of tools of training to meet the needs of learning styles of students).

Topics for Evaluation and Training

Terminology

There are many commonly used terms that are rather unique to aquatic therapy, e.g., buoyancy assisted, buoyancy resisted, buoyancy supported, vertical, prone, supine, finning, sculling, frontal surface, slicing, pressing, turbulence assisted, and turbulence resisted. Daily notes and progress reports will contain these terms to designate progress and programs, and thus the staff must have an understanding of them.

Do the aquatic therapy reports reflect the lexicon of aquatic therapy to denote appropriate goals, progressions, and variations? The therapy staff should spend time with the billing staff to explain the terminology and develop explanation letters for the general aquatic program and the specific techniques and programs to be sent out to physicians, insurance companies, and attorneys. This training will clarify the designation of skilled care for aquatic therapy and reduce denials for reimbursements. To demonstrate understanding of the terms of hydrotherapy, the therapist must apply this knowledge to the client through selection of water depth, exercise, direction of movement, verbal cues given, hand placement, and use of equipment to provide an individualized aquatic program to meet the client's characteristics and needs.

Understanding of Hydrodynamics

Hydrodynamics is thoroughly explained in Chapter 2. Are your staff applying hydrodynamics as they work with patients? The competency level in each technique can be determined using terms such as *no knowledge, limited knowledge, basic understanding, advanced knowledge,* and *extensive experience.* The International Council for Aquatic Therapy and Rehabilitation Industry Certifications (ICATRIC); (2829 South Manito Blvd., Spokane, WA 99203; phone: 425-444-2720; www.icatric.org) has a test for minimum standards within the field of aquatic therapy. There are currently no other tests for advanced knowledge. What terms have therapists heard, read, or learned? Do they understand that there are many techniques being used and that there truly is a difference between exercise in the water and on land? Courses being taught have certificates of attendance at each level.

Desire/Interest

Does the therapist have a passion for aquatic therapy? Developing a staff of enthusiastic, educated aquatic therapists will support your program and allow it to build to a more advanced level. Aquatic therapy is not a new technique, but, unfortunately, at this time it is an underdeveloped, undersupported technique. The staff will need to express their enthusiasm to physicians, insurance companies, and management. Unfortunately, many clinicians are never asked what they know, care about, believe in, are skilled in, or want to do with aquatic therapy. Often therapists are moved into aquatic therapy because someone else is leaving or because they know how to swim. Having staff who are truly committed to and believe in the use of aquatic therapy will provide the impetus needed for an aquatic therapy program to develop into one that is financially successful. The excitement will motivate patients, support staff, and physicians and referrals, and positive results will increase.

Asking staff members what their interests are and evaluating their current knowledge can save management time and money. Frequently the therapist who is sent to a conference and then is responsible for educating the rest of the staff leaves the program within 6 months! Client service will improve when the staff working in the pool is chosen from those most interested and skilled in the pool.

Some therapists have sensitive skin or have their own phobias or dislikes concerning swimming pools (e.g., chemicals, wearing a swimsuit, allergies, or asthma). These issues will influence the therapists' performance and their clients may not receive optimum care.

As a manager, support for your interested therapist creates enthusiasm for aquatic therapy that will incite the interest of other staff members. This will result in increased referrals, positive outcomes, and a financially profitable aquatic therapy program.

Risk Management

Risk management is a crucial topic when one works in an aquatic setting. Please review the issues related to risk management that are discussed elsewhere in this book in the chapters by Dr. Osinski and Ms. Clement. Many risks exist in the pool area; drowning is just one of these. The number of slips and falls can be reduced or prevented with an appropriate floor surface, drainage, and maintenance. Requiring soap showers before therapy, wearing of proper footwear, and appropriate dress can also influence pool maintenance. Knowledge of chemical balance in the pool to recognize when pool chemistry is imbalanced or air quality is not appropriate (humidity, temperature, and fumes) and having an action plan to follow to correct imbalances will reduce liability. Having the sensitivity to deal with fearful clients and having specific policies concerning precautions and contraindications (e.g., for patients with osteotomies and wounds and for those who are incontinent) will improve and clarify your referral base. Management should create a pool maintenance team consisting of a lead aquatic therapist, a maintenance professional, and a member of management, and send the team to participate in a certified pool operator training course. This will assure that pool maintenance is managed by a team of educated personnel. Long-term exposure to imbalanced pool water and poor air quality may result in significant adverse health problems for the staff.

With regard to who may be permitted to use the pool, there are absolute contraindications and there are precautions. Some facilities classify all concerns as contraindications, restricting pool use by clients who could truly benefit from aquatic therapy, often because of ignorance of pool maintenance and problem management strategies. There are many clinical concerns that can safely be managed through close monitoring, through the careful use of skin barrier products such as Tegaderm, through personal awareness of individual patient physiologic problems, and through the use of specialized products or techniques for toileting (bowel and bladder control schedules) and other concerns.

How does your staff deal with fearful clients? Staff with a strong understanding of and compassion for fearful clients combined with strong safety skills will produce a positive experience for a sector of clients who often never make it to the pool.

Prioritize Needs for Your Facility

Accreditation

The Joint Commission on Accreditation of Healthcare Organizations (JCAHO) will evaluate the pools and clinic space and records. Are your records ready for review? Do referrals reflect specific requests for aquatic therapy? Do therapy evaluations and progress notes denote the rationale for aquatic therapy and specific aquatic therapy progressions? Do the daily notes match the billing codes for services provided? Policies and procedures to address these issues must be clear and supported by the documentation.

Safety Standards

JCAHO and the Occupational Safety and Health Administration (OSHA) have standards as does your local health department. Do you have someone on staff who can evaluate your facility(ies) and determine what must be done to pass inspections? Do your city, county, or state regulations require you to have a lifeguard in your pool area? Are the basic water safety or new water safety procedures for health professionals adequate? What specific procedures do you need to develop to handle emergency situations (e.g., availability of 911 or codes)? Again, policy and procedure manuals need to reflect appropriate practice and local regulations.

Record Keeping

Records should be clear and concise, with forms stored on the computer to be revised as often as needed. Specific sheets for specific diagnosis groups with blank spaces to add individualized recommendations can be very helpful and timesaving. The staff can help to develop a set of abbreviations indicating specific exercises, equipment used, position of the body, and direction of movement to streamline record keeping.

Exercise Sheets

Exercise sheets with pictures and clear descriptions can be very helpful for clients, both at poolside (enlarged and laminated or printed on waterproof paper) and at home. Aquatic exercise card sets are available through Visual Health Informex (Tacoma, Wash).

Billing

Is there a streamlined method for billing? Is there a communication channel between the therapy department and the billing department that may be off site? Have the therapy staff offered an in-service program to the billing/claims staff so they know what the terminology means? Are daily notes sent with each bill? Are letters of information on the specific techniques and terminology of aquatic therapy used in the clinic available? The aquatic therapist must be aware of billing issues and be conscious of the need for clarity when writing aquatic therapy reports and daily notes. Education of billing department staff, insurance claims representatives, and referring physicians to maintain long-term referrals and reimbursements/payments for aquatic therapy is necessary. The therapist must clarify the use of a skilled level of aquatic therapy by noting specific methods, techniques, and progressions. Developing specific functional goals from your evaluation, followed by reassessment and resetting goals, creates the framework for a viable therapy program.

Pool Maintenance

The water in a well-maintained pool is crystal clear and not cloudy or green. The bottom drain of the pool, regardless of its depth, must be clearly visible. Staff should be instructed in the processes of checking the chemical balance of the pool water every 2 hours and in the performance of regular pool maintenance, including cleaning skimmer baskets, tiles, and gutters, backwashing or cleaning filters, and scheduled draining of the pool for maintenance and cleaning (annually, semiannually, quarterly, or monthly depending upon the volume of water, filter system, and usage rates). These tasks may be outsourced. Chemical levels, air quality, equipment cleaning and sanitizing, and maintenance should be the concern of each staff member exposed to the pool environment for obvious reasons. Depending upon the delegation of tasks, therapy staff may be trained to test the halogen system and the pH, alkalinity, and hardness of the pool water (being aware of individual color discrimination vision because these are often measured with color strips!).

Staff Scheduling

In the *ARN Network Newsletter*,[1] a discussion of scheduling illuminated the concerns of therapists who were using valuable time dressing and undressing rather than staying in the pool for one half or all of a day. Having additional staff in the pool (lifeguard, assistant, and aide) to watch clients may be essential so that time is available for the therapist to complete paperwork. Scheduling of staff is also based on the quality of the pool water and air and, hence, concerns for the amount of exposure of health and safety of staff are based on quality of pool water and air. In recent discussions on the Aquatic Therapy & Rehab Institute (ATRI) listserv, professionals were recommending no more than 3 hours of pool time each day with regular breaks to hydrate. However, some therapists are in the pool for 6 to 8 hours/day.

Handling Skills

The most common error seen when a therapist moves into aquatic therapy is underhandling or overhandling of clients. When assisting a client into a supine position, an unskilled practitioner may grasp the client's neck and pelvis or legs firmly and actually lift the client out of the water. Aquatic therapy training can be spent teaching a lightness of touch, body mechanics, and sensitivity to individual buoyancy levels and needs as well as an understanding of how to use the water to support the client in your arms. Other important elements of staff skill are to determine when flotation is needed and when it is not, how to assist clients in donning and doffing equipment, and how to provide verbal cues to the client to use breath to assist transition. The skilled and experienced staff member will be able to support the client as needed and know how to work with a fearful client in establishing trust and confidence in the therapist.

RESOURCES

In the next sections, a listing of currently available options to aid in staff development is provided. This list certainly will change over time, but because the field is growing dynamically and is still underpublicized, the author felt that a resource directory would be useful, even though it may become outdated.

University-Based Programs

UNCG has an aquatic leadership program option: aquatic instructional leadership and aquatics for therapy/rehabilitation specialty within the School of Health and Human Performance, Department of Exercise and Sport Science (www.uncg.edu). It is not affiliated with a therapy degree, and many of the standard techniques as well as safety and management issues are included. The aquatic curriculum provides entry-level professional preparation for students to competently assess and improve upon existing programs and to design and deliver effective programs for a wide range of aquatic settings.

Classes taught include the following:

ESS 150: Swimming for Non-Swimmers
ESS 151: Beginning Swimming
ESS 202: Water Aerobics
ESS 203: Fitness Swim
ESS 252: Low-Intermediate Swimming
ESS 255: Water Safety Education
ESS 259: Water Safety Instructor
ESS 262: Safety Training for Swim Coaches
ESS 280: Research and Evaluation in Exercise and Sport Science
ESS 459: Teaching Swimming to Individuals With Special Needs
ESS 559: Water Exercise for Therapy and Rehabilitation
ESS 560: Aquatic Therapeutic Modalities
ESS 594: Internship

The following courses are listed in the UNCG bulletin for further descriptions.

Instructional Aquatic Activities and Fitness:

ESS 150: Swimming for Non-Swimmers
ESS 151: Beginning Swimming
ESS 202: Water Aerobics
ESS 203: Fitness Swim
ESS 252: Low-Intermediate Swimming
ESS 254: High-Intermediate Swimming

ESS 256: Advanced Swimming
ESS 257: Synchronized Swimming*
ESS 260: Water Polo*
ESS 261: Springboard Diving*
ESS 268: Canoeing*
ESS 269: Sailing*
(*Not taught on a regular basis; taught by demand.)

Aquatic Management and Leadership:

ESS 255: Water Safety Education*
ESS 258: Lifeguard Training
ESS 259: Water Safety Instructor
ESS 262: Safety Training for Swim Coaches*
ESS 458: Aquatic Facility Management
(*Not taught on a regular basis; taught by demand.)

Aquatic Therapy:

ESS 459: Teaching Swimming to Individuals With Special Needs
ESS 460: Introduction to Therapeutic Aquatics
ESS 559: Water Exercise for Therapy and Rehabilitation
ESS 560: Aquatic Therapeutic Modalities

Paula Briggs, MS, ATRIC, Assistant Professor of West Virginia University, developed an aquatic therapy program at the university. The program is found in the WVU School of Medicine under the Division of Exercise Physiology (Department of Human Performance & Applied Exercise Science, School of Medicine, Robert C. Byrd Health Science Center, West Virginia University, P.O. Box 9227, Morgantown, WV 26506-9227; phone: 304-293-6509; home: 304-292-2937; fax: 304-293-7105; e-mail: pbriggs@hsc.wvu.edu). The Website for the aquatic therapy curriculum is: www.hsc.wvu.edu/som/ep/; click on "Degrees" and "Aquatic Therapy." The requirements for the curriculum are the same as those for the exercise physiology program.

Coursework for the aquatic therapy specialization includes the following:

EXPH 450: Theory of Aquatic Therapy (3 credits)
EXPH 451: Applications of Aquatic Therapy (3 credits)
EXPH 452: Aquatic Therapy Facility Management (3 credits)
EXPH 491/672: Professional Field Placement (6 credits)

This specialty has an enrollment of 30 students. The student is required to file an application with two letters of recommendation, an essay, the appropriate GPA, and an interview. Students normally would start the specialization during their junior year.

Nonuniversity Training

ATRI is a multidisciplinary group of aquatic professionals. ATRI has developed standards within the profession of aquatic therapy for basic qualifications and safety. ATRI hosts a national conference, usually in August, alternating between East Coast and West Coast locations, as well as regional conferences. The national conference lasts 4 days with 2 days of preconference specialty courses that include Aquatic Safety, Introduction to Aquatic Therapy, Aquatic Exercise Association (AEA) fitness instructor certification, ATRI rheumatology certification, ATRI examination, AEA personal training certification, Ai Chi basic certification, Aquatic Back Rehabilitation, Clinical Wassertanzen, and the Burdenko Method. The symposium covers a variety of topics from risk management, facility design, and techniques by name or by diagnoses. The regional conferences usually last 2 to 3 days and include a variety of topics such as back rehabilitation, shoulder rehabilitation, Watsu, and Ai Chi. Contact ATRI for more information (phone: 906-482-9500; e-mail: atri@up.net; www.atri.org).

Individuals and organizations also offer specific aquatic conferences. This is a short list of potential resources with current addresses as of publication:

American Physical Therapy Association (APTA), www.apta.org/bulletin/course_listings
Igor Burdenko, The Burdenko Institute; phone: 800-287-3365;
  e-mail: igor@burdenko.com; www.burdenko.com
Harold Dull, Worldwide Aquatic Bodywork Association (WABA);
  phone: 707-987-9638; www.waba.edu
Mary Essert, Essert Associates; e-mail: messert@mindspring.com;
  www.mindspring.com/~messert
Gwen Garrett, phone: 757-489-1371
Douglas Kinnaird, Kinnaird Seminars and Therapeutic Aquatics, Inc.;
  phone: 307-739-1835
Juliana Larsen, phone: 352-490-2345
Julia Meno, phone: 307-739-1835; e-mail: jmeno@wyoming.com;
  www.therapeutic-aquatics.com, www.aquaticcentral.com
Ruth Meyer, phone: 434-293-9987; e-mail: watsuva@aol.com
Minakshi, Minakshi's Aquatic Bodywork Island Studio; phone: 305-743-2624
Terri Mitchell, e-mail: texterri@Austin.rr.com
Marilou Moschetti, Aqua Technics Consulting Group; phone: 831-688-2696
Andrea Poteat-Salzman, Aquatic Resource Network, 302 160th Street Suite 200,
  Amery, WI 54001; www.aquaticnet.com
Rehab Institute of Chicago; phone: 312-238-6179
Peggy Schoedinger, Aquatic Therapy Innovations, Inc.; phone: 303-447-3256;
  e-mail: PegAquatic@aol.com
Laree Shanda, Constellate; www.constellate.com; 425-444-2720
Rosemary Shuler, MS, CTRS, Waterspice; phone: 919-556-1225;
  e-mail: waterspice@juno.com
Thomas Tierney, PT, Aquatic Physical Therapy Resources; phone: 630-810-1717

Within specific techniques, the originators teach their programs at a variety of locations:

American Alliance for Health Physical Education, Recreation and Dance (AAHPERD)
Arthritis Foundation, phone: 800-933-0032
Aquatic Consultants of Georgia: Harriet Adams, phone: 404-350-6185
Aquatic Council Adapted Aquatics Program
The Burdenko Method: Igor Burdenko
The Halliwick Method: Johann Lambeck, et al
Multiple Sclerosis Society
New Bad Ragaz Ring Method: Urs Gamper, PT, Johan Lambeck PT, Peggy
  Schoedinger, PT, Gwendolyn Garrett, OTR, et al
Task Training Method: Thomas Tierney
Watsu: Harold Dull, et al

Standards of the Industry

Aquatic Therapy & Rehab Institute (ATRI), www.atri.org. ATRI offers information on regulations, health and safety (cardiopulmonary resuscitation [CPR], first aid, and emergency action plan [EAP]), legal and ethical practices, professional responsibility, 30 hours of training, 6-month internship, client evaluations, prevention and treatment goals, contraindications, terminology, rational for therapy, and equipment.

American Alliance for Health, Physical Education, Recreation and Dance (AAHPERD) Aquatic Council. The position paper on Aquatic Therapy Safety Guidelines, third draft, 2001, covers the need for safety when working in an aquatic setting. The Aquatic Council recommends standards that include having knowledge of health of the participant, an EAP, a lifeguard on deck at all times or therapy staff with lifeguard or community water safety, CPR and first aid, water exercise, and swimming skills, facility safety (uncluttered deck, adherence to Americans with Disabilities Act (ADA) guidelines, correct chemical balance of water, and adequate lighting, heating, ventilation, and acoustics).

American Occupational Therapy Association (AOTA) Aquatic Section, 4720 Montgomery Lane, P.O. Box 31220, Bethesda, MD 20824-1220; phone: 301-652-2682; www.aota.org

American Physical Therapy Association (APTA) Aquatic Section, 111 North Fairfax St., Alexandria VA 22314-1488; phone: 703-684-APTA, 800-999-2782; www.apta.org, www.aquaticpt.org; 1351 members

Arthritis Foundation. The Arthritis Foundation offers a 1- to 2-day training course called the Arthritis Foundation/YMCA Aquatic Program, which is a recreational exercise program. Many hospital administrators have sent therapists to these courses because they are relatively inexpensive (depending upon where you live) and of short duration. This program has a prescribed number of exercises and recommends initially 3 to 5 repetitions, building up to 12 repetitions. There is an endurance component as well. The focus is on moving every joint every day as tolerated. This focus, while useful, is structured so that it may be used safely by all persons with arthritis in an independent environment, and thus may fall well short of an individualized therapeutic regimen under the supervision of a knowledgeable therapist.

Multiple Sclerosis Society. The Multiple Sclerosis Society has an aquatic exercise program that is offered regionally or locally. Training courses for instructors are not sponsored nationally and the Society Website does not provide any information on aquatic therapy for persons with multiple sclerosis.

National Swimming Pool Foundation, P.O. Box 495, Merrick, NY 11566; phone: 516-623-3447; www.nspf.com. Certified pool operator (CPO) courses are taught throughout the United States. Each state has its specific regulation, a number of states require that every pool have a CPO and lifeguard at all times. CPO courses have a varied duration with a written examination covering topics on water quality, mechanical systems, filters, and regulations.

State therapy laws—scope of practice. There are state practice acts that specifically mention aquatic therapy under the specific therapy practice. Fortunately there is a history for many therapy fields in the use of aquatic therapy within their scope of practice.

Worldwide Aquatic Bodywork Association (WABA). The requirements to allow calling oneself a Watsu practitioner have evolved over the past 5 years from approximately 100 hours of course work to 500 hours. WABA recognizes that students attending Watsu training courses have a variety of backgrounds and credentials and will review past course work that can be applicable to a certain number of hours. In keeping with California educational regulations, the only courses that are accredited by California are those taught in California. Many of the courses taught in Florida are recognized by the Florida Massage Therapy licensing board.

Training Topics

Basic Safety and Emergency Response

All employees will need documented training on the facility emergency codes and procedures through the human resources department or their direct management team. These codes must be reviewed for their specific application in the pool area. For example, when a code calls for fire evacuation, the clients are given towels and moved outside through the direct access door; they are not permitted to return to the locker room to get dressed. Because of extremes of weather, the clients are then directed to the nearest building that is clear of fire hazard to avoid overexposure to the weather. In contrast, if there is a tornado code, the clients are transferred into the locker room if it has been deemed to be a safe location.

Staff must be assessed for both didactic knowledge of safety procedures as well as practical skills through a combination of written tests and poolside drills. Drills with staged in-water events and emergency pool evacuations should be conducted. Other potential crises must be anticipated and appropriate procedures determined. Safety drills should be regularly scheduled as well as unannounced, and the staff briefed on the outcomes and suggested improvements. All of these events and the subsequent discussions must be documented. Pool facilities are required to have a method of communication: phone, intercom, or alert button; some pool facilities in retirement communities use a "nurse call" button with a long string on it which reaches the pool. The ongoing challenge is to be sure that electronics function well in the humid pool environment, so regular checks of the pool emergency equipment are necessary. A call button would alert the on-call staff in the building; a phone could be used to call 911 or the in-house emergency management team as deemed by the responder and the facility procedures.

Evacuation of all potential client populations served by the facility from the pool must be practiced, using single- and multiple-person techniques. This should include safe use of spine boards, in-water CPR assistance, etc.

An important issue to discuss with staff is the difference between distress and drowning and how they are handled. An individual in distress may have a cramp or may have slipped and gotten his or her face wet. Typically this person can be verbally assisted or minimally assisted to the side of the pool and checked for level of need, e.g., a towel, a drink of water, or the need for further medical attention. A near-drowning or drowning requires immediate response. The standard progression of the American Red Cross is reach, throw, tow, go, and then evaluate the need for CPR or artificial respiration.

Advanced safety procedures include life guarding, life support in water, and the presence of an accident and emergency department as needed within your facility.

Basic Handling Techniques

These classes cover the basic aquatic issues that will influence the therapy session. If the therapist does not have a background in aquatics, these issues will not be obvious to him or her. They must include the basics of client evaluation and individualized aquatic therapeutic program design. The initial evaluation should include assessment of a patient's skills for a positive and safe aquatic experience: mouth closure, nose clearing and breathing, eye blinking, need for ear plugs, head control and posture (need for flotation devices), rolling over (prone to supine position; rotation around the vertical axis), and recover to stand (rotation around the horizontal axis). What is the patient's body type/build and resultant ability to float or sink? Knowledge of these characteristics influences the therapist's choice of depth of water for therapy.

It is essential to know how to support, assist, and resist clients as they ambulate and exercise as well as what verbal, visual, and physical cues will be needed by clients as they enter the pool. Each client should receive information on the temperature (water and air), use of the handrails on the stairs, the depth of the steps, and the depths of the pool and where they change—point out depth markers and lines or ropes. Clients should be directed to stay by the wall and hold on to the railing or side of the pool until they are cleared for open pool activity.

Some other techniques include the following:

- Teaching clients to use their arms to assist or resist motion or to develop coordination using contralateral/reciprocal arm swing.
- Allowing for adjustment to the various depths of the pool.
- Testing buoyancy level by lifting one foot or squatting down to shoulder depth to determine whether, at 90% unloading, they maintain stability.
- Assisting in transitions: the use of cues—verbal, visual, and physical
- Progressing from vertical to horizontal (supine): stand in chest depth of water, squat down. Teaching sculling or finning to progress to the squat scull: Can the client scull hard enough to lift their feet off the bottom? Does the client's feet come off the bottom as he or she squats down?
- Changing position: stand to squat to lie back with inhalation and scull arms to float, extending legs and abducting arms as needed.
- Understanding the cues to assist in floating: arms overhead (abduct slowly) to hands out of water (fingers flex or wrist flexes), quick, deep inhalation with slow, partial exhalation (watch hyperventilation), bend knees, use abdominal muscles to draw leg toward the water surface.
- Recovering to stand: lift head, tuck knees toward chest, reach arms back into extension then sweep forward, push feet to bottom of pool simultaneously and stand up.
- Moving from vertical to horizontal (prone): practice the face-wet procedure and explain what is expected. Will the client lift his or her head up (cervical extension) to breathe, rotate (rhythmic breathing), or use a mask and snorkel? Thorough instruction in use of mask and snorkel is vital. Discuss recovery to stand before submerging the client: lift the client's head up using thoracic and cervical extension, push down on the water (shoulders extend from 90 to 180 degrees of shoulder joint flexion), flex knees toward chest, and then push both feet to the bottom of the pool. Again, it is helpful to inhale at the initiation to bring the chest up over the hips and to be patient with the time it takes for rotation around the horizontal axis depending upon the length of the individual's torso and legs.

- Supporting the client's head if he or she requires assistance moving from vertical to supine by using head-neck support: placing the hand on the occiput with the forearm aligned down the spine (head/chin hand support from the American Red Cross *Lifeguarding Today*),[2] when the client is sitting sideways on the therapist's knee, asking the client to inhale as he or she leans back and the therapist keeps the head as close to the water from the beginning so that it does not move into hyperextension as the therapist lifts the sacrum/float point to the surface.
- Using minimal support needed initially, proceeding to assistance, support, and resistance.
- Being able to describe and teach these skills to clients of all ages (children, teens, adults, elderly).
- Being responsible for instructing the client in the changes resulting from being in the water (standing in an aquatic environment): the influence of water on breathing, balance, movement, and exercise intensity; the effects of buoyancy such as stability, unloading; production of visual effects in water through refraction and reflection; the effects of water on the client's ability to walk; concerns about hydration, overheating, or chilling (hyperthermia and hypothermia); and an explanation of the use of rate of perceived exertion scale and an aquatic exercise heart rate chart.
- Being able to demonstrate transitioning of a client from the pool deck into pool with necessary verbal cues and assistance as he or she progresses through an education and therapy session and to demonstrate the ability to transition a client through various positions in the water using appropriate body mechanics for himself or herself and the client including vertical, supine (head/sacrum, cheek to cheek, pelvic hold), prone, and neutral float positions.
- Instructing a client in basic swimming skills for safety, exercise, and long-term skills.
- Screening for aquatic therapy referral (facility contraindications and precautions) including why to refer and why not to refer.
- Being personally aware: the in-water therapist must be aware of his or her own postures and responses in the water and know his or her relative density/buoyancy level to warrant the use of ankle weights for stabilization to prevent injury to the therapist and stability for the appropriate client treatment. Ankle weights to be used under water must be lead free (see www.waba.edu for ordering information).

Equipment Progression

It is essential for staff to know their equipment and what amount of resistance or assistance it creates. Douglas Bedgood, designer of Aquatoner, has completed research and offers a list of amounts of resistance created by the Aquatoner, depending upon how open it is (the amount of surface area) (Aquatherapeutics, Inc., Key West, Fla; phone: 305-295-7702, 800-237-0469). Staff need to look at buoyancy, surface area, and turbulence created by equipment. Knowing how to label equipment and educate clients on when and how to vary resistance is an essential part of the treatment program. A great variety of equipment that uses buoyancy to create resistance is available. The therapist needs to understand these factors to create a progressive aquatic therapy program.

Technique Application

There are several chapters in this book that address applying specific techniques to diagnosis or function. Based on the client base, specific techniques can be introduced to expand the services offered for specialty training by diagnosis (e.g., orthopedics, neuromuscular, fibromyalgia, or knee replacement).

Advanced Methods

Advanced handling is use of the lightest, softest support to proceed to assistance, support, and resistance. To allow therapists time to develop personalized methods based on ongoing education and prior knowledge of techniques (e.g., massage, myofascial release, craniosacral release, energy work, yoga, or Tai Chi) time in the pool should be allotted for creative play and practice by the therapists with each other. Experimenting with each other and communicating positive and negative concerns in a constructive manner helps therapists develop safe and logical methods that they can then apply to clients.

As an example, in New Hampshire and the Boston area aquatic therapy study groups met every other month or more often, with a specific topic for each meeting, most of which included in-pool time. Training courses, literature, and techniques were discussed, and techniques were actually practiced. The group recognized the need for a multidisciplinary approach and the fact that the more highly skilled everyone was the more likely physicians would refer patients and insurance carriers would reimburse.

Teaching Clients for Community-Based Programs

There is a growing trend for therapy practices to use pools within the community; e.g., at the YMCA and health clubs clients are acclimated to a lifestyle habit of attending the facility regularly, using the services, and being around apparently healthy individuals. Hospital corporations have been building these facilities over the past 10 years, often filling a need within a small community for a well-apportioned fitness facility that can cover its cost with its varied usage.

Otherwise therapists may form relationships with the local YMCA, health club, hotel fitness facility, or condominium association. Knowledge of what the fees are, who the instructors are, where the lifeguards are, what the pool temperatures and depths are, and what the pool quality is like is necessary so that patients can be transitioned into a long-term program. More rural communities are discovering the team approach and offer open membership to the pools and health clubs of their timeshare/condominiums or private club, or they lease the pool out to subcontractors offering transitional programs.

AQUATIC THERAPY AND REHABILITATION INDUSTRY CERTIFICATION PREREQUISITES

Before sitting for the examination, the candidate must document and submit the following prerequisites:

- The candidate must show current certification in CPR and first aid training within the last 4 years through documentation, certification, license, or education. (Some CPR certification may include first aid training.)

- The candidate must show documentation of basic water rescue skills, within the last 4 years.*
- The candidate must have 30 hours of documented **training** specific to aquatic therapy and rehabilitation, i.e., continuing education training specific to aquatic therapy, not practice in the field.†

The candidate must document one of the following:‡

- An undergraduate (including associate's) or graduate degree in exercise science, biology, premedicine, physical education, recreation, or a related field; **OR**
- An unrelated undergraduate degree, plus 3 years in the field working 25 to 30 hours a week (or 3000 hours total) in aquatic therapy or rehabilitation; **OR**
- Without a degree, an approved water fitness certification and 5 years (or 5000 hours) working in aquatic therapy or rehabilitation.‡

Candidates who do not have the prerequisites but expect to have them within 6 months of the examination date may sit for the examination. If prerequisite documentation is not attached to your certification registration, you must notify us when it will be submitted. Certification, if the examination is passed, will not be issued until proof of prerequisites is received.

REFERENCES

1. ARN Network Newsletter, Vol 6, No 2, p 8.
2. Lifeguarding Today (American Red Cross), 1990.

---

*Documentation must include rescue and immobilization, backboard skills, seizure intervention, basic swimming and rescue skills, recognition of emergency situations and activating emergency medical services, reaching and throwing, assists, rescue tube skills, removal of an injured client from the pool or accident site, and responding to and managing aquatic emergency situations. Copies of certification are valid documentation, although certification is not necessary to fulfill this prerequisite. If your documentation is in letter form, it must state that you have been taught and performed the skills mentioned above. This can be fulfilled by your lifeguard or similar aquatic professional.

†The courses must directly address teaching techniques and issues regarding water therapy. A syllabus may be required. Copies of certificate of completion, lists of events attended, continuing education unit (CEU) forms, letters from trainers, or college transcripts are valid documentation. Titles of courses, dates, locations, length, and trainer must be included. ATRI educational events such as Aquatic Therapy Specialty Institutes, Aquatic Therapy Symposiums, and Professional Development Days can apply toward your 30 hours. Please note that a course required for your related degree cannot count toward your 30 hours, as it is included in the degree requirement.

‡Documentation may be a copy of your diploma, license, college transcripts, certification, a letter from your supervisor/manager or other validating professional on letterhead. Approved certifications are those that have met the standards and procedures of the national regulatory organizations NOCA, CLEAR, and NCCA. Check with your certification organization if it is not listed. Currently approved water fitness certification is AEA.

Chapter 16

The Lyton Model: An Interdisciplinary Model of Care

Lynette Jamison,* MOT, OTR/L, CPO and
Charlotte Norton,* DPT, MS, ATC, CSCS

In the aquatic setting, an interdisciplinary team provides the continuum of care for patients and clients. The team includes the patient or client, physician, occupational therapist, physical therapist, aquatic exercise instructor, certified athletic trainer, exercise physiologist, kinesiologist, massage therapist, and certified recreation specialist. Each team member has a specific role in the continuum of care, although on occasion, the roles may overlap. For example, the roles of the physical therapist and occupational therapist are interchangeable for developing coordination with developmentally delayed children.

For this text, the Lyton Model is used to describe the aquatic team members. Licensed treatment, fitness, and wellness are the divisions of care and treatment of the model with the client at the center. The Lyton Model places the client at the center to illustrate the importance and consequences of decision-making and to indicate that the client is an active member of the team for the treatment plan or aftercare.

Professionals who maintain a license to practice in a particular state provide licensed treatment in this model. Licensed professionals are held accountable for following their state practice guidelines. Medicare guidelines state that reimbursed therapy services may be provided by a practitioner who maintains a license. Fitness refers to an apparently healthy client working toward a state of physical well-being as determined by measures such as $\dot{V}O_{2max}$. The professional working with this individual has a specialized background in water fitness. Wellness in the Lyton Model refers to the client who has a chronic disease, such as arthritis, and is trying to improve the quality of his or her life through the use of an aquatic medium. The professional working in the wellness arena also must have specialized training in water exercises for those with special needs.

LICENSURE, REGISTRATION, CERTIFICATION, AND TITLE ACTS

A state or jurisdiction grants licensure to medical professionals in 1 of the 50 states or 3 jurisdictions. Jurisdictions include Puerto Rico, District of Columbia, and

---

*Copyright Lynette Jamison and Charlotte Norton.

the U.S. Virgin Islands. A license allows the practitioner to work in that state or jurisdiction. The state practice act defines the scope of practice and the disciplinary action to be taken when violations occur. Although practice acts vary within the states for the disciplines, state boards have the authority to suspend or revoke a license as well as prohibit practice.

Registration by state or national organizations may or may not offer a scope of practice and disciplinary action. Registration is obtained after graduation from an accredited college or university program, completion of a registration application, and successful completion of the registration examination.

Certification is documentation for status and is used to document specific qualifications. Certification may be achieved after graduation from an accredited college or university program, completion of an internship, completion of the certification application, and passing of the certification examination. Regulation is monitored by the specific certifying agency.

Title acts and trademark laws are state and discipline specific. Requirements to practice vary from no formal education to graduation from an accredited college or university program. There is no regulatory agency to monitor conduct and no disciplinary action can be taken. Those who have not graduated from an allied health program may call themselves "therapists," but employment and reimbursement opportunities are limited for those without supporting education and licensure.

REGULATION AND EDUCATIONAL STANDARDS

National professional organizations and state agencies regulate allied health professionals and determine coursework and standards (if any); an examination is required for regulation by licensure. The allied health professions or agencies discussed in this section are the American Physical Therapy Association (APTA), the Federation of State Boards for Physical Therapy (FSBPT), the American Occupational Therapy Association (AOTA), National Boards for Certification in Occupation Therapy (NBCOT), the National Athletic Trainers Association (NATA), the National Council on Therapeutic Recreation (NCTR), the American College of Sports Medicine (ACSM), the American Kinesiotherapy Association (AKTA), and the American Massage Therapy Association (AMTA).

Aquatic therapy training does not have a consistent standard or base of any curriculum in the rehabilitation disciplines. Therefore, those who receive aquatic rehabilitative training must seek courses after graduation. Many courses in aquatic therapy and therapeutic techniques are not restricted to licensed physical and occupational therapists, and few are offered at the university level.

APTA/Physical Therapists and Assistants

Each state or jurisdiction uses the FSBPT examination to establish minimum licensure requirements for physical therapists and assistants. The FSBPT verifies and recognizes professional requirements that include graduation from an accredited master's physical therapy program, an internship, and the national physical therapy licensure examination. Physical therapist assistants graduate from an accredited associate's degree program. Licensure or registration is not required in all states for the physical therapy assistant to practice.

AOTA/Occupational Therapists and Assistants

Each state or jurisdiction uses the NBCOT examination to establish licensure requirements for occupational therapists and assistants. NBCOT offers registration for occupational therapists and certification for occupational therapy assistants. Requirements for an occupational therapist registered (OTR) include graduation from an accredited master's of occupational therapy program, 6 months of fieldwork, and passing the NBCOT examination. To maintain national registration, the OTR must submit a renewal application every 5 years, document the required number of continuing education hours, and attest to good character.

Certification for the occupational therapy assistant requires graduation from an accredited occupational therapy assistant program, 440 hours, or 12 weeks, of fieldwork, and passing the NBCOT examination for occupational therapy assistants.

NATA/Athletic Trainers

Education for athletic trainers has followed two paths: curriculum and internship. Curriculum programs are usually within the departments of exercise and sport science or physical education at a college or university. The Commission on Accreditation of Allied Health Education Programs is responsible for accreditation. In addition, curriculum students must be supervised by an certified athletic trainer (ATC) for 800 hours. The internship route is being phased out and will no longer meet the requirements for certification in 2004.

Athletic trainers are certified through the National Athletic Trainer Association Boards of Certification (NATABOC), an organization that monitors professional conduct and continuing education. To meet eligibility requirements for certification, the candidate must be a graduate from an accredited baccalaureate athletic training program, complete 800 contact hours supervised by an ATC, and pass the certification examination. Eight continuing education units are required every 3 years to maintain certification.

Thirty-nine states regulate athletic training. Twenty-one states require licensure for ATCs, 8 states require certification, 6 states require registration, and 4 states have exemptions. The remaining 11 states recognize, but do not require, national certification. There is variability in credentialing depending upon the state. All states, with the exception of Texas, recognize the certification of the athletic trainer as a requirement for credentialing.

NCTR/Therapeutic Recreation Specialists

Recreational therapists are certified by the NCTR. Requirements for certification are graduation from an accredited baccalaureate therapeutic recreation program, a 10-week internship, and a passing score on the NCTR certification examination. To maintain certification, the recreational therapist must submit proof of 50 continuing education units every 5 years. There is no state regulation for recreational therapists.

ACSM/Exercise Physiologists

There is no national certification or state regulation for exercise physiologists. It is estimated that more than 600 organizations offer certification to exercise physiologists; many do not require a specific education or fieldwork to be eligible to attend the certification courses. The ACSM offers three levels of certification for exercise physiologists in two specific tracks. One track is for those who practice in a clinical setting; the second is the health and fitness track. The requirements for the ACSM certification are a baccalaureate degree in an allied health field and a minimum of 600 hours of fieldwork in a clinical exercise program.

AKTA/Kinesiotherapist

National recognition for kinesiotherapists is provided by the AKTA. The requirements for professional recognition are graduation from a baccalaureate kinesiotherapy program, 1000 hours of clinical training under the direct supervision of a registered kinesiotherapist, a written and practical certification examination, and documentation of 50 continuing education units every 3 years. Ohio, New Hampshire, and Virginia recognize the profession of kinesiotherapy.

AMTA/Massage Therapist

There is no required national certification for massage therapists. Some states offer licensure, but regulation is inconsistent. Washington, DC, and 24 states require licensure, certification, or registration. Where licensing is available, massage therapists are required to complete a 500-hour curriculum.

Twenty-four states regulate massage therapy, 2 states have regulation laws in process, and 4 states have passed laws not yet in effect. The inconsistency is further complicated because state laws have precedence over local regulation, and there is a wide discrepancy in laws, ordinances, rules, and regulations governing massage therapy. Some professional massage associations are self-regulating bodies for the maintenance of registries and referral programs or to provide technique-specific certification.

Some agencies for massage therapists are the Worldwide Aquatic Bodywork Association (WABA), Aquatic Bodywork International (ABI), the Jahara Technique Central Office, the American Massage Therapy Association (AMTA), Associated Bodywork and Massage Professionals (ABMP), the International Massage Association (IMA), the American Oriental Bodywork Therapy Association (AOBTA), and the National Certification Board for Therapeutic Massage and Bodywork (NCBTMB).

Aquatic Exercise Instructors

Certification or course work is not required to teach aquatic exercise classes. There are no minimum standards, and validation of workshops attended varies from certificates of attendance/participation to certification from an organization such as the Aquatic Exercise Association.

The Aquatic Exercise Association offers a certification examination with requirements of high school graduation, 4 to 8 weeks of independent study, documentation of 6 months of teaching water fitness classes, cardiopulmonary resuscitation (CPR) certification, attendance of a 10-hour intensive review for the examination, and successful completion of the examination. Continuing education units are required for recertification.

CERTIFICATES OF PARTICIPATION FOR AQUATIC THERAPY—SPECIFIC SKILLS AND EDUCATION

During the last century, therapeutic aquatic techniques have evolved and continue to be developed and adapted from land-based techniques such as Feldenkrais, proprioceptive neuromuscular facilitation, shiatsu, and the Bobath Method. Previous educational requirements, licensure, or certification is not required to attend the aquatic therapy–specific skill courses, and certificates of participation are given for attendance of courses in the Bad Ragaz Ring Method, the Halliwick Method, and Watsu. The certificates offer documentation that an individual has attended a course that may be 1 hour or several days in length. There are no regulations or consequences for misconduct, poor or inaccurate instruction at the training, or incorrect performance of the techniques by the attendee after the workshop.

The Aquatic Therapy & Rehab Institute (ATRI) offers the ATRIC certification. It is multifaceted to accommodate those who wish to attain an aquatic certification. The candidate must know CPR and basic water rescue skills and have first aid training. The candidate must also provide certification, licensure, or educational alternatives with a minimum of 3000 hours of documented training specific to aquatic therapy and rehabilitation. Education or educational alternatives include the following:

- Undergraduate degree or graduate degree in exercise science, biology, premedicine, physical education, recreation, or a related field
- Unrelated undergraduate degree plus 3 years of field work for a total of 3000 hours in aquatic therapy or rehabilitation
- An approved water fitness certification and 5 years or 5000 hours of field work in aquatic therapy or rehabilitation

Finally, the candidate must achieve a passing score on the written examination.

ATRI also offers certification in special skill areas such as Ai Chi, BackHab, rheumatology, and others.

FUNCTION OF EACH TEAM MEMBER IN THE AQUATIC CONTINUUM

Aquatic Exercise Instructor

The aquatic exercise instructor leads classes to enhance the health-related components of fitness and/or wellness that are strength, flexibility, agility, range of motion, and endurance. The instructor generally teaches within group settings, or as a personal trainer may work with a client one on one for private payment. Instructors may specialize to instruct classes for special needs such as arthritis, fibromyalgia, and multiple sclerosis by attending workshops sponsored by the Arthritis Foundation/YMCA (AFYAP) or the National Multiple Sclerosis Society. Aquatic exercise instructors are independent contractors or employees.

Certified Athletic Trainer

ATCs work with active individuals to prevent or improve motor skills and motor performance after an injury. The ATC may also address cognitive, psychomotor, and affect of the individual.

Exercise Physiologist

The term *exercise physiologist*, once applied to the scientist and researcher with a doctor of philosophy degree, is now a common description for certain graduate-trained personnel who work in clinical settings such as hospitals, clinics, and some fitness facilities. The majority of these professionals are trained at the graduate level with experience specific to exercise physiology. These curricula are not standardized.

Kinesiotherapist

A kinesiotherapist treats the effects of disease, injury, and congenital disorders with therapeutic exercise and movement education. The kinesiotherapist uses movement patterns to increase one or more components of fitness.

Massage Therapist

The massage therapist uses touch to relax and nurture the body, mind, and spirit. Techniques employ the use of hands, knuckles, forearms, elbows, and feet to encourage and promote the body to function at an optimal level to facilitate health and well being. Techniques specific to the aquatic environment are Watsu, the Jahara Technique, and Water Dance.

Occupational Therapist

Occupational therapists assist patients to resume their daily occupation. Daily occupation refers to the activities during the course of a day that include bathing, dressing, eating, working at one's job, or playing if the patient is a child. Patients include those who suffer from physical or mental illness, injury, or disability.

Physical Therapist

Physical therapists rehabilitate patients who have experienced an interruption in normal functioning as a result of birth defect, injury, or illness. They use gross and fine motor activities to improve impairments including strength, flexibility, range of motion, balance, and coordination to minimize functional limitations and strength.

Certified Therapeutic Recreation Specialist (CTRS)

The CTRS provides leisure education and functional intervention to enable clients with disabilities to participate in the leisure and recreation aspects of life.

CASE STUDY REPRESENTING THE LYTON MODEL FOR THE AQUATIC CONTINUUM OF CARE

The patient is a 64-year-old female with a combination of osteoarthritis and rheumatoid arthritis. She weighs 205 pounds and is 5 feet tall. The initial diagnosis of arthritis was made at age 43. She was told she would need to lose weight and exercise 3 to 5 days per week. At age 56, the patient fell, broke her right hip, and received total hip replacement.

The patient lives in a ground-level house with her mother. They share the household responsibilities and grocery shopping. She finished the twelfth grade by taking special education classes. Her intellectual level is slightly impaired. She reads at the sixth grade level.

Current Medical Status

The patient is currently experiencing an exacerbation of rheumatoid arthritis. She has a perceived pain level of 7 on a scale of 1 to 10 (0 representing no pain).

Medications

She is taking an anti-inflammatory agent and a medication for pain.

Exam Findings

Range of Motion

Active right hip flexion is 90 degrees without pain, left hip flexion is 80 degrees with increased pain at end range of available motion. Right knee flexion is 80 degrees, left knee flexion is 75 degrees, and ankle dorsiflexion is limited to neutral and painful. Trunk rotation is painful and within functional limits. Shoulder flexion is 130 degrees bilaterally. Elbow flexion is within functional limits. Wrist and fingers are limited and painful with an ulnar deviation.

Strength

Upper extremity and trunk strength is 3/5, hip flexion 2+/5.

Sensation

Sensation is within normal limits throughout the upper and lower extremities, trunk, hands, and feet.

Mobility and Function

The patient demonstrates a bilateral Trendelenburg gait pattern. She ambulates with a wheeled walker during exacerbation of her arthritis. Transfers from sitting to standing are difficult, and standby assistance is necessary for bath bench transfers. She uses a step-to-gait pattern for ascending and descending stairs. She demonstrates appropriate hip precautions for limited right hip flexion, adduction, and internal rotation.

Activities of Daily Living

The patient is able to bathe and dress while sitting and using adaptive devices. Maximum assistance is necessary for heavy household chores, such as vacuuming and cleaning the shower.

Leisure Assessment

The patient lives a sedentary life. She enjoys bingo when she is able to get out. Prior to her hip replacement, she enjoyed water aerobics. She feels that the pain and her weight are barriers to her participation in leisure activities. She also demonstrates the depression and low self-esteem associated with chronic pain.

Fitness Assessment

The patient's mobility has been limited by pain; therefore, her overall endurance is very limited.

Resting heart rate: 75 beats per minute
Blood pressure: 138/88
Body composition: 39% body fat

Discipline-Specific Goals

Occupational Therapy

The patient will transfer on and off a shower bench independently and will increase participation with household chores to include vacuuming a 10 × 10–foot area.

Physical Therapy

The patient will strengthen bilateral hip abductors to minimize her Trendelenburg gait when she returns to walking without an assistive device. She will also demonstrate improved upper and lower extremity strength to increase the ease of sit-to-stand transfers.

Therapeutic Recreation

The patient will maintain her strength and abilities in water activity, transfers into the water, and comfort in the water to facilitate future leisure involvement in an arthritis aquatic program for pain reduction and weight loss.

Exercise Physiology

The patient will reduce her body fat by 3% per month. She will demonstrate how to exercise using the Borg Rate of Perceived Exertion scale.

Massage Therapy

The patient will experience decreased pain and increased range of motion.

Kinesiotherapy

The patient will perform exercises safely and correctly.

Application of the Lyton Model

The patient entered the Lyton Model at age 25 to lose weight. Her classes may have been taught by a combination of professionals including kinesiotherapists, aquatic exercise instructors, and exercise physiologists. After her total hip replacement, she participated in physical therapy and occupational therapy to address problems in range of motion, strength, gait, transfer between sitting and standing, and activities of daily living. Once discharged from an inpatient setting, the patient may continue with outpatient physical therapy and occupational therapy services to achieve her goals. Depending on the facility, an exercise physiologist may address issues related to body composition and exercise intensity for cardiovascular endurance. She may also see a certified therapeutic recreational specialist to address her leisure goals. Once discharged from an outpatient setting, the patient may be enrolled in an arthritis aquatic program taught by any of the professionals in the Lyton Model who possess the proper education, including kinesiotherapists, aquatic exercise instructors, and massage therapists.

The patient may move throughout the Lyton Model during different times in her life. She may require physical therapy and occupational therapy during exacerbation of her rheumatoid arthritis. Changes in her recreational activities and cardiovascular fitness may require additional input from the certified therapeutic recreational specialist and exercise physiologist. The other professionals in the Lyton Model continue to play an active role in the patient's wellness by providing opportunities for decreased pain and maintenance of mobility and function.

Chapter 17
Legal Aspect of Aquatic Therapy

Annie Clement, PhD, JD

Over the past decade the use of water or aquatic therapy for rehabilitation has become a mature industry. In addition to its genuine acceptance in the health care arena, aquatic therapy is popular among members of the general public who are seeking rehabilitation. Weightlessness achieved in the water enables participants to reach a high level of movement freedom. The privacy of the water rids them of the many inhibitions found in other exercise environments.

Professionals electing to work in aquatic therapy assume the risks of aquatic instructors and the liability of therapists. According to Andrea Salzman of the Aquatic Resources Network,[1] athletic trainers, exercise physiologists, kinesiotherapists, massage professionals, occupational therapists, physical therapists, and therapeutic recreation specialists are among those engaged in aquatic therapy.

A comprehensive search of court decisions involving aquatics failed to identify cases related to aquatic therapy. However, for aquatics in general, numerous incidents have resulted in court decisions. The National Safety Council identified drowning as the fourth leading cause of accidental death in the United States[2] and the third leading cause of accidental deaths internationally.[3] Four thousand deaths in aquatics were reported in the United States in 1999, a decrease of 5% from the 1998 figures. Consumer Product Safety researchers estimated that there were 151,233 swimming pool injuries that resulted in hospitalization in 1999. Although these injury figures were less than the injury figures for the sport activities of baseball/softball (339,775), basketball (597,224), cycling (614,549), and football (372,380), they were sufficiently large to send a warning to all aquatic professionals including aquatic therapists.[4]

Among senior populations, one of the target age groups for aquatic therapy, there has been a significant increase in swimming and diving incidents. Estimated incidents in 1990 were 1620 whereas in 1996 estimated incidents rose to 2623.[5]

In this chapter risks and liabilities that might be encountered by the aquatic therapist will be identified and explained, and methods of working successfully with them will be suggested. These will be discussed under the professional's concern for liability, joint responsibility with owners for facilities, and the business of aquatic therapy.

CONCERN FOR LIABILITY

Aquatic therapy is a form of human movement that occurs in the water; thus, the easiest areas to examine to predict the potential for incidents and possible litigation are human movement, exercise, swimming, and therapy. A rather unique situation in aquatic therapy is that the physician who prescribes the series of human movements is the one responsible or liable for the activity. This transfers the aquatic therapist's liability to the physician as long as the therapist is following the physician's guidance. In swimming and other sport activities, the swimming instructor selects and is liable for the events in the water. Under the circumstances described, the aquatic therapist will usually be held liable when the therapy provided has deviated from that prescribed by the physician. The therapist may or may not be liable in other situations. The nature of the liability could account for the very few court decisions found for the topic. The author has searched for decisions on medical cases in aquatic therapy with no success, thus supporting her view that only limited litigation exists. One reason for the low level of litigation is that because the field is so new, there has not been the opportunity for cases to proceed through the courts. Another potential reason is that the therapists have full knowledge of the participant's health history and may be using sophisticated risk management techniques, thus avoiding incidents. Further, most persons working in aquatic therapy have had considerable opportunity to learn about emergency action plans and to have experienced emergency situations and may be functioning efficiently at the first signs of an incident. Possibly even more important is the fact that aquatic therapy involves a one-to-one or one-to a small group session, thus enabling the therapist to maintain contact with the participant(s) at all times. Each of these factors contributes to a reduction in incidents causing injury. This is not to suggest that there is no need for professionals to strive for a high level of safety and to maintain a successful record in risk management.

LEGAL THEORIES

Knowledge of the following legal theories will be helpful to the aquatic therapist: standard of care, negligence, product liability, and risk management. Standard of care and negligence will be addressed in this section. Product liability and risk management are included in the discussion of facilities.

Standard of Care

A standard of care is the lowest level of conduct a professional is permitted to use while carrying out his or her job. It means that any behavior below that standard should result in the professional being removed from the position. This level of behavior is not to be confused with the ideal standards recommended and promoted by most professional organizations. Nearly all people strive to meet very high standards in their work. Again, the standard of care is the minimal standard essential to the task. Often, particularly in the medical profession, the standard is in writing and is readily available to all professionals. Aquatic therapists do not have a written standard; however, they do have a sufficient quantity of high-quality literature to enable a person to easily fashion his or her own standard. In addition to the literature, standards are derived from the academic and on-the-job training a professional has received. Knowledge of contemporary publications and the industry magazines will enhance one's understanding of change and innovations in the field.

The standard of care in aquatic therapy is based on the ability of the professional and the image the professional presents to the public. The latter includes the job description. Under the law, professionals are held to the skills and knowledge they have acquired for a particular job or task. In an investigation of an incident, the following questions will be asked: What are the professional's qualifications and knowledge, and did he or she meet the minimum standard of the profession? What is the content of the person's education? What is his or her level of experience? Is the professional certified? Failure to meet the acceptable standard of care is a significant factor in a court's decision to find liability.

The second area deals with what the public and employer expect from a person engaged in aquatic therapy. Are the professional's knowledge and skill adequate for the job described and the physician's prescription? Did he or she possess the skills and knowledge the physician and client expected? Is the job description appropriate to the service that was provided to the client on the day of the incident? If the professional's skills and knowledge, as presented either to the physician or the employer, are inadequate or inappropriate for the service that was provided, the physician or employer will become liable along with the professional for the incident. If the skills and knowledge presented to the physician and employer are adequate and appropriate but the professional is not able to carry them out, the professional may become liable.

So, how does the professional prepare or learn to manage risks? He or she should prepare a comprehensive statement of personal skills and knowledge and be ready to explain the statement to a nonprofessional. For example, an exercise physiologist or a physical therapist must not only list his or her degrees but also know what those degrees represent. Documented skills and knowledge must be contemporary. Records of in-service training, contents of courses, and texts to which one refers must be readily available.

Many opportunities for learning and updating aquatic therapy skills and knowledge exist. Some involve certification. When listing active certificates, one must remember that the owner will be held accountable for knowledge and skills acquired in obtaining each certificate. If the information acquired has not been used, the materials should be reviewed and assurances made that the owner can use them effectively, or the credential should be removed from the application.

Risk management specialists on occasion speculate about the possibility that serious incidents involving highly qualified professionals may be attributed to factors outside of the individual's reach or be directly related to the physical and mental capacity of the professional on the day of the incident. For example, evidence exists to suggest that general aquatic incidents occur more often in the early days of the opening of a facility to the public or on the first day of a client's new experience. Although professionals are urged to use extreme caution during these times, there is no way a person's first experience can be eliminated.

A professional's mental and physical capacity is best monitored by the professional. Adequate sleep, time for relaxation, and a positive work environment are essential to the success of all employees. Professionals are expected to monitor personal habits and experiences to be sure they are competent in the work environment. Employers are wise to maintain a high-quality work environment and to recognize an employee's willingness to share personal concerns that could lead to a problem in carrying out a task on a particular workday. Honest sharing of employee concerns can result in a few individuals gaining a day to play whereas the great majority of people will use a day off only to retain their mental and physical health. Employers should ignore the one or two persons who will take advantage of such a situation and recognize the sincerity of those willing to monitor their competence.

The professional's standard of care is his or her capacity to do those things that he or she documented could be done, meet the specifications identified in the job description, and achieve what the public, using common sense, would expect the aquatic therapist to do.

A Lawsuit

An incident occurs, and a client is damaged physically or psychologically. The client believes that the damage was caused or aggravated by the professional, the facility, or both. The client brings a cause of action against all potential defendants (persons and agencies that were involved in the incident). When the action is a tort for personal injuries it is usually one of the following: negligence, intentional tort, or product liability.

Negligence, the tort most often found in physical activity litigation, is that incident you never expected would happen. To cause the defendant to be found negligent, the plaintiff must prove that the professional had a duty, the duty was breached or not fulfilled, the failure to fulfill the duty was the direct cause of the injury, and the plaintiff sustained substantial damage.[6]

The duty is the standard of care in a particular situation. Professionals need to know what it is, be articulate in describing it to other professionals and lay people, and be able to identify competent professionals who would support their statements. Plaintiffs must then prove that the duty was not fulfilled. Often they will obtain experts who will investigate the existence of the standard of care on the day of the incident. Was the standard adequate and appropriate, and was it properly carried out? Depositions, under oath, will usually reveal the standard and whether it was maintained on the day of the incident. Direct or proximate cause of the injury or death and damages will receive considerable attention from legal and medical personal. The aquatic therapist's role in litigation tends to revolve around the standard and whether it was breached.

Defendants have a number of defenses that may become part of the case. Among those defenses are contributory negligence and assumption of risk. Contributory negligence involves the actions of the injured party that contributed to his or her injury, for example, if the injured party failed to follow the therapist's instructions or lied about his or her skills that may have contributed to the problem. Assumption of risk is the client's acceptance of general risks, for example, in entering and leaving a swimming pool and in the use of the water.

Contributory negligence and assumption of risk may be combined into a mathematical formula that allocates fault. Comparative fault or comparative negligence is the percentage of fault of the injured party compared with the defendant's percentage of fault. For example, under comparative fault, the injured party may be liable for 40% of the fault and the defendant for 60% of the fault. This means that 40% of a $100,000.00 award will become the responsibility of the injured person; 60% will remain the obligation of the defendant.

An intentional tort is a different cause of action and requires a different approach to an incident. An intentional tort means that the act was intended but not necessarily that it was intended to cause harm. For example, offensive touching is an intentional tort. Pushing a person who loses his or her balance, falls, and hits his or her head, sustaining a severe injury, can be the intentional action that was not expected to cause harm. Here, the defendant who was involved in the incident must be able to state his or her intentions at the time of the incident. Reports and interviews taken by investigators at the scene are also used to establish the facts of the incident. Often, eyewitnesses play a substantial role.

Defenses to intentional torts are consent, self-defense and defense of others, necessity, and discipline. Consent means that the injured party agreed to the action. Self-defense or defense of others enables a person under attack to fight for personal survival or the survival of others. Necessity covers situations in which the action was essential to protect the persons involved, and discipline is the use of a physical action when that is the only choice to maintain a person's safety. Physical contact is common in therapy and in teaching of beginning swimming skills. Care should be taken in defining appropriate and inappropriate actions and in sharing these definitions with clients.

JOINT RESPONSIBILITY WITH OWNERS FOR FACILITIES

When the facility and its permanently attached equipment play a primary or secondary role in the incident, the owner of the facility becomes liable. Also, owners of the building play an important role in the risk management and emergency action plans and responsibilities.

Codes and Regulations

State and local laws, national standards, and numerous sets of guidelines govern aquatic facilities. Often, designated aquatic therapy pools are outside regulations; others are within regulations. First, and foremost, the aquatic therapist must obtain the state and local codes and determine the type of pool he or she is working in. The following are examples of the content of the Florida and California Codes on swimming pools and supervision of participants.

Title XXXIII of the Florida Regulation of Trade, Commerce, Investments, and Solicitations, Chapter 514, Public Swimming and Bathing Facilities defines a swimming pool in the following way:

> A public swimming pool or public pool shall mean a conventional pool, spa-type pool, wading pool, special purpose pool, or water recreation attraction, to which admission may be gained with or without payment of a fee and includes, but is not limited to, pools operated by or serving camps, churches, cities, counties, daycare centers, group home facilities for eight or more clients, health spas, institutions, parks, state agencies, schools, subdivisions, or the cooperative living-type projects of five or more living units, such as apartments, boardinghouses, hotels, mobile home parks, motels, recreational vehicle parks, and townhouses.... "Private pool" means a facility used only by an individual, family, or living unit members and their guests which does not serve any type of cooperative housing or joint tenancy of five or more living units.[7]

Florida statute section 514.0115 "exempts private pools used for instruction and water therapy facilities from standard supervision regulations. The water therapy facility must be connected with a hospital or doctor's office or be a part of a licensed physical therapy unit."

The California Health and Safety Code defines *swimming pool* in the following ways:

> (a) "Swimming pool" or "pool" means any structure intended for swimming or recreational bathing that contains water over 18 inches deep. "Swimming pool" includes in-ground and above-ground structures and includes, but is not limited to, hot tubs, spas, portable spas, and nonportable wading pools.
> (b) "Public swimming pool" means a swimming pool operated for the use of the general public with or without charge, or for the use of the members and guests of a private club. Public swimming pool does not include a swimming pool located on the grounds of a private single-family home.[8]

Because the California Code does not exempt the aquatic therapy pool, it becomes necessary to examine California's statutes on supervision. *Lifeguard* means:

> The attendance at a public swimming pool during periods of use, of one or more lifeguards who possess, as minimal qualification, current Red Cross advanced lifesaving certificates or YMCA senior lifesaving certificates, or have equivalent qualifications and who are trained to administer first aid, including, but not limited to cardiopulmonary resuscitation...and who have no duties to perform other than to supervise the safety of participants in water-contact activities. Lifeguard services includes the supervision of the safety of participants in water-contact activities by lifeguards who are providing swimming lessons, coaching or overseeing water-contact sports, or providing water safety instruction to participants when no other persons are using the facilities unless those persons are supervised by separate lifeguard services.[8]

These two state codes present the divergent thinking on aquatic therapy pools and supervision. Florida has removed aquatic therapy pools from the code and places them in the hands of the owner of the pool; California leaves aquatic therapy pools out of the code and suggests that professionals might be wise to hold lifeguard certificates. For example, the Florida aquatic therapist must determine whether the pool he or she has selected to rent or buy is under the Florida code. If the pool is not under the code, the professional may have to adhere to public pool standards.

Major differences in aquatic therapy and standard or competitive pools are the temperature of the water, space required for activity, depth of water, therapist/client ratio, and length of time therapist/instructor remains in the water. These differences involve health and supervision or safety codes. Water and air temperature and the extended period of time they must spend in the water are the primary concerns of aquatic therapists. They are both health code concerns. Maintaining an acceptable water and air temperature for aquatic therapy in a pool jointly used by regular and speed swimmers is extremely difficult. Arrangements have to be made for the changes in temperature. Therapists and teachers of young children who spend many hours each day in 3 or more feet of water have been found to suffer from a range of health problems. With the exception of the writings of Alison Osinski, scant attention has been focused on these problems. There is a need for comprehensive research on the optimal time an instructor should spend in the water daily, weekly, or monthly. The results of the research should influence code changes.

Although the water depth and space required for aquatic therapy differ from those needed for instructional or competitive swimming, these differences will not require code changes. The therapist/client ratio, in contrast to standard swimmer/instructor ratios, needs to be researched to determine the appropriate supervision for each of these groups. In the past, many of these problems have been resolved by agencies; however, uniform standards do not exist. Any research conducted on aquatic therapy health or supervision must consider current methods used in resolving these problems.

Guidelines

In addition to the standards and codes, there are a number of guidelines, certificates, and courses governing swimming or activities in the water and pools in which swimming and diving occur. They address maintenance, use, supervision, and risk management.

The maintenance and use of aquatic facilities are found in the American College of Sports Medicine's *Health/Fitness Facility Standards and Guidelines*,[9] *Facilities Planning for Physical Activity and Sport*,[10] and *The Complete Swimming Pool Reference*.[11] Therapy pools are the subjects of *Aquatic Rehabilitation for Health Professionals*[12] and *Aquatics: The Complete Reference Guide for Aquatic Fitness Professionals*.[13] Supervision is best defined in the American Red Cross *Lifeguarding Today*[14] and the YMCA's *On the Guard*.[15] The American Red Cross[16] and the YMCA provide courses and certificates for completing extensive training in the instruction and supervision of all forms of aquatics. Also, aquatic therapists will become familiar with the needs of special populations and note that the pool and the facility in which it is housed accommodate clients. *Swimming Pool Accessibility* from the National Center on Accessibility[17] is a valuable source for these concerns.

If the aquatic therapist owns the pool, he or she must adhere to all codes covering the facility. If the aquatic therapist leases the facility, details of the code and who is liable for regulations and guidelines must be spelled out in the lease document. Although the facility owner and operator are liable for maintenance of the codes and regulations, an understanding of these requirements is useful to the aquatic professional in assessing the environment in which he or she is working. Also, persons holding aquatic teaching and life-guarding credentials are expected to understand these laws.

THE BUSINESS OF AQUATIC THERAPY

Types of employment, methods of organizing a business, contracts, and risk management will be discussed in this section.

Types of Employment

The aquatic therapy professional seeking employment has three choices: be self-employed and an independent contractor (IC), work for someone else, or work as a regular employee or a member of a leasing firm. The difference in these arrangements is the legal responsibility on the work site and for withholding and paying taxes.

In an IC relationship the IC agrees, under a contract, to accept a specific sum of money for providing a service or product or carrying out a task. The IC controls and supervises the work, assigns the tasks, and is responsible for wages, insurance, and payment of compensation and employee benefits. He or she is liable for personal torts and the torts of their employees. The employer is expected to provide a safe working environment. The employer cannot supervise, evaluate, or fire the IC's employees or alter the tasks to be accomplished. Requests for change by the employer is a request for a change in the contract and must be negotiated with the IC. If an employer assumes responsibility for the IC's personnel and the execution of tasks, he or she will assume liability for the employee's torts and responsibility to the government for taxes.

A regular employee relationship is an agreement between the employer and employee that the employer will pay a certain wage per week, month, or year for the employee's labor or work. The nature of the tasks and the role of labor unions, etc., are factors in the details of the identified tasks. Employers are responsible for evaluation and termination. They also assume responsibility for the torts of the employees, for federal taxes, and for providing a safe working environment. "A regular employment relationship exists when the parties agree to the relationship, know that the employee is acting on behalf of the employer, and that the employer has agreed to pay the employee."[18]

A leased employment relationship is a combination of the IC and the regular employee arrangements. The leasing company is an IC of the employer; the employees are regular employees of the leasing firm. On the job, the employees are ICs to the employer and regular employees of the leasing firm. This means that the leasing firm is liable for the employee's torts and responsible for wages, benefits, compensation, and the withholding and paying of appropriate taxes. The leasing firm also hires, evaluates, and terminates employees. The employer remains responsible for the safety of the work site.

Methods of Organization

When an aquatic therapist becomes an IC or self-employed, he or she must organize a business. Among the possible choices are sole proprietorship, partnership, and corporation. The major differences among these organizations are the tax responsibilities, legal liability, and sophistication of records and applications. A sole proprietorship is a business started when a person opens a bank account and hangs out a shingle saying he or she is in business. The new owner uses his or her personal credit and money to launch the business. Business taxes are part of the owner's personal income tax return and are paid at the owner's tax level. The owner is liable to the extent of all personal assets for the expenses of the business. Many businesses are started this way and move to a more sophisticated organization as the business grows.

In light of the potential risk in businesses associated with physical activity, the sole proprietorship is not considered a good organization. If this model is to be used, the owner is encouraged to make insurance a high priority. The real advantage of this organization is that the owner makes all decisions and is able to run the business as he or she wishes.

A partnership is a business similar to the sole proprietorship but is owned by two or more people. A written statement of ownership is recommended, but not required, and can be filed in a number of states. The values of a written statement are that the co-owners' promises and details of how the business would be run or terminated after the demise of a partner or the necessity on the part of all partners to terminate the venture are affirmed.

Under the law, all partners are treated as equals. If one person provides more assets or time and expects to be compensated appropriately at the time of tax or termination, these differences must have been placed in writing. Liability for business expenses and incidents or accidents is joint among the owners, and any one owner can be held liable for the debts of the entire business. All personal assets of each owner are subject to liability. The advantages of a partnership are the ease of establishing the business, the ability to contribute labor as well as capital or in lieu of capital, and the efficiency of a small team in making decisions.

Corporation, the business formed under the authority of state government, is usually the recommended organization for a potentially thriving business. It is established by the filing of articles of incorporation with the secretary of a state. There are a number of requirements that this business must adhere to, including holding an annual meeting and maintaining of government requirements. A corporation is an entity. It can sue or be sued. Under a corporation, the owner's assets are no longer liable for the debts of the business. The owners are shareholders and are liable only to the extent of each owner's investment in the business. Corporations are either S or C businesses. Under an S corporation, designed for small businesses, the profit/loss tax liability passes to the individual owner's tax return. This is the same as for the sole proprietorship and partnership. Under a C corporation, the entity files income tax returns and pays a standard corporate tax that may or may not be less than an individual's level of taxation.

The above is a superficial review of business organizations to alert the new entrepreneur to these structures. All decisions involving the creation of business organizations should be made with the guidance of an attorney. Attorneys will provide owners with information and will draft and file the documents. The attorney will work with the owner's accountant in structuring the tax consequences.

Contracts

Aquatic therapy professionals will most often be involved in employment and leasing contracts. Contracts are agreements between parties to do something or refrain from doing something. They include an offer by one party, an acceptance by the party to whom the offer was made, and a consideration, which is usually a sum of money. All three factors—offer, acceptance, and consideration—must exist. These agreements may be verbal or written. Information in verbal agreements is often difficult to prove.

When one party fails to live up to the contract, the contract is breached and the party that has been harmed by the breach may choose to sue. Under contract law, the courts will attempt to enforce the contract according to the will of the parties on the date of the agreement.

A regular employment contract usually covers the following components:

1. Parties involved in the contract
2. Date on which the agreement was made
3. Date the agreement is to begin and date it will end
4. Services or job description: This may be a vague statement or a detailed list. Often, the statement will refer to and incorporate into the document the employee's handbook. Sometimes it will merely be a job title but one in which there is a consensus among professionals as to what that title means.

5. Qualifications required of the candidate
6. Compensation, including salary and benefits, and when and how the fees will be paid
7. Amount of time on the job or work time
8. Requirements of the employer, e.g., loyalty oaths, confidential requirements, protection of trade secrets, and ownership of intellectual property
9. Promises of the employer, including a safe working environment and sick and personal leave
10. Not-to-compete clauses and appropriate compensation for such clauses
11. Grounds for termination
12. Arbitration clause

Contracts for the leasing of a facility must consider the elements of contract, state and local statutes governing facilities, the rights and requirements of the owner, and the rights and requirements of the person to whom the facility is leased. The contract must clearly specify what is being leased including the pool, adjoining locker rooms, entry to the building, parking, and all other topics addressed.

The contract must contain the date and time the facility is to be used. Whether the lease is for the building or just for the pool must be determined. Adequate change and dressing time for clients must be requested. Determine whether the leased pool is in an open ongoing facility or a closed facility. When the pool is in an open facility, inquire whether clients will be permitted in the lounge or other open parts of the building. The term *lessor* for the following statements refers to the owner or manager who is leasing the building and/or the pool. The *lessee* is the aquatic therapist who is renting the facility and/or pool. Answers to the following questions will guide the professional in designing a lease.

Facility

1. Facility or amount of facility to be leased
2. Condition of the facility at acceptance and return
3. Method of entry to the facility: escort or keys. If escort, identify exact time and location of person. If keys, specify when and where will the key be obtained and returned. Be sure all entry and exit procedures meet local, state, and federal codes (e.g., safety and Americans with Disabilities Act).[19,20]
4. Total time in facility

Pool and Equipment

1. Pool must meet federal, state, and local health and aquatic codes, including those of the Occupational Safety and Health Administration (OSHA).
2. Pool size is appropriate for activity.
3. Building, locker rooms, and pool meet American with Disabilities Act requirements and additional requirements specified in the lease as needed for aquatic therapy.
4. Safety equipment is in the pool room and has been checked prior to lease date and time (including all emergency equipment).
5. Specific emergency numbers are available for immediate help should the facility not meet agreed-to standards.
6. Pool is a safe and healthy work environment for professionals.

Supervision

1. Supervision is both a safety and public relations component. Clients must be safe in the building and in the pool. An incident can be a public relations disaster for the lessee and the owner of the building.
2. Level of supervision of the activity, including who will provide supervisors, and the credentials, including background checks, that will be considered appropriate is defined.
3. On-site maintenance, including unexpected human accidents, will be the responsibility of the lessor or lessee.
4. Owner of the pool will provide the emergency action plan. The written plan should be attached to the lease and should specify the last date it was rehearsed and checked. The existence, membership, and date of the owner's or manager's last safety committee meeting is part of the swimming pool lease. (For a detailed explanation of OSHA regulations, see Clement[21].)
5. Lessee should be required to teach the plan to and rehearse the plan with his or her personnel. If owner's or manager's personnel are the supervisors, lessor should specify dates of their training and content of the program.
6. Agreement is made about accident reports, release of information to the media, notification of owner, and other concerns.

Insurance

1. Both parties will probably carry insurance.
2. Indemnification clauses are very popular and need to be carefully considered. Indemnification means that one party agrees that his or her business insurance will cover the other party. Each party and its insurance company needs to be aware of the liabilities assumed in these clauses. Seek legal advice in drafting or accepting this responsibility. Be sure to present to counsel a clear case of your professional liability. Do not expect the lawyer to know all the details of pool safety and client attention.

Risk Management

Risk management is the identification, evaluation, and control of loss.[22] Identification of risks results in an audit or list of written statements in which the professional, using his or her background, relies upon sources, background, and contents of guidelines and certificates to create a comprehensive list of risks involving safety and best business practices. Each item on the list is evaluated in the context of probability of it happening, severity, or the extent of the loss should it happen, and magnitude or the number of people or sum of money lost if it did happen.

After the evaluation is complete, professionals agree on methods of control, which can include altering the activity to reduce the risk, eliminating the risk, or retaining the risk and covering with insurance. Sources of help in carrying out risk management are *Risk Management in Sport*[23] and *Legal Responsibility in Aquatics*.[18]

REFERENCES

1. Salzman A: Aquatic Resource Network Newslett 6(2):3, 2001.
2. National Safety Council: Injury Facts. Itasca, Ill: National Safety Council, 2000, p 8.
3. National Safety Council: International Accident Facts. Itasca, Ill: National Safety Council, 1999, pp 10–11.
4. United States Consumer Product Safety Commission: Consumer Product Safety Review, 2000, Vol 5, No 2, pp 4, 5.
5. United States Consumer Product Safety Commission: Consumer Product Safety Review, 1998, Vol 3.
6. Clement A: Law in Sport and Physical Activity. Cape Canaveral, Fla: Sport and Law Press, 1998, pp 27, 28.
7. Florida Statutes. Title XXXIII Regulation of Trade, Commerce, Investments, and Solicitations, Chapter 514 Public Swimming and Bathing Facilities, 2000, Section 514.01–514.08.
8. Deering's California Code Annotated. California Health & Safety Code, 2001, Section 115921–116055.
9. Tharrett ST, Peterson JA: Health/Fitness Facility Standards and Guidelines. Champaign, Ill: Human Kinetics, 1997.
10. Sawyer T (ed): Facilities Planning for Physical Activity and Sport. Dubuque, Iowa: Kendall/Hunt, 1999.
11. Griffith T: The Complete Swimming Pool Reference. St Louis: Mosby Lifeline, 1994.
12. Ruoti RG, Morris DM, Cole AJ (eds): Aquatic Rehabilitation for Health Professionals. Philadelphia: Lippincott, 1997.
13. Sova R: Aquatics: The Complete Reference Guide for Aquatic Fitness Professionals. Boston: Jones & Bartlett, 1991.
14. American Red Cross: Lifeguarding Today. St Louis, Mosby Yearbook, 1995.
15. YMCA of the USA: On the Guard. Champaign, Ill: Human Kinetics, 2001.
16. American Red Cross: Swimming and Diving. St Louis: Mosby Yearbook, 1996.
17. National Center on Accessibility: Swimming Pool Accessibility. Martinsville, Idaho: National Center on Accessibility, 1996.
18. Clement A: Legal Responsibility in Aquatics. Cape Canaveral, Fla: Sport and Law Press, 1997, p 379.
19. Americans with Disabilities Act of 1990, Public Law No. 101-336, 104 Stat. 327 (codified at 42 USCA 1202–1213).
20. Equal Employment Opportunities Commission and the U. S. Department of Justice: Americans with Disabilities Act Handbook. Washington, DC: US Government Printing Office, 1991.
21. Clement A: Aquatics and the law. In Appenzeller H (ed): Risk Management in Sport. Durham, NC: Carolina Academic Press, 1998.
22. Clement A: Children and water injuries. In Frost JL (ed): Children and Injuries. San Francisco: Lawyers & Judges, 2001.
23. Appenzeller H: Risk Management in Sport. Durham, NC: Carolina Academic Press, 1998.

Index

A

Abulation. *See* Social bathing
Aerobic conditioning, 218–219
Ai chi, 122, 258
Aldosterone, 46–47
American Physical Therapy Association (APTA), 14
Americans with Disabilities Act, 68
Ankle rehabilitation, 228–229
Antidiuretic hormone (ADH), 46–47
Aquadance. *See* Watsu
Aquatic Exercise Association (AEA), 14
Aquatic therapy
  in America, history
    early Twentieth Century, 8–9
    Great Depression era, 9–11
    Nineteenth Century, 6–8
    post World War II, 12–13
    renaissance, 16
    World War II era, 11–12
  ankle, 228–229
  for arthritis
    active exercises, 214
    benefit, 209–212
    functional reeducation, 218–219
    maintenance programs, 220–221
    passive techniques, 213–214
    resistive exercises, 214–217
  biologic effects, 19–20
  for children (*see* Pediatric aquatic therapy (PAT))
  circulatory system, 33–38
  CNS, 50–51, 153
  commonly treated ailments, 115
  conditioning
    effectiveness, 35–36, 43–44
    history, 14–15
    kinetic chain issues, 44
    RPE and, 38–39
  endrocrine system, 44, 46–48
  equipment
    basic principles, 116–118
    materials used, 119–120
    options, 120–123
    W.A.T.E.R scale, 120–123
  facilities, 290–292

Aquatic therapy (*continued*)
  knees, 229–233
  logical approach, 159–161
  medical standards, 8–9
  musculoskeletal system, 43
  origins of, 1–2
  PNS, 50–51
  principles, 137
  pulmonary system, 39–42
  rehabilitation, 1
  renal system, 44, 46–48
  shoulders, 233–237
  standard of care, 352–354
  thermoregulation, 48–50
  weight control, 51–52
Armstrong, Neil, 13
Arthritis
  acute phase management, 212–213
  definition, 207
  demographics, 208
  disease effects, 208–208
  exercise benefits, 209–212
  juvenile rheumatoid, case study, 275–277
  subacute phase management
    aerobic conditioning, 218
    exercises, 214–217
    functional reeducation, 218–219
    joint mobilization, 213
    maintenance programs, 220–221
    passive techniques, 213–214
    patient education, 219–221
  types, 207
Arthritis Foundation YMCA Program (AFYAP)
  class planner worksheet, 222
  description, 220–221
  exercises, 223–224
  for juvenile arthritis, 224–225
Athletic trainers, 343, 345
Autonomic nervous system (ANS), 48, 103–105

B

Bad Ragaz Ring Method (BRRM)
  description, 159–160
  equipment options, 121
  for neurologic disorders, 160–161
  pediatrics, 258

Balance
  center of, 23
  control
    basic movement, 85–86
    combined rotation, 83–84
    description, 78–79
    longitudinal rotation, 81–82
    mental inversion, 84–85
    movement, 85
    sagittal rotation, 79–81
    simple progression, 85
    in stillness, 85
    transverse rotation, 81
    turbulent gliding, 85
    upthrust, 84–85
Baruch, Bernard M., 9
Baruch, Simon, 8
Becker, Bruce, 13
Bicycling, 79
Bilateral movements, 155
Billing, 329–330
Borg Scale, 144
Breath control, 77–78, 263–265
Brennan Scale, 144–146
British thermal units (BTU), 31
Buoyancy
  center of, 23
  depth of water and, 155
  description, 22–23
  in Halliwick concept, 75
  joint loading and, 23–25
Burdenko method, 122
Burns, from whirlpool therapy, 314
Burt, Bernard, 14
Business, organization of, 358–359

C

Calorie, 30–31
Cardiopulmonary fitness, 227–228
Cardiovascular system, 33–38, 315
Catecholamines, 48
Central nervous system (CNS), 50–51, 153
Cerebral palsy
  PAT program, case study
    background, 270–271
    impairments, related goals/activities, 274
    long-term program, 272–275
    relevant problems, 271–272
Certifications, 338–339, 341–342
Children
  aerobic power, 240
  breath control, 263–265
  disabled, fitness levels, 240–241
  respiratory function, 239–240
  temperature response, 241–242
Chronic heart failure (CHF), 42
Circulatory system, 33–38
Conduction, 31–33
Contracts, 359–361
Convection, 31–33
Coulter, John S., 10, 11

D

Deep-water environments, 292
De Leon, Ponce, 6
De Normandie, John, 6
De Soto, Hernando, 6
Drag force, 138
Dull, Harold, 99, 157

E

Edema reduction, 211
Eising, Lucille, 12
Emergency procedures, 70
Employees. *See* Staff
Endrocrine system, 44, 46–48
Energy transfer, thermal, 31–33
Equipment
  basic principles, 116–118
  materials used, 119–120
  options, 120–123
  resources, 129–134
  standards, 360
  W.A.T.E.R scale, 120
Erdman, William, 12
Exercise instructors, 344, 345
Exercise physiologists, 343–344, 346
Expiratory reserve volume (ERV), 39–40

F

Fantus, Bernard, 11
Feldenkrais, 122
Fibromyalgia, 105
Fishbein, Morris, 11
Fitch, W.E., 9
Fitness, aquatic
  aerobic training, 36
  effectiveness, 35–36, 43–44
  history, 14–15
  kinetic chain issues, 44
  RPE and, 38–39
Flax, Herman, 12
Fletcher, George B., 10
Flotation, 283–285
Flow motion, 26
Fluid Moves. *See* Feldenkrais
Foster, Sigmund, 12

G

Galen, 4, 307
General System Theory (GST), 74
Giedion, Sigfried, 1–2
Goode, Thomas, 6
Gove-Nichols, Mary, 6
Greek spa culture, 2, 4–5
Groedel, Franz, 9
Gubner, Richard, 12

H

Halliwick concept
  development, 73–74
  elements, 73
  equipment options, 121

Halliwick concept *(continued)*
  instructional application (*see* Ten-point program)
  for neurologic disorders, 162–163, 165
  pediatric applications, 257
  in WST
    assessment, 86, 88
    case history, 96–97
    elements, 87
    exercise patterns, 93
    modes of treatment, 93–96
    rotational axis, 88–89
    treatment objectives, 88
    treatment techniques, 91–92
    water depth, 90
    working positions, 89
Heat, 30–33, 138
Henriksen, Jens, 12
Hinsdale, Guy, 8
Hippocrates, 307
Hopkins, Frank, 9
Hormones. *See* Endrocrine system
Hot tubs, 292
Hubbard, LeRoy, 9
Hydrodynamics, staff understanding of, 327
Hydrology, medical, 19
Hydrostatic pressure
  description, 21–22
  edema and, 211
Hydrotherapy. *See* Aquatic therapy
Hypothermia, from whirlpool therapy, 314

I
Immersion, 19
Infections, 313–314, 318–319
Inspiratory reserve volume (IRV), 39

J
Jahara experiential method, 122
Jarman, Melitus, 9
Jefferson, Thomas, 6
Joint
  loading, buoyancy and, 23–25
  mobilization, 213
  protection, 219–220

K
Kellogg, John Harvey, 8
Kidney, 46–48
Kinesiotherapists, 344, 346
King, Nelda, 10
Knee
  diagnosis, 231
  functional anatomy, 229–231
  rehabilitation, 231–233
  ROM progression, 233
Kneeling, 89
Kneipp, Father, 15
Krusen, Frank H., 11–12
Kyphosis, 201–202

L
Laminar flow, 27–28
Liability
  concerns, 352
  lawsuits, 354–355
  standard of care and, 352–354
Licensure, 341–342
Licht, Sidney, 2, 12
Lowman, Charles LeRoy, 8–9, 10, 12
Lungs, effects of hydrotherapy, 39–42
Lyton model
  application, 349
  case study, 347–348
  description, 341

M
Manual therapy, 122
Martin, Louis G., 10
Massage therapists, 344, 346
Masunaga, 102
McClellan, Walter S., 2, 9
McFarland, J. Wayne, 12
McMillan, James, 73–75, 78, 86, 162, 241–242
Medieval spa culture, 2, 4–6
Moorman, John Jennings, 6
Motor control models, 152–153
Motor skills training, children, 269
Muscular dystrophy, 42

N
Neurologic disorders
  aquatic neurorehabilitation
    BRRM, 159–161
    case study, 170–174
    general guidelines, 155–156
    Halliwick method, 162–163, 165
    TTTA, 167–170
    water shiastu, 157–159
  associated impairments, 152
  description, 152
  rehabilitation models, 153–154
  Watsu sessions for, 108–110

O
Occupational therapists, 343, 346
Orthopedic impairments, 110–111
Osteoarthritis, 207
Ott, V.R., 13

P
Pain. *See under* Spine
Pain modulation, 51
Paracelsus, 5
Parkinson's disease, 107
Pascal, Blaise, 21
Peale, Albert Charles, 7
Pediatric aquatic therapy (PAT)
  breath control, 263–265
  for cerebral palsy, case study
    background, 270–271

Pediatric aquatic therapy (PAT) *(continued)*
    impairments, related goals/activities, 274
    long-term program, 272–275
    relevant problems, 271–272
  clinical applications, 258–259
  common practice settings, 245
  contraindications, 248
  daily living, training for, 280
  description, 239
  emphasis, 243
  evaluation form, 250
  family-centered care, 244–245
  functional task differences, 242
  handling techniques
    considerations, 249
    prone, 252–254
    supine, 254–255
    vertical, 249, 252
  interdisciplinary aspects, 243
  interventions, 257–258
  land therapies, combining with, 245
  mental adjustment, 260–263
  motor skill training, functional, 269
  outcomes/goals, 256–257
  pool locations, 246
  precautions, 247–248
  progression, 265–269
  referral criteria, 246–247
  for rheumatoid arthritis, case study
    function level, 276
    history/referral, 275–276
    impairments, related goals/activities, 277
    progress, 277
    treatment programs, 276
  safety considerations, 255–256
  for sensory processing problems, 280–282
  skill evaluations, 248–249
  for sports injuries, 277–278
  swimming skill training, 282–285
  water temperature, 241–242
  weight training, 278–280
People with Arthritis Can Exercise (PACE), 220
Peripheral nervous system (PNS), 50–51
Peto, Andras, 257
Physical therapists, 342, 346
Poliomyelitis, 12
Polyarticular disease, 275
Pools
  accreditation, 329
  building, case studies
    background, 292–295
    barriers, 302–303
    documentation, 296, 298
    facilitators, 302–303
    program integration, 298–302
    strategic planning, 303–304
  codes/regulations, 355–357
  community, 291–292
  designing
    common errors, 66–69
    construction documents, 61–63
    construction phase, 64
    contracts, 64

Pools *(continued)*
    demographic survey, 59
    feasibility studies, 59–60
    permitting process, 63–64
    prefabricated, 65–66
    preliminary design, 59–60
    pre-opening inspection, 64–65
    process, 57
    programming requirements, 59
    site analysis, 58–59
    team, functions, 60–61
    trends, 57
  documentation, 69–71
  guidelines, 357
  health facility, 291
  maintenance, 330
  standards, 360
Pregnancy, 50
Pressure ulcers
  adjuvant treatments, 308
  prevalence, 307
  pulsatile lavage therapy
    description, 315–316
    effects on debris, 318
    effects on wound infection, 318–319
    pressures produced by, 316–318
    side effects, 320–321
    use of antibiotics, 319
    use of antiseptic agents, 319–320
  whirlpool therapy
    adverse effects, 313–315
    analgesic effects, 313
    bacterial load, 309–310
    frequency, 311
    guidelines, 308
    immersion duration, 311
    local tissue perfusion, 312–313
    use of antiseptic agents, 311–312
    water agitation, 310
    water temperature, 310–311
    wound débridement, 309
    wound rinsing, 310
Proprioceptive neuromuscular facilitation (PNF), 122, 159–160
Propulsion, 30
Prostaglandin E, 47
Pulsatile lavage therapy
  description, 315–316
  effects on debris, 318
  effects on wound infection, 318–319
  pressures produced by, 316–318
  side effects, 320–321
  use of antibiotics, 319
  use of antiseptic agents, 319–320

Q
Quadruped exercise, 188–190

R
Range of Movement, effects of water, 155–156
Rating of perceived exertion, 144
Recording keeping, 329

Refraction, 25–26
Registrations, 341–342
Relative perceived exertion (RPE), 38–39
Renin, 46–47
Resistance effects, 29–30
Respiratory problems, 239–240
Reynolds, Joshua, 28
Reynolds number, 28–29
Rheumatic diseases. *See* Arthritis
Risk management, 328–329, 352, 361
Roberts, H.H., 8
Roman spa culture, 2, 4–6
Roosevelt, Franklin D., 9
Roszak, Theodore, 15
Running, aqua
 benefits, 137
 biomechanics, 138–140
 description, 137
 exercise response to, 140–143
 form, maintaining, 139–140
 guidelines for clinicians, 146
 intensity grading
  cadence, 144–146
  heart rate, 143–144
  RPE, 144
 special populations, 148
Rush, Benjamin, 6

S

Safety
 basic procedures, 335
 PAT programs, 255–257
 standards, 329
 underwater activity, children, 265
Scaer, 103
Scheuermann's kyphosis, 201–202
Schoedinger, Peggy, 99
Scoliosis, idiopathic, 202
Sculling, supine, 186–188
Sensory processing problems, children, 280–282
Shiatsu. *See* Zen Shiatsu
Shoulder
 diagnosis, 234–235
 functional anatomy, 233–234
 rehabilitation, 236–237
Sigerist, Henry, 11
Smith, Euclid, 10
Social bathing, 2
Spas
 concept of, 2
 cultures, historical, 2, 4–6
 design, 9–11
 facilities, 292
 research, 9–11
 ten domains, 15–16
 term, etymology, 2
 universal features, 10
Spinal cord injury, 42
Spine
 pain
  aquatic stabilization techniques
   log-roll swim, 190, 193–195

Spine *(continued)*
   modified superman, 182–183
   prone swimming, 195–197
   quadruped exercise, 188–190
   supine sculling, 186–188
   supine swimming, 198–199
   wall crunch, 187–189
   wall sit, 181–182
   water walking backward, 185–186
   water walking forward, 183–185
  diagnosis, 177–180
  incidence, 177
  rehabilitation programs, 180
  swimmers, 198, 199–201
  treatment, 177–180
 stabilization, equipment options, 121
 traction, equipment options, 121
Sports injuries, children, 277–278
Stabilization techniques
 distal, 155
 log-roll swim, 190, 193–195
 modified superman, 182–183
 prone swimming, 195–197
 quadruped exercise, 188–190
 supine sculling, 186–188
 supine swimming, 198–199
 wall crunch, 187–189
 wall sit, 181–182
 water walking backward, 185–186
 water walking forward, 183–185
Staff. *See also* training
 certifications, 338–339, 341–342
 evaluation, 326–327
 function, 345–346
 handling skills of, 330–331
 policies/procedures, 69
 positions, description, 345–346
 scheduling, 330
 standard of care requirements, 352–354
 supervisions, 361
Starlings law, 34
Stroke volume, 34–35
Superman, modified, 182–183
Surface tension, 26
Suspended sitting, 80
Swimming
 flotation, 283–285
 log-roll, 190, 193–195
 PAT program, 282–285
 prone, 195–197
 spinal injury, biomechanics, 199–202
 spinal pain from, 197, 199–202
 stroke training, 122
 supine, 198–199
Systemic disease, 275

T

Task-type training approach (TTTA), 167–170, 173–174
Temperature
 core body, children, 241–242
 regulation, 138

Temperature *(continued)*
    response to, 241–242
    water, whirlpool, 310–311
Ten domains, 15–16
Ten-point program. *See also* Halliwick concept
    balance control
        basic movement, 85–86
        combined rotation, 83–84
        description, 78–79
        longitudinal rotation, 81–82
        mental inversion, 84–85
        movement, 85–86
        sagittal rotation, 79–81
        simple progression, 85
        in stillness, 85
        transverse rotation, 81
        turbulent gliding, 85
        upthrust, 84–85
    mental adjustment/disengagement, 76–78
Theophrastus of Hohenheim. *See* Paracelsus
Therapeutic recreation specialist, 343, 346
Thermal energy transfer, 31–33
Thermodynamics, 30–33
Thermoregulation, 48–50
Title acts, 341–342
Training
    certificates of participation, 345
    community programs, 338
    in equipment progression, 337
    in handling techniques, 336–337
    industry standards, 334–335
    nonuniversity programs, 332–333
    options, 325–326
    regulation/standards, 342–344
    in safety, 335
    topics for, 327–329
    university-based programs, 331–332
Trall, Russell, 6
Turbulent flow, 28

U
Ulcers. *See* Pressure ulcers
Unilateral movements, 155

V
Venous pressures, 33–38
Viscosity, 27, 29–30

W
Wallace, Albert W., 10
Wall crunch, 187–189
Wall sit exercise, 181–182
Walton, George G., 6–7
Wassertanzen. *See* Watsu
Water
    body positions in, 156
    buoyancy, 22–25
    composition, 20
    density, 20–21
    depth, 90
    gravity, 20–21
    hydrostatic pressure, 21–22

Water *(continued)*
    refraction, 25–26
    specific therapy (*see also* Halliwick concept)
        assessment, 86, 88
        case history, 96–97
        elements, 87
        exercise patterns, 93
        modes of treatment, 93–95
        rotational axis, 88–89
        treatment objectives, 88
        treatment techniques, 91–92
        water depth, 90
        working positions, 89
    surface tension, 26
    temperature, heart rate and, 34–35
    thermodynamics, 30–33
    time-dependent properties, 26–30
    walking backward, 185–186
    walking forward, 183–185
W.A.T.E.R. scale
    classification system outline, 123–124
    for flotation devices, 126
    function, 120
    for resistive devices, 127
    for tethers/portable stations, 128
Watsu
    in acute rehabilitation, 105
    advantages, 172
    description, 157
    development, 101–102
    effectiveness, underlying principles, 99–101
    equipment options, 121
    inspired bodywork, 101–102
    for neurologic disorders, 108–109, 158–159
    for orthopedic impairments, 110–111
    pediatric applications, 258
    physiologic effects, 102–105
    in acute rehabilitation, 105
    precautions, 111–113
    psychological effects, 105
    session essentials, 108
    underwater techniques, 123
Weight control, 51–52
Weight training, children, 278–280
Weil, Andrew, 15
Whirlpool therapy
    adverse effects, 313–315
    analgesic effects, 313
    bacterial load, 309–310
    benefits, 211–212
    frequency, 311
    guidelines, 308
    immersion duration, 311
    local tissue perfusion, 312–313
    use of antiseptic agents, 311–312
    water agitation, 310
    water temperature, 310–311
    wound débridement, 309
    wound rinsing, 310
Wright, Rebekah, 10

Z
Zen Shiatsu, 102